Antisense Oligodeoxynucleotides and Antisense RNA

Novel Pharmacological and Therapeutic Agents

Pharmacology and Toxicology: Basic and Clinical Aspects

Mannfred A. Hollinger, Series Editor
University of California, Davis

Forthcoming Titles

Anabolic Treatment for Osteoporosis, James F. Whitfield and Paul Morley
Basis of Toxicity Testing, Second Edition, Donald J. Ecobichon
CNS Injuries: Cellular Responses and Pharmacological Strategies, Martin Berry and Ann Logan
Lead and Public Health: Integrated Risk Assessment, Paul Mushak
Molecular Bases of Anesthesia, Eric Moody and Phil Skolnick
Receptor Characterization and Regulation, Devendra K. Agrawal

Published Titles

Antibody Therapeutics, 1997, William J. Harris and John R. Adair
Muscarinic Receptor Subtypes in Smooth Muscle, 1997, Richard M. Eglen
Antisense Oligodeonucleotides as Novel Pharmacological Therapeutic Agents, 1997, Benjamin Weiss
Drug Delivery Systems, 1996, Vasant V. Ranade and Mannfred A. Hollinger
Experimental Models of Mucosal Inflammation, 1996, Timothy S. Gaginella
Brain Mechanisms and Psychotropic Drugs, 1996, Andrius Baskys and Gary Remington
Receptor Dynamics in Neural Development, 1996, Christopher A. Shaw
Ryanodine Receptors, 1996, Vincenzo Sorrentino
Therapeutic Modulation of Cytokines, 1996, M.W. Bodmer and Brian Henderson
Pharmacology in Exercise and Sport, 1996, Satu M. Somani
Placental Pharmacology, 1996, B. V. Rama Sastry
Pharmacological Effects of Ethanol on the Nervous System, 1996, Richard A. Deitrich
Immunopharmaceuticals, 1996, Edward S. Kimball
Chemoattractant Ligands and Their Receptors, 1996, Richard Horuk
Pharmacological Regulation of Gene Expression in the CNS, 1996, Kalpana Merchant
Human Growth Hormone Pharmacology: Basic and Clinical Aspects, 1995, Kathleen T. Shiverick and Arlan Rosenbloom
Placental Toxicology, 1995, B. V. Rama Sastry
Stealth Liposomes, 1995, Danilo Lasic and Frank Martin
TAXOL®: Science and Applications, 1995, Matthew Suffness

Pharmacology and Toxicology: Basic and Clinical Aspects

Published Titles Continued

Endothelin Receptors: From the Gene to the Human, 1995, Robert R. Ruffolo, Jr.
Alternative Methodologies for the Safety Evaluation of Chemicals in the Cosmetic Industry, 1995, Nicola Loprieno
Phospholipase A_2 in Clinical Inflammation: Molecular Approaches to Pathophysiology, 1995, Keith B. Glaser and Peter Vadas
Serotonin and Gastrointestinal Function, 1995, Timothy S. Gaginella and James J. Galligan
Chemical and Structural Approaches to Rational Drug Design, 1994, David B. Weiner and William V. Williams
Biological Approaches to Rational Drug Design, 1994, David B. Weiner and William V. Williams
Direct Allosteric Control of Glutamate Receptors, 1994, M. Palfreyman, I. Reynolds, and P. Skolnick
Genomic and Non-Genomic Effects of Aldosterone, 1994, Martin Wehling
Peroxisome Proliferators: Unique Inducers of Drug-Metabolizing Enzymes, 1994, David E. Moody
Angiotensin II Receptors, Volume I: Molecular Biology, Biochemistry, Pharmacology, and Clinical Perspectives, 1994, Robert R. Ruffolo, Jr.
Angiotensin II Receptors, Volume II: Medicinal Chemistry, 1994, Robert R. Ruffolo, Jr.
Beneficial and Toxic Effects of Aspirin, 1993, Susan E. Feinman
Preclinical and Clinical Modulation of Anticancer Drugs, 1993, Kenneth D. Tew, Peter Houghton, and Janet Houghton
In Vitro *Methods of Toxicology*, 1992, Ronald R. Watson
Basis of Toxicity Testing, 1992, Donald J. Ecobichon
Human Drug Metabolism from Molecular Biology to Man, 1992, Elizabeth Jeffreys
Platelet Activating Factor Receptor: Signal Mechanisms and Molecular Biology, 1992, Shivendra D. Shukla
Biopharmaceutics of Ocular Drug Delivery, 1992, Peter Edman
Pharmacology of the Skin, 1991, Hasan Mukhtar
Inflammatory Cells and Mediators in Bronchial Asthma, 1990, Devendra K. Agrawal and Robert G. Townley

Antisense Oligodeoxynucleotides and Antisense RNA

Novel Pharmacological and Therapeutic Agents

Edited by

Benjamin Weiss

Cheif, Division of Neuropsychopharmacology
Department of Pharmacology
MCP◊Hahnemann School of Medicine
Allegheny University of the Health Sciences
Philadelphia, Pennsylvania

CRC Press
Boca Raton New York

Senior Acquiring Editor: Paul Petralia
Project Editor: Helen Linna
Marketing Manager: Susie Carlisle
Direct Marketing Manager: Becky McEldowney
Cover design: Denise Craig
PrePress: Kevin Luong
Manufacturing: Sheri Schwartz

Library of Congress Cataloging-in-Publication Data

Antisense oligodeoxynucleotides and antisense RNA novel pharmacological and
therapeautic agents / edited by Benjamin Weiss
p. cm. — Pharmacology and Toxicology
Includes bibliographical references and index.
ISBN 0-8493-8552-0
1. Pharmacology and Toxicology. 2. Pharmacology — Clinical Aspects.
I. Weiss, Benjamin. II. Series.
QR749.H64G78 1997
616′.0149—dc20
DNLM/DLC
for Library of Congress

97-68923
CIP

International Standard Book Number 0-8493-8552-0
Library of Congress Card Number 97-68923
Printed in the United States of America 1 2 3 4 5 6 7 8 9 0
Printed on acid-free paper

Dedication

"To Joyce, without whose genes I would not have such great children and grandchildren."

Table of Contents

Series Preface

The series, *Pharmacology and Toxicology: Basic and Clinical Aspects,* has been created in recognition of the fact that, from time to time, a new area of interest within a discipline matures to a critical mass that merits organization and integration of the respective observations into a free-standing monograph. In order for such an undertaking to be successful, each editor and/or author must be qualified to identify and select sources best suited to communicate essential aspects of that subject. Such is the case with *Antisense Oligodeoxynucleotides and Antisense RNA: Novel Pharmacological and Therapeutic Agents.* Dr. Benjamin Weiss has assembled a list of contributors whose expertise in their respective areas is well known.

Mannfred A. Hollinger, Ph.D.
Series Editor
Professor and Chair
Department of Medical Pharmacology and Toxicology
University of California, Davis

PREFACE

A revolution is taking place in pharmacology. Whereas in the past, drugs were designed to mimic or antagonize the actions of proteins, we now have the opportunity to selectively inhibit the synthesis of those proteins. That is, we are able through the use of antisense strategies, to alter the expression of specific genes encoding vital proteins.

The use of antisense strategies to modify biological events will usher in a new era of pharmacotherapy, for pharmacologists will now be able to design agents that are more predictable and selective in their actions. These new compounds, which can be targeted to specific genes or gene transcripts, can be readily synthesized and can be examined in a variety of *in vitro* and *in vivo* biological systems, all in relatively short periods of time when compared with the time required for the development of conventional pharmacotherapeutics. The specific molecular mechanisms by which these new agents act and correlations between alterations in biological events and the molecular changes that they induce can also be readily discerned. All this is possible because of another revolution: the explosion of molecular biological discoveries.

The initial excitement and high expectations in this field has, however, now been tempered by the evidence that not all antisense agents are necessarily acting through a antisense mechanism. Nevertheless, we should not be discouraged by finding that antisense agents are not as selective as we had originally hoped. This field of endeavor is akin to the first flight at Kitty Hawk field. It was unreasonable to expect that initial flight would take us to the moon. That it only traveled a few hundred yards was sufficient to point the way toward far reaching flights in the future. So it is with this field of antisense strategies. The pioneers, several of whom are represented in this volume, have just begun the journey. As we travel this path, there will be many exciting advances and as yet undreamed of discoveries, and unfortunately, but inevitably, there will also be many setbacks, disappointments and false trails.

This monograph will be a practical, state-of-the-art treatise on antisense oligodeoxynucleotide technology and the potential application of these strategies in therapeutics. It also includes critical analyses of the specificity of these agents, addressing the possibility that some of the actions of antisense oligomers may be acting through sequence-specific but non-antisense mechanisms.

We begin with a chapter on the history of the early development of antisense oligodeoxynucleotides by Toulmé. This will be followed by a chapter by Crooke reviewing how oligodeoxynucleotides have been chemically modified to increase their stability, delivery and penetration into cells. These issues are of extreme practical importance and will serve as a stepping-off point to the subsequent chapters. The next chapter by Agrawal and Zhang will review the pharmacokinetic properties of antisense oligodeoxynucleotides and will serve as a bridge between the chemistry and subsequent chapters on the biological effects of antisense oligodeoxynucleotides.

The subsequent chapter by Neckers and Iyer will concentrate on the non-antisense effects of antisense oligodeoxynucleotides.

The latter chapters, which involve the use of both *in vitro* and *in vivo* model systems, and which include the results of some early clinical trials, consider the varied actions of these agents and their potential for treating certain clinical disorders. These include chapters on the use of antisense oligodeoxynucleotides to study reproductive behavior (McCarthy), pain perception (Rossi and Pasternak), hypertension (Phillips and Gyurko), and cancer (Wickstrom). We conclude with chapters on the use of non-viral and viral expression vectors that encode antisense RNA sequences and their potential therapeutic applications in treating disorders involving abnormal cell growth (Oberstrass and Nellen), in inhibiting replication of the human immunodeficiency virus (Bunnell and Morgan), and in treating a variety of neurobiological disorders, including mental illness (Davidkova, Zhang, Zhou, Nichols and Weiss).

Antisense RNA-generating vectors have the advantages of antisense oligodeoxynucleotides insofar as their rational design, specificity, and ease of synthesis is concerned, but have the added advantages in that they may have a longer duration of action, and they may be made to selectively target the antisense to specific cell types and to be selectively expressed in certain cell types. The use of these approaches has the potential of providing a selectivity of action that would be an unprecedented advance in the study and treatment of diseases.

We hope this volume adds not only to our knowledge of basic biological mechanisms but also to our quest for novel, more selective pharmacotherapeutic agents. Equally important, we hope it stimulates the critical analysis of existing studies and progress toward new discoveries in this exciting field.

The Editor

Benjamin Weiss, Ph.D., is Professor of Pharmacology and Psychiatry, and Chief of the Division of Neuropsychopharmacology, Department of Pharmacology, Allegheny University of the Health Sciences, Medical College of Pennsylvania ♦ Hahnemann University School of Medicine, Philadelphia, PA.

Dr. Weiss graduated in 1958 from the Philadelphia College of Pharmacy and Science, Philadelphia, PA with a B.Sc. in Pharmacy (with Distinction), where he also received his Master's degree in 1960. He obtained his Ph.D. from the Philadelphia College of Pharmacy and Science, Philadelphia, PA in 1963. Dr. Weiss was a Postdoctoral Fellow at the National Institutes of Health from 1963–1966, a Research Associate at the College of Physicians and Surgeons, Columbia University from 1966–1968 and was Chief of the Section on Neuroendocrinology at the National Institute of Mental Health from 1968–1972 before joining the Department of Pharmacology at the Medical College of Pennsylvania in 1972 as Professor of Pharmacology.

Dr. Weiss is a member of the American Society for Neurochemistry, Americal Society for Pharmacology and Experimental Therapeutics, American College of Neuropsychopharmacology, International Brain Research Organization, American Association of University Professors, Society for Neuroscience, British Brain Research Association, European Brain Behavior Society, and the International Society for Neurochemistry.

Among his numerous awards, he has received the Gold Medal for achieving the highest scholastic average of all the college graduates in his class, the Joseph W. E. Harrison Award for Excellence in Pharmacology, the Frederick William Haussman Memorial Prize, the Dobbins Scholarship, the Rexall Award, the Bordon Award, the Rho Chi Honorary Pharmaceutical Society Award, the Christian R. and Mary F. Lindback Award for Distinguished Teaching, a Research Medal awarded by the University of Milan, Milan, Italy, a Merit Award from the National Institute of Mental Health, and an Outstanding Scientist Award from the China Bureau of Foreign Experts Affairs, Suzhou Medical College, Suzhou, China.

Dr. Weiss serves on several Editoral Advisory Boards and consults for the National Institute of Mental Health, the National Institute of Aging, the National Science Foundation, the Manitoba Health Research Council, the Franklin Research Center and various pharmaceutical companies. Dr. Weiss has organized a number of scientific symposia and conferences, has chaired about two dozen scientific sessions at national and international meetings and conferences, has been an invited speaker at more than 60 national and international scientific conferences and symposia and has presented more than 100 guest lectures at universities and institutions. He has been the recipient of numerous grants from the National Institutes of Health, including grants from the National Cancer Institute, National Institute of Aging, National Institute of Neurological and Communicative Disorders and Stroke, National Institute of Mental Health, and National Institute of General Medical Sciences. He has also received grants from the Nato Advanced Study Institute, Scottish Rite Schizophrenia Research Program, and the Allegheny-Singer Research Insitute.

Dr. Weiss has edited a book entitled *Cyclic Nucleotides in Diseases* and has published 170 research papers and review articles. His current major research interests include the development of novel molecular biological strategies to alter biological processes.

Contributors

Sudhir Agrawal, Ph.D.
Hybridon, Inc.
Cambridge, Massachusetts

Bruce A. Bunnell, Ph.D.
Clinical Gene Therapy Branch
National Center for Human Genome Research
National Institutes of Health
Bethesda, Maryland

Stanley T. Crooke, M.D., Ph.D.
ISIS Pharmaceuticals
Carlsbad Research Center
Carlsbad, California

Genoveva Davidkova, M.D., Ph.D.
Department of Pharmacology
MCP◊Hahnemann School of Medicine
Allegheny University of the Health Sciences
Philadelphia, Pennsylvania

Robert Gyurko, M.D.
Cardiovascular Research Center
Harvard Medical School
Massachusetts General Hospital
Charlestown, Massachusetts

Kanak Iyer, M.D.
Medicine Branch
National Cancer Institute
National Institutes of Health
Bethesda, Maryland

Margaret M. McCarthy, Ph.D.
Department of Physiology
Center for Studies in Reproduction
University of Maryland
Baltimore, Maryland

Richard A. Morgan, Ph.D.
Clinical Gene Therapy Branch
National Center for Human Genome Research
National Institutes of Health
Bethesda, Maryland

Leonard M. Neckers, Ph.D.
Medicine Branch
National Cancer Institute
National Institutes of Health
Bethesda, Maryland

Wolfgang Nellen, Ph.D.
Department of Genetics
University of Kassel
Kassel, Germany

Robert A. Nichols, Ph.D.
Department of Pharmacology
MCP◊Hahnemann School of Medicine
Allegheny University of the Health Sciences
Philadelphia, Pennsylvania

Jürgen Oberstrass, Ph.D.
Department of Genetics
University of Kassel
Kassel, Germany

Gavril W. Pasternak, M.D., Ph.D.
Department of Neurology
The Cotzias Laboratory of Neuro-Oncology
Memorial Sloan-Kettering Cancer Center
New York, New York

M. Ian Phillips, M.D.
Department of Physiology
College of Medicine
University of Florida
Gainesville, Florida

Grace C. Rossi, Ph.D.
Department of Neurology
The Cotzias Laboratory of Neuro-Oncology
Memorial Sloan-Kettering Cancer Center
New York, New York

Jean-Jacques Toulmé, Ph.D.
INSERM U386
IFR Pathologies Infectieuses
Université Victor Segalen Bordeaux II
Bordeaux, France

Benjamin Weiss, M.D.
Department of Pharmacology
MCP◊Hahnemann School of Medicine
Allegheny University of the Health Sciences
Philadelphia, Pennsylvania

Ruiwen Zhang, M.D., Ph.D.
Department of Pharmacology and Toxicology
University of Alabama
Birmingham, Alabama

Eric Wickstrom, Ph.D.
Department of Microbiology and Immunology
Kimmel Cancer Center
Thomas Jefferson University
Philadelphia, Pennsylvania

Sui-Po Zhang, M.D.
Department of Pharmacology
MCP◊Hahnemann School of Medicine
Allegheny University of the Health Sciences
Philadelphia, Pennsylvania

Long-Wu Zhou, M.D.
Department of Pharmacology
MCP◊Hahnemann School of Medicine
Allegheny University of the Health Sciences
Philadelphia, Pennsylvania

Acknowledgments

I wish to acknowledge with deep appreciation the valuable editorial contributions of Genoveva Davidkova and Joyce Weiss and the excellent secretarial and administrative assistance of Theresa Delgado.

Chapter 1

Historical Aspects of Antisense Oligodeoxynucleotides

Jean-Jacques Toulmé

CONTENTS

I. INTRODUCTION

Antisense nucleic acids are sequences complementary to a sense one, strictly speaking, an RNA bearing genetic information. In the early days of the field, messenger RNA was very generally targeted; hence the term anti-messenger was used for a while.[1] Actually, any kind of RNA can be a target: pre-RNA, mRNA, or viral RNA, the goal being to perturb the "reading" of the encoded information by the antisense-sense hybrid.

To recognize their target, antisense nucleic acids make use of chemical interactions involved in double helices. The composition of the antisense is dictated by the sequence of the RNA with which it is designed to interact, according to the Watson-Crick pairing rules. Therefore, any gene whose sequence is known can be targeted. The selectivity of the binding is primarily achieved by the uniqueness of the target, allowing one to specifically turn off the expression of only one given gene. This

0-8493-8552-0/97/$0.00+$.50

constitutes an invaluable tool for genetic studies and may lead to the development of new therapeutic agents. Blocking the synthesis of a predetermined protein will produce a phenotype to investigate the function of the cognate gene in cells or in live plants or animals. This is particularly attractive for eukaryotic organisms that are not suitable for classical genetic studies because of long generation time or genome complexity. One major interest of the antisense strategy is related to the design of drugs to reduce the expression of any dysfunctional or undesired gene responsible for major pathologies (oncogenes, viral genes, etc.).

Interestingly nature makes use of antisense sequences to regulate gene expression at different levels. In the early 1980s, it was demonstrated that the control of plasmid copy number in bacteria involved natural antisense RNA (see Reference 2 for a review). The most famous example is probably the regulation of ColE1 DNA replication. The primer is generated from an RNA species (RNA II) by RNase H cleavage of RNA II-DNA heteroduplex. This process is negatively controlled by RNA I, a small untranslated RNA, complementary to RNA II. The formation of the RNA I-RNA II complex precludes the hybridization of the nascent RNA II transcript with its DNA template, preventing RNase H to generate the primer.[3,4] Natural antisense RNAs have been also shown to play a role in the translational regulation of prokaryotic genes. The balanced expression of the *Escherichia coli* major outer proteins OmpC and OmpF is regulated in response to the osmolarity of the growth medium. The osmoregulation process involves in particular a 174-base long transcript termed *micF* RNA, exhibiting 70% complementarity to the *OmpF* message, including the Shine-Dalgarno sequence and the translation initiation codon. The association of the two RNA species was shown to inhibit the production of OmpF.[5] Several other examples of regulation of bacterial or phage gene expression by antisense RNA are available.[6,7]Numerous RNAs complementary to transcribed regions have been identified in eukaryotes. However, only in a very limited number of cases has an indication been provided that these "counter-transcripts" may play a role in the regulation of gene expression.[8-10]

These studies have stimulated the engineering of artificial antisense RNA. This is achieved in two different ways. In the first one, the RNA is produced *in situ* from an "antisense gene" placed in an inverted orientation with respect to the natural situation, thus the non-coding strand is transcribed. The expression of many genes has been reduced using this strategy, both in prokaryotes and in cultured eukaryotic cells.[11,12] (See Reference 13 for a review.) A limited number of successful results have been reported *in vivo*.[14-16] Alternatively, antisense RNA can be synthesized *in vitro* from an appropriate construct. The antisense transcript is then delivered to the target organism by means of microinjection. This technique has been widely used in *Drosophila* or mouse embryos and *Xenopus* oocytes or eggs.[17,18]

The use of transcripts generated *in vitro* has a principal very similar to the use of synthetic oligonucleotides. In both cases the antisense sequence has to be taken up by the cell or be introduced by microinjection or by a carrier. Artificial regulation of gene expression by antisense RNA turned the light on the chemical side of the stage. The nature of the regulatory sequence is not restricted to RNA; any chemistry is convenient for antisense sequences as far as the molecules are able to selectively bind the target with a sufficiently high affinity. Nucleic acid chemists working on oligonucleotide analogs had proposed interfering with the function of mRNA long before the discovery of natural antisense RNA. In a prophetic paper published in 1967, Grineva and co-workers[19] suggested using short oligodeoxynucleotides functionalized with an alkylating group for "complementary addressed" modification of nucleic acids:

"Modification of a monomer unit of the polymer chain with some reagent and subsequent study of the activity of the modified biopolymer is one of the possible approaches to elucidate the role of this unit in the activity under investigation. To realize this approach it is necessary to modify selectively determined monomer unit of the biopolymer molecule without touching other similar residues. A more general approach would be provided by reagents, specially devised to discriminate between similar monomer units having different intramolecular environment due to interaction with neighbour lying residues of the polymer chain. **In the case of nucleic acids it seems promising for the purpose to obtain compounds, containing a reactive group bound to oligonucleotide residue capable of specific base pairing with the complementary nucleotide sequence.**"

By the mid-1970s major contributions from the laboratory of Ts'o and Miller demonstrated the potential interest of chemically modified oligonucleotides to probe the structure and the function of nucleic acids. They showed that ethylphosphotriester tri- and tetra-oligodeoxynucleotides, complementary to either the 3′ terminus or to the anticodon region of the $tRNA^{Phe}$ from *E. coli* inhibited the *in vitro* reaction catalyzed by aminoacyl-tRNA synthetase.[20] Such compounds are resistant to serum nucleases and are taken up by hamster embryo cells. Their addition to cultured fibroblasts resulted in a decreased protein synthesis.[21] The reversibility of the effect was likely due to the degradation of the oligonucleotide within the cell. Due to the short size of the sequence used, no selective effect could be expected, but Miller et al. recognized that their "observations ... lay the groundwork for continued investigation into the use of neutral oligonucleotide analogues as probes and regulators of nucleic acid function within living cells."[21]

Indeed, hybrid-arrest of translation by complementary DNA fragments was used to identify mRNAs.[22,23] One of the key contributions on antisense oligonucleotides was published by Zamecnik and Stephenson.[24,25] Due to the development of DNA synthesis in solution they were able to prepare a tridecamer complementary to the reiterated sequence which was recently identified at both ends of the RNA of the Rous sarcoma virus (RSV). They were able to inhibit viral mRNA translation in cell-free extracts in a sequence-dependent manner.[24] They also performed *in vitro* assays with infected chick embryo fibroblasts, speculating that the complementary 13-mer could interfere with the production of RSV.[25] The development of the virus, monitored by the reverse transcriptase activity, was inhibited by the addition of the antisense oligomer at 10 μg/ml (about 2 μ*M*). The authors considered the problem of degradation by exonucleases and used an oligonucleotide terminally protected by isourea derivatization. They also suggested alternative possibilities for hybridization interference (translation initiation block, transcription block, etc.) and concluded about the potential of oligonucleotide hybridization "to inhibit oncogenic viral integration, multiplication and cell transformation." For these authors,

"...the possible future general chemotherapeutic potentiality of oligonucleotide hybridization depends first on sequencing RNAs (or DNAs) from oncogenic viruses to which particular animal species are susceptible, and then synthesizing deoxyribo- or ribo-oligonucleotides that are of sufficient length to hybridize well with a segment of viral RNA or DNA, and are sufficiently specific for the virus in question (non-oncogenic as well as oncogenic) to avoid hybridizing well with normal cellular nucleic acids. For example, if the primary sequence of a unique small segment of a negative strand RNA virus such as influenza, measles, or rabies were known, it would be possible to synthesize and test its oligonucleotide complement as a possible virus inhibitor".[25]

Today it is not easy to understand why the pioneering work of oligonucleotide chemists in the late 1970s did not awaken a significant interest, as there were very few papers published in the field from 1979 to 1985.[26-38] Their contribution was actually acknowledged after the discovery of natural regulation of gene expression by antisense RNA. The availability of automated oligonucleotide synthesis allowed the development of the antisense strategy using chemically modified oligomers.

During the last ten years numerous oligonucleotide analogs have been synthesized which display improved antisense properties compared to unmodified regular DNA or RNA. Molecular mechanisms responsible for the inhibition of gene expression by complementary oligomers have been elucidated. Experiments with synthetic oligonucleotides are no longer restricted to cell-free assays or tissue culture; *in vivo* assays in animals have been reported and clinical trials are underway. The design of regulatory sequences has been extended by new concepts like DNA being targeted by triple-helix forming oligomers susceptible to interfere with transcription,[39] and nucleic acid-binding proteins responsible for gene regulation that can be trapped by short oligomers mimicking the natural binding site of these regulatory proteins, thus acting as decoys.[40] Even if one excludes these so-called triplex (or anti-gene) and sense approaches for which RNA is not the target of the regulatory oligonucleotide, the antisense strategy offers new possibilities. The use of circular clamps or double-hairpin-forming oligomers involves the formation of local triple helices.[41-43] Last, beyond rational design, *in vitro* selection of aptamers offers a new way to identify regulatory oligonucleotide sequences.[44] This chapter will highlight the key steps of the short but fruitful history of antisense oligonucleotides.*

II. MOLECULAR MECHANISMS RESPONSIBLE FOR THE INHIBITION OF GENE EXPRESSION BY ANTISENSE OLIGONUCLEOTIDES

Antisense oligonucleotides complementary to mRNA were initially viewed as steric blockers. The sense-antisense duplex was supposed to prevent the translation by direct competition with the macromolecular complex translating the message, hence the name hybrid-arrested translation to characterize this process. However, this accounted for only part of the effects induced by complementary oligonucleotides. Physical blocking did not provide an explanation for the inhibition of translation by antisense oligomers targeted to the 3′ end of the message downstream of the stop codon.[33] Moreover, in several cases it appeared that the target RNA did not remain intact in the process. This suggested that oligodeoxynucleotides could induce the degradation of the message by ribonuclease H (RNase H). Indeed, the addition of *E. coli* RNase H to reticulocyte lysate led to the inhibition of translation of tobacco mosaic virus mRNA by cDNA fragments, which were inefficient antisense sequences in the absence of the bacterial enzyme.[45] In contrast, no addition of exogenous RNase H was required to inhibit protein synthesis in wheat germ extract. This latter cell-free medium exhibited a higher level of endogenous RNase H, active under *in vitro* translation conditions, than reticulocyte lysate.[46]

It turned out that antisense oligonucleotide studies, stimulated the interest for RNases H, together with the fact that such an activity plays a key role in the development of retroviruses, including the human immunodeficiency virus (HIV).

* Ribozymes (RNA sequences catalyzing the cleavage of a target RNA chain) will not be discussed here, although their effect is primarily mediated through the binding of "antisense motifs," flanking the catalytic core, to the "sense" sequence surrounding the cleavage site. Chemically synthesized ribozymes have been prepared and evaluated which share some characteristics with true antisense oligonucleotides.

Although the crystal structure of both the *E. coli* HI enzyme and of the p15 domain of the reverse transcriptase of HIV-1 have been solved,[47-49] very little is known about eukaryotic enzymes, which are of prime interest for therapeutic applications of antisense oligonucleotides in mammals.

Ribonucleases H are enzymes which cleave the RNA strand of RNA-DNA complexes. They were discovered in calf thymus in 1969 by Stein and Hausen[50] and are ubiquitous enzymes found in every cell from bacteria to higher eukaryotes. In *E. coli* the HI enzyme was shown to be involved in DNA replication by selective removal of Okazaki fragments, which prime the synthesis of the lagging strand. In retroviruses, RNase H is involved in the degradation of the retroviral RNA and in the removal of the tRNA primer, prior to the integration of the viral genome in the host genome (see References 51 and 52 for reviews). In higher eukaryotes much less is known. Two types of activity, termed HI and HII, have been characterized in bovine tissues[53] and more recently, in those of humans.[54,55] They differ by their molecular weight and their biochemical properties. RNase HII is active exclusively in the presence of Mg^{2+} (and inhibited by Mn^{2+}) whereas RNases HI are activated by either cations.[56] RNases HI are likely involved in replication and RNases HII in transcription.[51,52]

Thus, at least two mechanisms are responsible for the inhibition of translation by antisense oligonucleotides. In the first one, the binding of the oligonucleotide to its target RNA is strong enough to prevent either the scanning of the message by the translating complex or its binding to RNA. In other words, the antisense sequence acts as a road block by physically preventing the "reading" of the genetic information. In the second process the oligonucleotide mediates the cleavage of the complementary portion of the target RNA by RNase H. Therefore, the important difference between the two mechanisms is that the first one is reversible and stoichiometric, while the second one is irreversible and can be catalytic. As the oligonucleotide remains intact in the RNase H-dependent process, it can re-bind to a second RNA molecule once freed from the first duplex, following RNA cleavage. Therefore, RNase H acts as an amplifier of antisense effects. The combination of this enzymatic activity with complementary oligodeoxynucleotides can lead to the destruction of multiple targets.

It is important to note that only the RNase H-dependent mechanism is operative for inhibiting the elongation of a polypeptide chain. In the absence of RNase H, an oligomer complementary to the coding region is displaced from the target RNA by the ribosome. In contrast, physical arrest can be observed with oligonucleotides bound to the 5′ region of the message (from the cap site to about 15 nucleotides downstream of the AUG), as demonstrated both with cDNA fragments and with synthetic oligomers.[57,58]

The involvement of RNase H in antisense oligonucleotide-mediated effects has been demonstrated for cell-free translation assays[45,59,60] and for microinjected *Xenopus* oocytes.[60,61] It is assumed that the same mechanisms are responsible for the effects of oligonucleotides observed in higher eukaryotic cells. However, mostly indirect indications suggest that RNase H is involved. Several reports have mentioned that the level of target mRNA was decreased upon treatment of cultured cells with oligonucleotides[62,63] and that cells devoid of RNase H are not sensitive to antisense oligomers.[64] However, oligonucleotide derivatives that do not elicit RNase H were also reported to lead to decreased mRNA levels.[65] Direct evidence for the involvement of RNase H was provided recently for embryonic lung fibroblasts[66] and for myelogenous leukemia cells.[67] Generally, although clevage products generated by RNase H cannot be detected as they are immediately trimmed by intracellular

RNases, in these cases RNA fragments were visualized by ribonuclease protection analysis and reverse-ligation mediated polymerase chain reaction (PCR).

The two mechanisms (hybrid arrest and RNase H-mediated cleavage) responsible for the antisense effect of oligonucleotides are not restricted to the inhibition of translation. RNase H has a predominant nuclear location, and oligonucleotides are known to distribute in both nuclear and cytoplasmic compartments.[68,69] As the target sequence is usually present both on the mature mRNA and on the pre-RNA, antisense oligomers could prevent either splicing or transport of the RNA from the nucleus to the cytoplasm. Indeed, splicing inhibition has been unambiguously demonstrated using oligonucleotides targeted to intron-exon junctions or to intron sequences.[70-72] The inhibition of reverse transcription by antisense oligonucleotides has also been demonstrated to take place through these two different processes.[73,74] This might be of interest for controlling the development of retroviruses.[75]

Besides these two major mechanisms, oligonucleotides can mediate additional effects. The binding of an antisense oligomer can induce a conformation change of the target, subsequently interfering with a biological process (protein binding, lifetime, etc.). Such an effect has been suggested to explain the inhibition of translation of ICAM-1 mRNA in human lung carcinoma cell lines.[76] It was recently demonstrated that antisense oligomers triggered drastic conformational changes of a DNA hairpin, altering its cleavage by a restriction enzyme.[77] Finally, unexpected effects of oligonucleotides, either sequence-dependent or sequence-independent, have been described which mainly rest upon the association of oligonucleotides with proteins (see Chapter 4).

III. DESIGNING AN ANTISENSE OLIGONUCLEOTIDE

Naked unmodified DNA or RNA oligomers are of limited interest for antisense applications in living organisms or even in cultured cells. The need for chemically modified derivatives was recognized in the pioneering works of Miller and Ts'o[20] and of Zamecnik and Stephenson,[25] who used ethylphosphotriester and isourea conjugates, respectively, to slow down the degradation of antisense oligonucleotides by endo- and exonucleases. Protection against nucleases is not the only parameter to take into account in the design of oligomers of improved efficiency. Antisense oligonucleotides have to compete with proteins for binding to RNA. This requires that their affinity is sufficiently high. (However, as discussed below, this should be carefully adjusted in order to get specific effects.) The oligonucleotides should be taken up by cells and should reach the compartment where the sense sequence is located. Due to the likely key role played by RNase H, the ability of modified oligomers to induce RNA degradation should also be considered. Pairing with the sense strand requires that the target is available, i.e., not engaged in a stable secondary or tertiary RNA structure. Finally, for biological purposes the compound should be devoid of toxicity. Before briefly discussing these different points, it is important to understand that the introduction of any chemical modification will perturb the overall physical and biochemical properties of the oligonucleotide and therefore will make necessary the complete evaluation of the antisense behavior of the analog.

Nuclease sensitivity was the easiest problem to solve. Numerous compounds have been prepared which show an increased metabolic stability.[78] Phosphorothioates, in which a nonbridging oxygen of an internucleosidic group has been substituted by a sulfur, are by far the most frequently used analog, both *in vitro* and *in vivo*, including in human beings.[79] However, they display nonspecific affinity for many proteins. This might be of interest, for instance, in the case of AIDS as antisense phosphorothioate oligonucleotides are inhibitors of the HIV reverse transcriptase and prevent the binding of the retrovirus to the host cell. These sequence-independent effects are discussed in Chapter 4. Methylphosphonates have been used for years by the groups of Miller and Ts'o, and in contrast to unmodified and phosphorothioate oligomers, they are uncharged molecules.[80] They display a rather low affinity for RNA under physiological conditions. This might be due, at least in part, to the fact that methylphosphonate oligomers are obtained as a mixture of compounds as the substitution of a nonbridging oxygen of the internucleoside link by a methyl group generates a chiral phosphorus atom and, consequently, two stereoisomers with different binding constants. Therefore, a methylphosphonate sequence n units long will be a mixture of 2^n different molecules, a property shared by phosphorothioate analogs.

More recently, several nuclease resistant derivatives namely 2'-*O*-methyl oligoribonucleotides,[81] N3'-P5' phosphoramidates,[82] and peptide nucleic acid (PNA),[83] have received particular attention, essentially because they have a greater affinity for RNA than unmodified oligomers. One can therefore expect to observe biological effects at lower concentrations. However, it remains to be proved that this actually provides any advantage to these compounds in living systems, because, as stated above, the antisense efficiency results from the balance between several parameters: lifetime, binding constant, and uptake, in particular. For instance, PNA is not taken up by cells and should be administered by electroporation or via a carrier. Last, it should be mentioned that the chemically modified oligomers listed above, except phosphorothioate analogs, do not elicit RNase H activity.

Antisense properties are related to the fraction of the target site covered by the oligonucleotide, whereas the specificity derives from the relative amount of oligomer bound to its target and to any partially complementary sites (nontarget sites). Therefore, the selectivity index of antisense oligonucleotides is directly related to the binding constants for the perfect complementary site and for the mismatched sequences, on the one hand, and to the concentration of the different partners, on the other hand, according to the law of mass action. On a statistical basis, an AT sequence 19 nucleotides long and a GC sequence 15 nucleotides long are unique in the human genome at the DNA level.[84] Uniqueness at the RNA level is achieved using 15- and 11-mer for AT and GC targets, respectively.

In contrast to what one would intuitively conclude, increasing the length of the antisense sequence will result in a decreased rather than in an increased specificity. Indeed, longer sequences will generate a larger number of partially complementary sequences, leading to complexes that are stable under the experimental conditions. In other words, a long antisense oligonucleotide will tolerate more mismatches than a short one and, therefore, form hybrids with multiple nontarget sites. The interdependence of affinity and specificity has been clearly demonstrated for antisense sequences targeted to the point-mutated region of the Ha-ras gene; whereas a 17-mer showed discrimination between the mutated and the wild-type sequence, a 19-mer did not, and a 15-mer showed a very low efficiency.[85]

Similar observations have been reported for sandwich oligomers. Two chemistries were combined in an antisense sequence to take advantage of different properties. For instance, methylphosphonate/phosphodiester/methylphosphonate chimeras are resistant to exonucleases and allow RNase H cleavage if the unmodified stretch is larger than four nucleotides. It was demonstrated that such molecules display enhanced selectivity in cell-free translation assays[86,87] and in cultured cells.[88,89] A chimeric methylphosphonate/phosphodiester sandwich type oligomer displayed a better discrimination between its target site on the α-globin mRNA and partially complementary sites on the β-globin message than did the unmodified antisense sequence.[86] This was related to a reduced RNase H sensitivity of the nonperfect hybrids formed with methylphosphonate chimeras. This was essentially dictated by the affinity of the antisense oligomer for the target and nontarget sites. The homologous 2′-*O*-alkyl/phosphodiester sandwich oligomer, which binds stronger to RNA than the methylphosphonate chimera, did not show any selectivity.[87]

One of the major problems which still remains to be solved is delivering oligonucleotides into the cell and to having them reach their target. The numerous positive results obtained with oligomers added in the cell growth medium or used *in vivo* definitely demonstrate that they are able to cross the plasma membrane. However, oligonucleotides and their analogs, including methylphosphonates which are neutral, do not diffuse freely through the phospholipid bilayer.[90] They are rather taken up through energy-dependent mechanisms, primarily absorptive endocytosis and fluid phase pinocytosis. Part of the uptake could be mediated through the interaction with an 80-kDa membrane protein; this protein has been identified on the surface of different cell types.[91,92] Larger proteins have also been characterized.[93] Oligonucleotide conjugates have been prepared in order to improve the uptake of antisense derivatives by live cells. The early attempts made use of polycations and hydrophobic tails. Polylysine was shown to improve the antisense efficiency of oligomers targeted to the initiation region of the N protein from the vesicular stomatitis virus (VSV) by about two orders of magnitude.[94] Cholesteryl conjugates also led to increased uptake[95] and better anti-HIV-1 activity in Molt-3 cells.[96] These chemical modifications, aimed at improving the cell penetration, can also yield nuclease resistant oligomers; tethering the ligand to the 3′ end of the oligonucleotide protects it from 3′ exonuclease which is the most abundant exonuclease form. More recently, oligonucleotides have been linked to fusogenic peptides[97] or to a peptide derived from the homeodomain of the *Drosophila antennapedia* protein.[98] In both cases this resulted in improved biological properties compared to the free oligonucleotide. Alternatively, carriers such as liposomes,[69] lipoproteins,[99] nanospheres,[100] or polyethyleneimine[101] were used to deliver antisense oligomers to live cells. Recent studies have shown interest in the so-called cationic lipids to deliver polyanions, i.e., DNA and oligonucleotides. Lipofectin, a combination of dioleyloxypropyltrimethyl ammonium (DOTMA) and dioleylphosphatidylethanolamine (DOPE) was used successfully.[102] Lewis et al.[103] were able, using phosphorothioate oligonucleotides combined with a noncationic lipid formulated with DOPE, to observe sequence specific antisense effects on HeLa cells in the nanomolar range. In addition to being beneficial for the uptake, this kind of carrier protects the oligomer from nucleases and restricts the interaction between the oligonucleotide and the cell membrane, for instance, decreasing the sequence-independent effects of phosphorothioate analogs.[104]

Two points related to uptake should also be considered: cell targeting and compartmentalization inside the cell. In order to decrease the amount of oligonucleotides used in antisense experiments and to reduce side effects, it is desirable to restrict the distribution of oligomers only to those cells expressing the target gene. This has been achieved using cell surface receptors as markers recognized by the cognate ligand, conjugated to the antisense sequence. For this purpose, immunoliposomes,[104] neoglycoproteins,[105] and folate[106] have been used.

Following endocytosis, the bulk of oligonucleotide accumulates into the lysozomal compartment. However, the occurrence of biological effects such as inhibition of gene expression clearly indicates that part of the oligonucleotide escapes and reaches its target, either in the cytoplasm[107] or in the nucleus,[108] as both cytoplasmic (VSV development) and nuclear events (splicing of herpesvirus early messages) have been blocked. Presently, very little is known about oligonucleotide trafficking between the different cell compartments. The intracellular distribution of the oligonucleotides and their biological effects depend on the means by which they have been administered. For instance, antisense oligomers complementary to p53 mRNA were shown to be active only on streptolysine-permeabilized cells but not on intact ones.[89]

For an oligonucleotide to bind to an RNA and to induce antisense effects, the target sequence should be available for base-pairing. The presence of folded regions, as well as the association of the RNA with proteins, can restrict the binding of the complementary oligonucleotide, resulting in a weak antisense effect.[109,110] Predicting tertiary and secondary structure of RNA is not an easy task even for isolated molecules in solution. Therefore, selecting a target for antisense studies is more of a hit-or miss-process than a rational one. Different approaches have been considered to circumvent this problem (see Reference 111 for a review). The identification of an open region for hybridization can be achieved through general screening of antisense oligomers against a target message, from the 5′ to the 3′ end.[112-114] Increasing the affinity of the oligomer for the complementary RNA sequence will allow the antisense oligomer to compete more efficiently with the intramolecular RNA structure. This can be achieved by increasing the length of the oligonucleotide[115] or by tethering it to an intercalating agent, for instance.[84] However, the specificity will decrease as the binding constant to partially complementary sites will also be increased (see above). To reduce the thermodynamic cost for melting the structure, one can take advantage of unpaired bases in loops or bulges.[116] Alternatively, strategies have been proposed to accommodate the folded motif in the complex. This was achieved through the formation of local triple helices[117,127] or by *in vitro* selection of oligomers able to interact with the structured RNA.[118,119]

IV. CONCLUSION

Antisense oligonucleotides have proven to be valuable tools for molecular genetic studies. The large number of successful *in vitro* studies in the 1980s, along with the developments in oligonucleotide chemistry which allowed the synthesis of multigram quantities at reduced costs, as well as the urgent need of nonconventional drugs for major human pathologies, led to *in vivo* trials at the beginning of this decade. The first study on animals using a synthetic oligonucleotide was published in 1992 by Rosenberg et al.[120] They reported on the inhibition of the proliferation of intimal artery smooth muscle cell in rat carotid. The phosphorothioate oligomer, complementary to *c-myc*, was delivered locally by a pluronic gel. This constituted a model for the treatment of restenosis following coronary artery angioplasty. Several reports were then published on different animals including mouse, rat, rabbit, and duck. Oligonucleotides were delivered by various means: local delivery by catheter or by subcutaneously implanted osmotic pumps and intravenous or intraperitoneal injection. Different classes of genes have been targeted, indicating that antisense oligonucleotides are of potential interest for major human pathologies including cancer, infectious diseases, neuropsychiatric disorders, and restenosis. Most of the antisense oligonucleotides used *in vivo* in animal models were phosphorothioate analogs. This is also the case for the sequences presently under investigation in human clinical trials for acute or chronic myelogenous leukemia, genital warts, and AIDS-related retinitis due to cytomegalovirus (CMV) infection.[121] Although it is presently too early for conclusions to be drawn regarding the efficacy of these molecules, it is fascinating to see how fast the field evolved from *in vitro* cultured cell assays to a phase III human clinical trial (for CMV retinitis). Less than ten years ago many people thought that oligonucleotides would not enter live cells!

Besides the antisense approach, several related strategies are being explored that take advantage of the unique properties of nucleic acids for designing new tools for research in molecular biology and potential new therapeutic agents. These include triplex- or "antigene"-forming oligomers, sense oligonucleotides, and aptamers. Targeting double-stranded DNA to generate triple-stranded structures that could interfere with transcription or replication is an attractive solution. In this case, a single sequence has to be inhibited by the oligonucleotide, in contrast to multiple transcripts in the antisense strategy. Therefore, one might expect biological effects at lower oligonucleotide concentration for triplex-forming sequences than for antisense ones. The present major hurdle for this approach is the limited repertoire of target sequences, as triple helices can be formed essentially from duplexes made of pyrimidines on one strand and purines on the second strand.[39] Although different ways to accommodate inverted base pairs in triple helices have been described (i.e., reading a pyrimidine in a purine stretch), we are far from being able to form triple-stranded structures with any double strand. However, pyrimidine-purine motifs are much more frequent in eukaryotic genomes than are expected on a statistical basis. More importantly, such sequences prone to triple helical formation are encountered in promoter regions. Indeed, artificial regulation of transcription has been reported in cultured cells, mostly with oligopurines or G.T oligomers. Triple helices have also been generated for antisense purposes; in this case a single-stranded RNA sequence is targeted by circular or so-called clamp oligonucleotides.[41,42,122,123] A similar approach has also been used to target hairpin structures.[43,117]

In the sense approach, the target is neither RNA nor DNA but a nucleic acid-binding protein. Proteins which exhibit sequence-specificity will bind to synthetic oligomers with this sequence. This has been amply used to characterize the binding sites of transcription factors by electrophoretic mobility shift assays and to inhibit *in vitro* transcription controlled by different factors such as SP1.[124] One may think that delivery of double-stranded oligonucleotides into cells would allow the cell to trap the cognate protein, thus allowing it to artificially modulate the transcription of the genes under its control. Indeed, microinjection of such decoys with the cAMP response element into 3T3 fibroblasts inhibited the induction of *c-fos* by cyclic AMP.[125] Chemically modified oligomers have also been used; double-stranded phosphorothioate oligonucleotides have been shown to specifically prevent the transcription of reporter constructs[126] in transfected cells. Sense oligomers should be delivered as double-stranded molecules. This led to the design of the so-called dumbbell oligomers which are circular covalently closed sequences exhibiting a short duplex region. Dumbbell oligomers inhibited the effect of the transcription factor HNF1 in human epithelial cells.[40] It should be possible to use such an approach to titrate out regulatory RNA binding proteins. In this case the sense oligomer should mimic an RNA fragment.

Recently a new strategy took advantage of the physical properties of nucleic acid chains to design specific ligands against various kinds of targets, wherein sequences of interest are extracted by *in vitro* selection from large libraries of random oligomers. Therefore, in contrast to the aforementioned approaches (antisense, triplex, sense), the oligonucleotide is not rationally designed on the basis of known interactions between the target and the ligand, but selected according to a given criteria (affinity, activity, etc.). Due to the propensity of nucleic acids to fold into rigid organized structures, oligonucleotide libraries will generate multiple shapes exhibiting many binding properties, some of them being exquisitely adapted to the target of interest. Indeed, aptamers, the generic name for the selected oligomers, have been identified for a large variety of molecules, ranging from small organic constituents, such as amino acids or nucleotides, to macromolecules.[44] If one targets an element (a protein or a nucleic acid sequence) involved in gene expression, aptamers could modulate the synthesis of the related protein.

These oligonucleotides (antisense, triplex-forming, sense, aptamers) share a number of characteristics. Improvement of efficiency is expected by using nuclease-resistant derivatives or analogs that are taken up more easily by live cells. However, they are profoundly different regarding their mode of action, the biochemical nature of the target, and the cell compartment they should reach. Rather than rival, these different strategies should be considered as complementary. One approach might prove better than another depending on the gene sequence, the level of expression, the lifetime of the gene products (RNA, protein), or the regulatory circuits. Nucleic acids now offer a wide range for designing new therapeutic agents.

ACKNOWLEDGMENTS

The author's laboratory is supported by the Direction des Recherches Etudes et Techniques, the Conseil Régional d'Aquitaine, the Agence Nationale de Recherche sur le SIDA, and the Association pour la Recherche contre le Cancer.

REFERENCES

1. Toulmé, J. J. and Hélène, C, Antimessenger oligodeoxynucleotides: an alternative to antisense RNA for artificial regulation of gene expression — a review, *Gene*, 72, 51, 1988.
2. Simons, R. W., Naturally occurring antisense RNA control — a brief review, *Gene*, 72, 35, 1988.
3. Itoh, T. and Tomizawa, J.-I., Formation of an RNA primer for initiation of replication of ColE1 DNA by ribonuclease H, *Proc. Natl. Acad. Sci. U.S.A.*, 77, 2450, 1980.
4. Polisky, B., ColE1 replication control cicuitry: sense from antisense, *Cell*, 55, 929, 1988.
5. Mizuno, T., Chou, M. Y., and Inouye, M., A unique mechanism regulating gene expression: translational inhibition by a complementary RNA transcript (micRNA), *Proc. Natl. Acad. Sci. U.S.A.*, 81, 1966, 1984.
6. Simons, R. W. and Kleckner, N., Biological regulation by antisense RNA in prokaryotes, *Ann. Rev. Genet.*, 22, 567, 1988.
7. Takayama, K. M. and Inouye, M., Antisense RNA, *Crit. Rev. Biochem. Mol. Biol.*, 25, 155, 1990.
8. Bester, A. J., Kennedy, D. S., and Heywood, S. M., Two classes of translational control RNA: their role in the regulation of protein synthesis, *Proc. Natl. Acad. Sci. U.S.A.*, 72, 1523, 1975.
9. Stevens, J. G., Wagner, E. K., Devi-Rao, G. B., Cook, M. L., and Feldman, L. T., RNA complementary to a herpes virus α gene mRNA is prominent in latently infected neurons, *Science*, 235, 1056, 1987.
10. Volloch, V., Schuweitzer, B., and Rits, S., Antisense globin RNA in mouse erythroid tissues: structure, origin, and possible function, *Proc. Natl. Acad. Sci. U.S.A.*, 93, 2476, 1996.
11. Coleman, J., Hirashima, A., Inokuchi, Y., Green, P. J., and Inouye, M., A novel immune system against bacteriophage infection using complementary RNA (micRNA), *Nature*, 315, 601, 1985.
12. Izant, J. G. and Weintraub, H., Inhibition of thymidine kinase gene expression by anti-sense RNA: a molecular approach to genetic analysis, *Cell*, 36, 1007, 1984.
13. Murray, J. A. H., *Antisense RNA and DNA*, 11, Wiley-Liss, New York, 1992, 401.
14. Katsuki, M., Sato, M., Kimura, M., Yokoyama, M., Kobayashi, K., and Nomura, T., Conversion of normal behavior to shiverer by myelin basic protein antisense cDNA in transgenic mice, *Science*, 593, 1988.
15. Kitajima, I., Shinohara, T., Bilakovics, J., Brown, D. A., Xu, X., and Nerenberg, M., Ablation of transplanted HTLV-I Tax-transformed tumors in mice by antisense inhibition of NF-kappaB, *Science*, 258, 1792, 1992.
16. Fakhrai, H., Dorigo, O., Shawler, D. L., Lin, H., Mercola, D., Black, K., Royston, I., and Sobol, R. E., Eradication of established intracranial rat gliomas by transforming growth factor B antisense gene therapy, *Proc. Natl. Acad. Sci. U.S.A.*, 93, 2909, 1996.

17. Melton, D. A., Injected anti-sense RNAs specifically block messenger RNA translation *in vivo*, *Proc. Natl. Acad. Sci. U.S.A.*, 82, 144, 1985.
18. Rosenberg, U. B., Preiss, A., Seifert, E., Jäckle, H., and Knipple, D. C., Production of phenocopies by Krüppel antisense RNA injection into *Drosophila* embryos, *Nature*, 313, 703, 1985.
19. Belikova, A. M., Zarytova, V. F., and Grineva, N. I., Synthesis of ribonucleosides and diribonucleoside phosphates containing 2-chloroethylamine and nitrogen mustard residues, *Tetrahedron Lett.*, 37, 3557, 1967.
20. Barrett, J. C., Miller, P. S., and Ts'o, P. O. P., Inhibitory effect of complex formation with oligodeoxynucleotide ethyl phosphotriesters on transfer ribonucleic acid aminoacylation, *Biochemistry*, 13, 4897, 1974.
21. Miller, P. S., Braiterman, L. T., and Ts'o, P. O. P., Effects of a trinucleotide ethyl phosphotriester, Gmp(Et)Gmp(Et)U on mammalian cells in culture, *Biochemistry*, 16, 1988, 1977.
22. Paterson, B. M., Roberts, B. E., and Kuff, E. L., Structural gene identification and mapping by DNA-mRNA hybrid-arrested cell-free translation, *Proc. Natl. Acad. Sci. U.S.A.*, 74, 4370, 1977.
23. Hastie, N. D. and Held, W. A., Analysis of mRNA populations by cDNA-mRNA hybrid-mediated inhibition of cell-free protein synthesis, *Proc. Natl. Acad. Sci. U.S.A.*, 75, 1217, 1978.
24. Stephenson, M. L. and Zamecnik, P. C., Inhibition of Rous sarcoma viral RNA translation by a specific oligodeoxyribonucleotide, *Proc. Natl. Acad. Sci. U.S.A.*, 75, 285, 1978.
25. Zamecnik, P. C. and Stephenson, M. L., Inhibition of Rous sarcoma virus replication and cell transformation by a specific oligodeoxynucleotide, *Proc. Natl. Acad. Sci. U.S.A.*, 75, 280, 1978.
26. Summerton, J., Intracellular inactivation of specific nucleotide sequences: a general approach to the treatment of viral diseases and virally-mediated cancers, *J. Theor. Biol.*, 78, 77, 1979.
27. Miller, P. S., McFarland, K. B., Jayaraman, K., and Ts'o, P. O. P., Biochemical and biological effects of nonionic nucleic acid methylphosphonates, *Biochemistry*, 20, 1874, 1981.
28. Jayaraman, K., McFarland, K., Miller, P., and Ts'o, P. O. P., Selective inhibition of *Escherichia coli* protein synthesis and growth by nonionic oligonucleotides complementary to the 3′ end of 16S rRNA, *Proc. Natl. Acad. Sci. U.S.A.*, 78, 1537, 1981.
29. Trudel, M., Dondon, J., Grunberg-Manago, M., Finelli, J., and Buckingham, R. H., Effect of oligonucleotide AGAGGAGGU on protein synthesis *in vitro*, *Biochimie*, 63, 235, 1981.
30. Winkler, M. E., Mullis, K., Barnett, J., Stroynowski, I., and Yanofsky, C., Transcription termination at the tryptophan operon attenuator is decreased *in vitro* by an oligomer complementary to a segment of the leader transcript, *Proc. Natl. Acad. Sci. U.S.A.*, 79, 2181, 1982.
31. Grachev, M. A., Zaychikov, E. F., Ivanova, E. M., Komarova, N. I., Kutyavin, I. V., Sidelnikova, N. P., and Frolova, I. P., Oligonucleotides complementary to a promoter over the region -8...+2 as transcription primers for *E. coli* RNA polymerase, *Nucleic Acids Res.*, 12, 8509, 1984.
32. Krämer, A., Keller, W., Appel, B., and Lührmann, R., The 5′ terminus of the RNA moiety of U1 small nuclear ribonucleoprotein particles is required for the splicing of messenger RNA precursors, *Cell*, 38, 299, 1984.
33. Kawasaki, E. S., Quantitative hybridization-arrest of mRNA in *Xenopus* oocytes using single-stranded complementary DNA or oligonucleotide probes, *Nucleic Acids Res.*, 13, 4991, 1985.
34. Blake, K. R., Murakami, A., Spitz, S. A., Glave, S. A., Reddy, M. P., Ts'o, P. O. P., and Miller, P. S., Hybridization arrest of globin synthesis in rabbit reticulocyte lysate and cells by oligodeoxyribonucleoside methylphosphonates, *Biochemistry*, 24, 6139, 1985.
35. Miller, P. S., Agris, C. H., Aurelian, L., Blake, K. R., Murakami, A., Reddy, M. P., Spitz, S. A., and Ts'o, P. O. P., Control of ribonucleic acid function by oligonucleoside methylphosphonates, *Biochimie*, 67, 769, 1985.
36. Gupta, K. C. and Kingsbury, D. W., Translation modulation *in vitro* of a eukaryotic viral mRNA encoding overlapping genes: ribosome scanning and potential roles of conformational changes in the P/C mRNA of Sendai virus, *Biochem. Biophys. Res. Commun.*, 131, 91, 1985.
37. Hélène, C., Montenay-Garestier, T., Saison, T., Takasugi, M., Toulmé, J. J., Asseline, U., Lancelot, G., Maurizot, J. C., Toulmé, F., and Thuong, N. T., Oligodeoxynucleotides covalently linked to intercalating agents: a new class of gene regulatory substances, *Biochimie*, 67, 777, 1985.
38. Knorre, D. G., Vlassov, V. V., and Zarytova, V. F., Reactive oligonucleotide derivatives and sequence-specific modification of nucleic acids, *Biochimie*, 67, 785, 1985.
39. Thuong, N. T. and Hélène, C., Sequence specific recognition and modification of double-helical DNA by oligonucleotides, *Angew. Chem. Int. Ed. Engl.*, 32, 666, 1993.
40. Clusel, C., Ugarte, E., Enjolras, N., Vasseur, M., and Blumenfeld, M., *Ex vivo* regulation of specific gene expression by nanomolar concentration of double-stranded dumbbell oligonucleotides, *Nucleic Acids Res.*, 21, 3405, 1993.
41. Kool, E. T., Molecular recognition by circular oligonucleotides — increasing the selectivity of DNA binding, *J. Am. Chem. Soc.*, 113, 6265, 1991.

42. Giovannangeli, C., Montenay-Garestier, T., Rougée, M., Chassignol, M., Thuong, N. T., and Hélène, C., Single-stranded DNA as a target for triple-helix formation, *J. Am. Chem. Soc.*, 113, 7775, 1991.
43. Brossalina, E. and Toulmé, J. J., A DNA hairpin as a target for antisense oligonucleotides, *J. Am. Chem. Soc.*, 115, 796, 1993.
44. Gold, L., Polisky, B., Uhlenbeck, O., and Yarus, M., Diversity of oligonucleotide functions, *Ann. Rev. Biochem.*, 64, 763, 1995.
45. Minshull, J. and Hunt, T., The use of single-stranded DNA and RNase-H to promote quantitative hybrid arrest of translation of mRNA/DNA hybrids in reticulocyte lysate cell-free translations, *Nucleic Acids Res.*, 14, 6433, 1986.
46. Cazenave, C., Frank, P., and Büsen, W., Characterization of ribonuclease H activities present in two cell-free protein synthesizing systems, the wheat germ extract and the rabbit reticulocyte lysate, *Biochimie*, 75, 113, 1993.
47. Katayanagi, K., Miyagawa, M., Matsuhima, M., Ishikawa, M., Kanaya, S., Matsuzaki, T., and Morikawa, K., Three-dimensional structure of ribonuclease H from *E. coli*, *Nature*, 347, 306, 1990.
48. Yang, W., Hendrickson, W. A., Crouch, R. J., and Satow, Y., Structure of ribonuclease H phased at 2 Å resolution by MAD analysis of the selenomethionyl protein, *Science*, 249, 1398, 1990.
49. Davies, J. F., Hostomska, Z., Hostomsky, Z., Jordan, S., and Mathews, D. A., Crystal structure of the RNase H domain of HIV-1 reverse trranscriptase, *Science*, 252, 88, 1991.
50. Stein, H. and Hausen, P., Enzyme from calf thymus degrading the RNA moiety of RNA-DNA hybrids: effect on DNA-dependent RNA polymerase, *Science*, 166, 393, 1969.
51. Crouch, R. J., Ribonuclease H: from discovery to 3D structure, *New Biologist*, 2, 771, 1990.
52. Wintersberger, U., Ribonucleases H of retroviral and cellular origin, *Pharmacol. Ther.*, 48, 259, 1990.
53. Vonwirth, H., Frank, P., and Büsen, W., Serological analysis and characterization of calf thymus ribonuclease HIIb, *Eur. J. Biochem.*, 184, 321, 1989.
54. Eder, P. S. and Walder, J. A., Ribonuclease-H from K562 human erythroleukemia cells — purification, characterization, and substrate specificity, *J. Biol. Chem.*, 266, 6472, 1991.
55. Frank, P., Albert, S., Cazenave, C., and Toulmé, J. J., Purification of human RNase HII, *Nucleic Acids Res.*, 22, 5247, 1994.
56. Toulmé, J. J., Boiziau, C., Larrouy, B., Frank, P., Albert, S., and Ahmadi, R., *Ribonuclease H: From Enzymes to Antisense Effects of Oligonucleotides*, in *DNA and RNA Cleavers and Chemotherapy of Cancer and Viral Diseases*, Meunier, B., Kluwer, Dordrecht, The Netherlands, 1996, 271.
57. Liebhaber, S. A., Cash, F. E., and Shakin, S. H., Translationally associated helix-destabilizing activity in rabbit reticulocyte lysate, *J. Biol. Chem.*, 259, 15597, 1984.
58. Boiziau, C., Kurfurst, R., Cazenave, C., Roig, V., Thuong, N. T., and Toulmé, J. J., Inhibition of translation initiation by antisense oligonucleotides via an RNase-H independent mechanism, *Nucleic Acids Res.*, 19, 1113, 1991.
59. Haeuptle, M. T., Frank, R., and Dobberstein, B., Translation arrest by oligodeoxynucleotides complementary to mRNA coding sequences yields polypeptides of predetermined length, *Nucleic Acids Res.*, 14, 1427, 1986.
60. Cazenave, C., Loreau, N., Thuong, N. T., Toulmé, J. J., and Hélène, C., Enzymatic amplification of translation inhibition of rabbit β-globin mRNA mediated by anti-messenger oligodeoxynucleotides covalently linked to intercalating agents, *Nucleic Acids Res.*, 15, 4717, 1987.
61. Dash, P., Lotan, I., Knapp, M., Kandel, E. R., and Goelet, P., Selective elimination of mRNAs *in vivo*: complementary oligodeoxynucleotides promote RNA degradation by an RNase-H-like activity, *Proc. Natl. Acad. Sci. U.S.A.*, 84, 7896, 1987.
62. Harel-Bellan, A., Durum, S., Muegge, K., Abbas, A. K., and Farrar, W. L., Specific inhibition of lymphokine biosynthesis and autocrine growth using antisense oligonucleotides in Th1 and Th2 helper T cell clones, *J. Exp. Med.*, 168, 2309, 1988.
63. Teichman-Weinberg, A., Littauer, U. Z., and Ginzburg, I., The inhibition of neurite outgrowth in PC12 cells by tubulin antisense oligodeoxyribonucleotides, *Gene*, 72, 297, 1988.
64. Boiziau, C. and Toulmé, J. J., Modified oligonucleotides in rabbit reticulocytes: uptake, stability and antisense properties, *Biochimie*, 73, 1403, 1991.
65. Gryaznov, S., Skorski, T., Cucco, C., Skorska, M. N., Chiu, C. Y., Lloyd, D., Chen, J. K., Koziolkiewicz, M., and Calabretta, B., Oligonucleotide N3′–P5′ phosphoramidates as antisense agents, *Nucleic Acids Res.*, 24, 1508, 1996.
66. Strauss, M., Hering, S., Lieber, A., Herrmann, G., Griffin, B. E., and Arnold, W., Stimulation of cell division and fibroblast focus formation by antisense repression of retinoblastoma protein synthesis, *Oncogene*, 7, 769, 1992.
67. Giles, R. V., Spiller, D. G., and Tidd, D. M., Detection of ribonuclease H-generated mRNA fragments in human leukemia cells following reversible membrane permeabilization in the presence of antisense oligodeoxynucleotides, *Antisense Res. Dev.*, 5, 23, 1995.

68. Clarenc, J. P., Lebleu, B., and Léonetti, J. P., Characterization of the nuclear binding sites of oligodeoxyribonucleotides and their analogs, *J. Biol. Chem.*, 268, 5600, 1993.
69. Léonetti, J. P., Degols, G., Clarenc, J. P., Mechti, N., and Lebleu, B., Cell delivery and mechanisms of action of antisense oligonucleotides, in *Prog. Nucleic Acid Res. Mol. Biol.*, 44, Cohn, W. E. and Moldave, K., Eds., Academic Press, San Diego, CA, 1993, 143.
70. Kean, J. M., Kipp, S. A., Miller, P. S., Kulka, M., and Aurelian, L., Inhibition of herpes simplex virus replication by antisense oligo-2′-*O*-methylribonucleoside methylphosphonates, *Biochemistry*, 34, 14617, 1995.
71. Dominski, Z. and Kole, R., Restoration of correct splicing in thalassemic pre-messenger RNA by antisense oligonucleotides, *Proc. Natl. Acad. Sci. U.S.A.*, 90, 8673, 1993.
72. Ramazeilles, C., Mishra, R. K., Moreau, S., Pascolo, E., and Toulmé, J. J., Antisense phosphorothioate oligonucleotides: selective killing of the intracellular parasite *Leishmania amazonensis*, *Proc. Natl. Acad. Sci. U.S.A.*, 91, 7859, 1994.
73. Loreau, N., Boiziau, C., Verspieren, P., Shire, D., and Toulmé, J. J., Blockage of AMV reverse transcriptase by antisense oligodeoxynucleotides, *FEBS Lett.*, 252, 53, 1990.
74. Boiziau, C., Thuong, N. T., and Toulmé, J. J., Mechanisms of the inhibition of reverse transcription by antisense oligonucleotides, *Proc. Natl. Acad. Sci. U.S.A.*, 89, 768, 1992.
75. Bordier, B., Perala-Heape, M., Degols, G., Lebleu, B., Litvak, S., Sarih-Cottin, L., and Hélène, C., Sequence-specific inhibition of human immunodeficiency virus (HIV) reverse transcription by antisense oligonucleotides: comparative study in cell-free assays and in HIV-infected cells, *Proc. Natl. Acad. Sci. U.S.A.*, 92, 9383, 1995.
76. Chiang, M. Y., Chan, H., Zounes, M. A., Freier, S. M., Lima, W. F., and Bennett, C. F., Antisense oligonucleotides inhibit intercellular adhesion molecule-1 expression by two distinct mechanisms, *J. Biol. Chem.*, 266, 18162, 1991.
77. Brossalina, E., Demchenko, E., Demchenko, Y., Vlassov, V., and Toulmé, J. J., Antisense oligonucleotide trigger conformation changes of a target sequence. Modulation of restriction nuclease activity, *Nucleic Acids Res.*, 24, 3392, 1996.
78. Milligan, J. F., Matteucci, M. D., and Martin, J. C., Current concepts in antisense drug design, *J. Med. Chem.*, 36, 1923, 1993.
79. Stein, C. A. and Cheng, Y. C., Antisense oligonucleotides as therapeutic agents — Is the bullet really magical?, *Science*, 261, 1004, 1993.
80. Miller, P. S., Oligonucleoside methylphosphonates as antisense reagents, *BioTechnology*, 9, 358, 1991.
81. Lamond, A. I. and Sproat, B. S., Antisense oligonucleotides made of 2′-*O*-alkylRNA — their properties and applications in RNA biochemistry, *FEBS Lett.*, 325, 123, 1993.
82. Gryaznov, S. M., Lloyd, D. H., Chen, J. K., Schultz, R. G., DeDionisio, L. A., Ratmeyer, L., and Wilson, W. D., Oligonucleotide N3′→P5′ phosphoramidates, *Proc. Natl. Acad. Sci. U.S.A.*, 92, 5798, 1995.
83. Egholm, M., Buchardt, O., Christensen, L., Behrens, C., Freier, S. M., Driver, D. A., Berg, R. H., Kim, S. K., Norden, B., and Nielsen, P. E., PNA hybridizes to complementary oligonucleotides obeying the Watson-Crick hydrogen-bonding rules, *Nature*, 365, 566, 1993.
84. Hélène, C. and Toulmé, J. J., Control of gene expression by oligodeoxynucleotides covalently linked to intercalating agents and nucleic acid cleaving reagents, in *Oligodeoxynucleotides: Antisense Inhibitors of Gene Expression*, 12, Cohen, J. S., Ed., Macmillan Press, London, 1989, 137.
85. Monia, B. P., Johnston, J. F., Ecker, D. J., Zounes, M. A., Lima, W. F., and Freier, S. M., Selective inhibition of mutant ha-ras messenger RNA expression by antisense oligonucleotides, *J. Biol. Chem.*, 267, 19954, 1992.
86. Larrouy, B., Blonski, C., Boiziau, C., Stuer, M., Moreau, S., Shire, D., and Toulmé, J. J., RNase-H mediated inhibition of translation by antisense oligodeoxynucleotides: a way to improve specificity, *Gene*, 121, 189, 1992.
87. Larrouy, B., Boiziau, C., Sproat, B., and Toulmé, J. J., High affinity or selectivity: a dilemma to design antisense oligodeoxynucleotides acting in RNase H-containing media, *Nucleic Acids Res.*, 23, 3434, 1995.
88. Giles, R. V. and Tidd, D. M., Increased specificity for antisense oligodeoxynucleotide targeting of RNA cleavage by RNase-H using chimeric methylphosphonodiester/phosphodiester structures, *Nucleic Acids Res.*, 20, 763, 1992.
89. Giles, R. V., Ruddell, C. J., Spiller, D. G., Green, J. A., and Tidd, D. M., Single base discrimination for ribonuclease H-dependent antisense effects within intact human leukaemia cells, *Nucleic Acids Res.*, 23, 954, 1995.
90. Akhtar, S., Basu, S., Wickstrom, E., and Juliano, R. L., Interactions of antisense DNA oligonucleotide analogs with phospholipid membranes (liposomes), *Nucleic Acids Res.*, 19, 5551, 1991.

91. Loke, S. L., Stein, C. A., Zhang, X. H., Mori, K., Nakanishi, M., Subasinghe, C., Cohen, J. S., and Neckers, L. M., Characterization of oligonucleotide transport into living cells, *Proc. Natl. Acad. Sci. U.S.A.*, 86, 3474, 1989.
92. Yakubov, L. E., Deeva, E. A., Zarytova, V. F., Ivanova, E. M., Ryte, A. S., Yurchenko, L. V., and Vlassov, V. V., Mechanism of oligonucleotide uptake by cells: involvement of specific receptors?, *Proc. Natl. Acad. Sci. U.S.A.*, 86, 6454, 1989.
93. Yao, G. Q., Corrias, S., and Cheng, Y.-C., Identification of two oligodeoxyribonucleotide binding proteins on plasma membranes of human cell lines, *Biochem. Pharmacol.*, 51, 431, 1996.
94. Lemaître, M., Bayard, B., and Lebleu, B., Specific antiviral activity of a poly(L-lysine)-conjugated oligodeoxyribonucleotide sequence complementary to vesicular stomatitis virus N protein mRNA initiation site, *Proc. Natl. Acad. Sci. U.S.A.*, 84, 648, 1987.
95. Boutorin, A. S., Guskova, L. V., Ivanova, E. M., Kobetz, N. D., Zarytova, V. F., Ryte, A. S., Yurchenko, L. V., and Vlassov, V. V., Synthesis of alkylating oligonucleotide derivatives containing cholesterol or phenazidium residue at the 3′ termini and their interaction with DNA within mammalian cells, *FEBS Lett.*, 254, 129, 1989.
96. Letsinger, R. L., Zhang, G., Sun, D. K., Ikeuchi, T., and Sarin, P. S., Cholesteryl-conjugated oligonucleotides: synthesis, properties and activity as inhibitors of replication of human immunodeficiency virus in cell culture, *Proc. Natl. Acad. Sci. U.S.A.*, 86, 6553, 1989.
97. Bongartz, J. P., Aubertin, A. M., Milhaud, P. G., and Lebleu, B., Improved biological activity of antisense oligonucleotides conjugated to a fusogenic peptide, *Nucleic Acids Res.*, 22, 4681, 1994.
98. Allinquant, B., Hantraye, P., Mailleux, P., Moya, K., Bouillot, C., and Prochiantz, A., Downregulation of amyloid precursor protein inhibits neurite outgrowth *in vitro*, *J. Cell Biol*, 128, 919, 1995.
99. Mishra, R. K., Moreau, C., Ramazeilles, C., Moreau, S., Bonnet, J., and Toulmé, J. J., Improved leishmanicidal effect of phosphorothioate antisense oligonucleotides by LDL-mediated delivery, *Biochem. Biophys. Acta*, 1264, 229, 1995.
100. Chavany, C., Le Doan, T., Couvreur, P., Puisieux, F., and Hélène, C., Polyalkylcyanoacrylate nanoparticles as polymeric carriers for antisense oligonucleotides, *Pharm. Res.*, 9, 441, 1992.
101. Boussif, O., Lezoualc'h, F., Zanta, M. A., Mergny, M. D., Scherman, D., Demeneix, B., and Behr, J. P., A versatile vector for gene and oligonucleotide transfer into cells in culture and *in vivo*: polyethylenimine, *Proc. Natl. Acad. Sci. U.S.A.*, 92, 7297, 1995.
102. Wagner, R. W., Matteucci, M. D., Lewis, J. G., Gutierrez, A. J., Moulds, C., and Froehler, B. C., Antisense gene inhibition by oligonucleotides containing C-5 propyne pyrimidines, *Science*, 260, 1510, 1993.
103. Lewis, J. G., Lin, K. Y., Kothavale, A., Flanagan, W. M., Matteucci, M. D., DePrince, R. B., Mook, R. A., Hendren, R. W., and Wagner, R. W., A serum resistance cytofectin for cellular delivery of antisense oligodeoxynucleotides and plasmid DNA, *Proc. Natl. Acad. Sci. U.S.A.*, 93, 3176, 1996.
104. Zelphati, O., Imbach, J. L., Signoret, N., Zon, G., Rayner, B., and Leserman, L., Antisense oligonucleotides in solution or encapsulated in immunoliposomes inhibit replication of HIV-1 by several different mechanisms, *Nucleic Acids Res.*, 22, 4307, 1994.
105. Midoux, P., Mendes, C., Legrand, A., Raimond, J., Mayer, R., Monsigny, M., and Roche, A. C., Specific gene transfer mediated by lactosylated poly-L-lysine into hepatoma cells, *Nucleic Acids Res.*, 21, 871, 1993.
106. Wang, S., Lee, R., Cauchon, G., Gorenstein, D. G., and Low, P. S., Delivery of antisense oligodeoxyribonucleotides against the human epidermal growth factor receptor into cultured KB cells with liposomes conjugated to folate via polyethylene glycol, *Proc. Natl. Acad. Sci. U.S.A.*, 92, 3318, 1995.
107. Léonetti, J. P., Mechti, N., Degols, G., Gagnor, C., and Lebleu, B., Intracellular distribution of microinjected antisense oligonucleotides, *Proc. Natl. Acad. Sci. U.S.A.*, 88, 2702, 1991.
108. Kulka, M., Smith, C. C., Aurelian, L., Fishelevich, R., Meade, K., Miller, P., and Ts'o, P. O. P., Site specificity of the inhibitory effects of oligo(nucleosidemethylphosphonate)s complementary to the acceptor splice junction of herpes simplex virus type I immediate early mRNA 4, *Proc. Natl. Acad. Sci. U.S.A.*, 86, 6868, 1989.
109. Verspieren, P., Loreau, N., Thuong, N. T., Shire, D., and Toulmé, J. J., Effect of RNA secondary structure and modified bases on the *in vitro* inhibition of trypanosomatid protein synthesis by antisense oligodeoxynucleotides, *Nucleic Acids Res.*, 18, 4711, 1990.
110. Vickers, T., Baker, F., Cook, P. D., Zounes, M., Buckheit, R. W., Germany, J., and Ecker, D. J., Inhibition of HIV-LTR gene expression by oligonucleotides targeted to the TAR element, *Nucleic Acids Res.*, 19, 3359, 1991.
111. Toulmé, J. J., Le Tinévez, R., and Brossalina, E., Targeting RNA structures by antisense oligonucleotides, *Biochimie*, 78, 663, 1996.

112. Goodchild, J., Agrawal, S., Civeira, M. P., Sarin, P. S., Sun, D., and Zamecnik, P. C., Inhibition of human immunodeficiency virus replication by antisense oligodeoxynucleotides, *Proc. Natl. Acad. Sci. U.S.A.*, 85, 5507, 1988.
113. Peyman, A., Helsberg, M., Kretzschmar, G., Mag, M., Grabley, S., and Uhlmann, E., Inhibition of viral growth by antisense oligonucleotides directed against the IE110 and the UL30 mRNA of herpes simplex virus type-1, *Biol. Chem. Hoppe Seyler*, 376, 195, 1995.
114. Ho, S. P., Britton, D. H. O., Srone, B. A., Behrens, D. L., Leffet, L. M., Hobbs, F. W., Miller, J. A., and Trainor, G. L., Potent antisense oligonucleotides to the human multidrug resistance-1 mRNA are rationally selected by mapping RNA-accessible sites with oligonucleotide libraries, *Nucleic Acids Res.*, 24, 1901, 1996.
115. Pascolo, E., Hudrisier, D., Sproat, B., Thuong, N. T., and Toulmé, J.-J., Relative contribution of photo-addition, helper oligonucleotide and RNase H to the antisense effect of psoralen-oligonucleotide conjugates, on *in vitro* translatioin of *Leishmania* mRNAs, *Biochim. Biophys. Acta*, 1219, 98, 1994.
116. Ecker, D. J., Vickers, T. A., Bruice, T. W., Freier, S. M., Jenison, R. D., Manoharan, M., and Zounes, M., Pseudo-half-knot formation with RNA, *Science*, 257, 958, 1993.
117. Brossalina, E., Pascolo, E., and Toulmé, J. J., The binding of an antisense oligonucleotide to a hairpin structure via triplex formation inhibits chemical and biological reactions, *Nucleic Acids Res.*, 21, 5616, 1993.
118. Mishra, R. K. and Toulmé, J. J., *In vitro* selection of antisense oligonucleotides targeted to a hairpin structure, *C. R. Acad. Sci. Paris*, 317, 977, 1994.
119. Mishra, R. K., Le Tinévez, R., and Toulmé, J. J., Targeting of nucleic acid secondary structures by antisense oligonucleotides designed through *in vitro* selection, *Proc. Natl. Acad. Sci. U.S.A.*, 93, 10679, 1996.
120. Simons, M., Edelman, E. R., Dekeyser, J. L., Langer, R., and Rosenberg, R. D., Antisense c-myb oligonucleotides inhibit intimal arterial smooth muscle cell accumulation *in vivo*, *Nature*, 359, 67, 1992.
121. Zon, G., Brief overview of control of genetic expression by antisense oligonucleotides and *in vivo* applications — prospects for neurobiology, *Mol. Neurobiol.*, 10, 219, 1995.
122. Wang, S. H. and Kool, E. T., Relative stabilities of triple helices composed of combinations of DNA, RNA and 2′-*O*-methyl-RNA backbones: chimeric circular oligonucleotides as probes, *Nucleic Acids Res.*, 23, 1157, 1995.
123. Giovannangeli, C., Thuong, N. T., and Hélène, C., Oligonucleotide clamps arrest DNA synthesis on a single-stranded DNA target, *Proc. Natl. Acad. Sci. U.S.A.*, 90, 10013, 1993.
124. Wu, H., Holcenberg, J. S., Tomich, J., Chen, J., Jones, P. A., Huang, S. H., and Calame, K. L., Inhibition of *in vitro* transcription by specific double-stranded oligodeoxyribonucleotides, *Gene*, 89, 203, 1990.
125. Berkowitz, L. A., Riabowol, K. T., and Gilman, M. Z., Multiple sequence elements of a single functional class are required for cyclic AMP responsiveness of the mouse c-fos promoter, *Mol. Cell. Biol.*, 9, 4272, 1989.
126. Bielinska, A., Shivdasani, R. A., Zhang, L., and Nabel, G. J., Regulation of gene expression with double-stranded phosphorothioate oligonucleotides, *Science*, 250, 997, 1990.
127. Pascolo, R. and Toulmé, J. J., Double hairpin complexes allow accomadation of all four base pairs in triple helices containing both DNA and RNA strands, *J. Biol. Chem.*, 271, 24187, 1996.

Chapter **2**

Advances in Understanding the Pharmacological Properties of Antisense Oligonucleotides

Stanley T. Crooke

CONTENTS

0-8493-8552-0/97/$0.00+$.50

I. INTRODUCTION

During the past few years, interest in developing antisense technology and in exploiting it for therapeutic purposes has been intense. Although progress has been gratifyingly rapid, the technology remains in its infancy and the questions that remain to be answered still outnumber the questions for which there are answers. Appropriately, considerable debate continues about the breadth of the utility of the approach and about the type of data required to "prove that a drug works through an antisense mechanism."

The objectives of this review are to provide a summary of recent progress, to assess the status of the technology, to place the technology in the pharmacological context in which it is best understood, and to deal with some of the controversies regarding the technology and the interpretation of experiments.

II. PROOF OF MECHANISM

A. Factors that May Influence Experimental Interpretations

Clearly, the ultimate biological effect of an oligonucleotide will be influenced by the local concentration of the oligonucleotide at the target RNA, the concentration of the RNA, the rates of synthesis and degradation of the RNA, type of terminating mechanism, and the rates of the events that result in termination of the RNAs activity. At present, we understand essentially nothing about the interplay of these factors.

1. *Oligonucleotide Purity*

Currently, phosphorothioate oligonucleotides can be prepared consistently and with excellent purity.[1] However, this has only been the case for the past three to four years. Prior to that time, synthetic methods were evolving and analytical methods were inadequate. In fact, our laboratory reported that different synthetic and purification procedures resulted in oligonucleotides that varied in cellular toxicity[2] and that potency varied from batch to batch. Though these are no longer synthetic problems with phosphorothioates, they, undoubtedly, complicated earlier studies. More importantly, with each new analog class and new synthetic, purification and analytical challenges are encountered.

2. *Oligonucleotide Structure*

Antisense oligonucleotides are designed to be single-stranded. We now understand that certain sequences, e.g., stretches of guanosine residues, are prone to adopt more complex structures.[3] The potential to form secondary and tertiary structures also varies as a function of the chemical class. For example, higher affinity 2′ modified oligonucleotides have a greater tendency to self-hybridize, resulting in more stable oligonucleotide duplexes than would be expected based on rules derived from oligodeoxynucleotides (Freier, unpublished results).

3. *RNA Structure*

Each RNA molecule has a unique sequence of nucleotides and a characteristic secondary structure. The structure of the RNA has a profound influence on the affinity of the oligonucleotide and on the rate of binding of the oligonucleotide to its RNA target.[4-5] Moreover, RNA structure produces asymmetrical binding sites that then result in very divergent affinity constants depending on the position of oligonucleotide in that structure.[5-7] This, in turn, influences the optimal length of an oligonucleotide needed to achieve maximal affinity. We understand very little about how RNA structure and RNA protein interactions influence antisense drug action.

4. *Variations in* In Vitro *Cellular Uptake and Distribution*

Studies in several laboratories have clearly demonstrated that cells in tissue culture may take up phosphorothioate oligonucleotides via an active process, and that the uptake of these oligonucleotides is highly variable depending on many conditions.[2,8] Cell type has a dramatic effect on total uptake, kinetics of uptake, and pattern of subcellular distribution. At present, there is no unifying hypothesis to explain these differences. Tissue culture conditions, such as the type of medium, degree of confluence, and the presence of serum can all have enormous effects on uptake.[8] The chemical class of oligonucleotides obviously influences the characteristics of uptake as well as the mechanism of uptake. Within the phosphorothioate class of oligonucleotides, uptake varies as a function of length, but not linearly. Uptake varies as a function of sequence, and stability in cells is also influenced by sequence.[8-9]

Given the above, it is obvious that conclusions about *in vitro* uptake must be very carefully made, and generalizations are virtually impossible. Thus, before an oligonucleotide could be said to be inactive *in vitro,* it should be studied in several cell lines. Furthermore, while it may be absolutely correct that receptor-mediated endocytosis is a mechanism of uptake of phosphorothioate oligonucleotides,[10] it is obvious that a generalization that all phosphorothioates are taken up by all cells *in vitro,* primarily by receptor mediated endocytosis, is simply unwarranted.

Finally, extrapolations from *in vitro* uptake studies to predictions about *in vivo* pharmacokinetic behavior are entirely inappropriate and, in fact, there are now several lines of evidence in animals and man that, even after careful consideration of all *in vitro* uptake data, one cannot predict *in vivo* pharmacokinetics of the compounds.[8,11-13]

5. *The Binding to and Effects of Binding to Non-Nucleic Acid Targets*

Phosphorothioate oligonucleotides tend to bind to many proteins, and those interactions are influenced by many factors. The effects of binding can influence cell uptake, distribution, metabolism, and excretion. They may induce non-antisense effects that can be mistakenly interpreted as antisense or complicate the identification of an antisense mechanism. By inhibiting RNase H, protein binding may inhibit the antisense activity of some oligonucleotides. Finally, binding to proteins can certainly have toxicological consequences.

In addition to proteins, oligonucleotides may interact with other biological molecules, such as lipids or carbohydrates, and such interactions, like those with proteins, will be influenced by the chemical class of oligonucleotide studied. Unfortunately, essentially no data bearing on such interactions are currently available.

An especially complicated experimental situation is encountered in many *in vitro* antiviral assays. In these assays, high concentrations of drugs, viruses, and cells are often co-incubated. The sensitivity of each virus to non-antisense effects of oligonucleotides varies depending on the nature of the virion proteins and the characteristics of the oligonucleotides.[14-15] This has resulted in considerable confusion. In particular, for HIV, herpes simplex viruses, cytomegaloviruses (CMV), and influenza virus the non-antisense effects have been so dominant that identifying oligonucleotides that work via an antisense mechanism has been difficult. Given the artificial character of such assays, it is difficult to know whether non-antisense mechanisms would be as dominant *in vivo* or result in antiviral activity.

6. *Terminating Mechanisms*

It has been amply demonstrated that oligonucleotides may employ several terminating mechanisms. The dominant terminating mechanism is influenced by RNA receptor site, oligonucleotide chemical class, cell type, and probably many other factors.[16] Obviously, as variations in terminating mechanism may result in significant changes in antisense potency, and studies have shown significant variations from cell type to cell type *in vitro,* it is essential that the terminating mechanism be well understood. Unfortunately, at present, our understanding of terminating mechanisms remains rudimentary.

7. *Effects of "Control Oligonucleotides"*

A number of types of control oligonucleotides have been used including randomized oligonucleotides. Unfortunately, we know little to nothing about the potential biological effects of such "controls", and the more complicated a biological system and test the more likely that "control" oligonucleotides may have activities that complicate interpretations. Thus, when a control oligonucleotide displays a surprising activity, the mechanism of that activity should be explored carefully before concluding that the effects of the control oligonucleotide prove that the activity of the putative antisense oligonucleotide are not due to an antisense mechanism.

8. *Kinetics of Effects*

Many rate constants may affect the activities of antisense oligonucleotides, e.g., the rate of synthesis and degradation of the target RNA and its protein, the rates of uptake into cells, the rates of distribution, extrusion and metabolism of an oligonucleotide in cells, and similar pharmacokinetic considerations in animals. Despite this, relatively few time courses have been reported, and *in vitro* studies have been reported that range from a few hours to several days. In animals, we have a growing body of information on pharmacokinetics, but in most studies reported to date the doses and schedules were chosen arbitrarily and, again, little information on duration of effect and onset of action has been presented.

Clearly, more careful kinetic studies are required and rational *in vitro* and *in vivo* dose schedules must be developed.

B. Recommendations

1. *Positive Demonstration of Antisense Mechanism and Specificity*

Until more is understood about how antisense drugs work, it is essential to positively demonstrate effects consistent with an antisense mechanism. For RNase H activating oligonucleotides, Northern blot analysis showing selective loss of the target RNA is the best choice, and many laboratories are publishing reports *in vitro* and *in vivo* of such activities.[17-20] Ideally, a demonstration that closely related isotypes are unaffected should be included. In brief, then, for proof of mechanism, the following steps are recommended:

1. Perform careful dose response curves *in vitro* using several cell lines and methods of *in vitro* delivery.
2. Correlate the rank order potency *in vivo* with that observed *in vitro* after thorough dose-response curves are generated *in vivo.*

3. Perform careful "gene walks" for all RNA species and oligonucleotide chemical classes.
4. Perform careful time courses before drawing conclusions about potency.
5. Directly demonstrate proposed mechanism of action by measuring the target RNA and/or protein.
6 Evaluate specificity and therapeutic indices via studies on closely related isotypes and with appropriate toxicological studies.
7. Perform sufficient pharmacokinetics to define rational dosing schedules for pharmacological studies.
8. When control oligonucleotides display surprising activities, determine the mechanisms involved.

III. MOLECULAR MECHANISMS OF ANTISENSE DRUGS

A. Occupancy-Only Mediated Mechanisms

Classic competitive antagonists are thought to alter biological activities because they bind to receptors preventing natural agonists from binding the inducing normal biological processes. Binding of oligonucleotides to specific sequences may inhibit the interaction of the RNA with proteins, other nucleic acids, or other factors required for essential steps in the intermediary metabolism of the RNA or its utilization by the cell.

1. *Inhibition of Splicing*

A key step in the intermediary metabolism of most mRNA molecules is the excision of introns. These "splicing" reactions are sequence specific and require the concerted action of spliceosomes. Consequently, oligonucleotides that bind to sequences required for splicing may prevent binding of necessary factors or physically prevent the required cleavage reactions. This then would result in inhibition of the production of the mature mRNA. Although there are several examples of oligonucleotides directed to splice junctions, none of the studies present data showing inhibition of RNA processing, accumulation of splicing intermediates, or a reduction in mature mRNA; nor are there published data in which the structure of the RNA at the splice junction was probed and the oligonucleotides demonstrated to hybridize to the sequences for which they were designed.[21-24] Activities have been reported for anti-c-myc and antiviral oligonucleotides with phosphodiester, methylphosphonate, and phosphorothioate backbones. Very recently, an oligonucleotide was reported to induce alternative splicing in a cell-free splicing system and, in that system, RNA analyses confirmed the putative mechanism.[25]

In our laboratory, we have attempted to characterize the factors that determine whether splicing inhibition is effected by an antisense drug.[26] To this end, a number of luciferase-reporter plasmids containing various introns were constructed and transfected into HeLa cells. Then the effects of antisense drugs designed to bind to various sites were characterized. The effects of RNase H-competent oligonucleotides were compared to those of oligonucleotides that do not serve as RNase H substrates. The major conclusions from this study were first, that most of the earlier studies from which splicing inhibition was reported were probably due to nonspecific effects. Second, less effectively spliced introns are better targets than those with strong consensus splicing signals. Third, the 3′ splice site and branchpoint are usually the best sites to target the oligonucleotide to inhibit splicing. Fourth, RNase H-competent oligonucleotides are usually more potent than even higher affinity oligonucleotides that inhibit by occupancy only.

2. *Translational Arrest*

A mechanism for which the many oligonucleotides have been designed is to arrest translation of the targeted protein by binding to the translation initiation codon. The positioning of the initiation codon within the area of complementarity of the oligonucleotide and the length of oligonucleotide used have varied considerably. Again, unfortunately, only in relatively few studies have the oligonucleotides, in fact, been shown to bind to the sites for which they were designed, and data that directly support translation arrest as the mechanism has been lacking.

Target RNA species that have been reported to be inhibited by a translational arrest mechanism include HIV, vesicular stomatitis virus (VSV), n-myc, and a number of normal cellular genes.[27-33]

In our laboratories, we have shown that a significant number of targets may be inhibited by binding to translation initiation codons. For example, ISIS 1082 hybridizes to the AUG codon for the UL13 gene of herpesvirus types 1 and 2. RNase H studies confirmed that it binds selectively in this area. *In vitro* protein synthesis studies confirmed that it inhibited the synthesis of the UL13 protein, and studies in HeLa cells showed that it inhibited the growth of herpes type 1 and type 2 with an IC_{50} value of 200 to 400 n*M* by translation arrest.[34] Similarly, ISIS 1753, a 30-mer phosphorothioate complementary to the translation initiation codon and surrounding sequences of the E2 gene of bovine papilloma virus, was highly effective and its activity was shown to be due to translation arrest. ISIS 2105, a 20-mer phosphorothioate complementary to the same region in human papilloma virus, was shown to be a very potent inhibitor. Compounds complementary to the translation initiation codon of the E2 gene were the most potent of the more than 50 compounds studied that were complementary to various other regions in the RNA.[35] We have shown inhibition of translation of a number of other mRNA species by compounds designed to bind to the translation initiation codon as well.

In conclusion, translation arrest represents an important mechanism of action for antisense drugs. A number of examples purporting employment of this mechanism have been reported, and recent studies on several compounds have provided data which unambiguously demonstrate that this mechanism can result in potent antisense drugs. However, very little is understood about the precise events that lead to translation arrest.

3. *Disruption of Necessary RNA Structure*

RNA adopts a variety of three-dimensional structures induced by intramolecular hybridization, the most common of which is the stem loop. These structures play crucial roles in a variety of functions. They are used to provide additional stability for RNA and as recognition motifs for a number of proteins, nucleic acids, and ribonucleoproteins that participate in the intermediary metabolism and activities of RNA species. Thus, given the potential general activity of the mechanism, it is surprising that occupancy-based disruption of RNA structure has not been more extensively exploited.

As an example, we designed a series of oligonucleotides that bind to the important stem-loop present in all RNA species in HIV, the *trans*-activating response or TAR element. We synthesized a number of oligonucleotides designed to disrupt TAR, showed that several indeed did bind to TAR, disrupt the structure, and inhibit TAR-mediated production of a reporter gene.[36] Furthermore, general rules useful in disrupting stem-loop structures were developed as well.[7]

Although designed to induce relatively nonspecific cytotoxic effects, two other examples are noteworthy. Oligonucleotides designed to bind to a 17-nucleotide loop in *Xenopus* 28 S RNA, which is required for ribosome stability and protein synthesis inhibited protein synthesis when injected into *Xenopus* oocytes.[37] Similarly, oligonucleotides designed to bind to highly conserved sequences in 5.8 S RNA inhibited protein synthesis in rabbit reticulocyte and wheat germ systems.[38]

B. Occupancy-Activated Destabilization

RNA molecules regulate their own metabolism. A number of structural features of RNA are known to influence stability, various processing events, subcellular distribution, and transport. It is likely that, as the intermediary metabolism of RNA is better understood, many other regulatory features and mechanisms will be identified.

1. 5′ Capping

A key early step in RNA processing is 5′ capping (Figure 1). This stabilizes pre-mRNA and is important for the stability of mature mRNA. It also is important in binding to the nuclear matrix and transport of mRNA out of the nucleus. As the structure of the cap is unique and understood, it presents an interesting target.

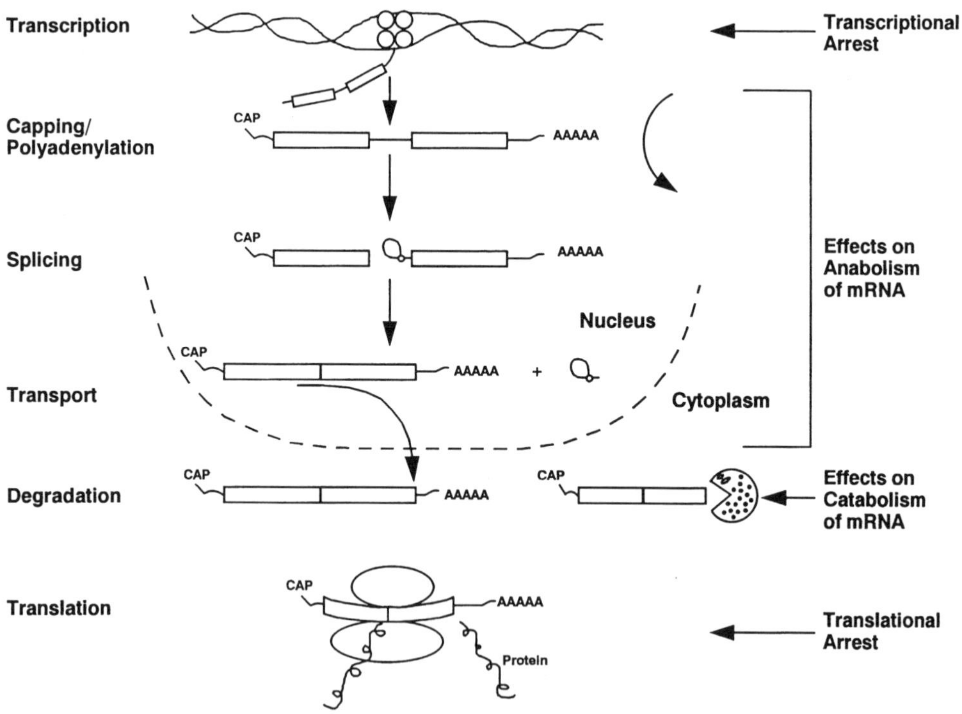

FIGURE 1
RNA processing

Several oligonucleotides that bind near the cap site have been shown to be active, presumably by inhibiting the binding of proteins required to cap the RNA. For example, the synthesis of SV40 T-antigen was reported to be most sensitive to an oligonucleotide linked to polylysine and targeted to the 5′ cap site of RNA.[39] However, again, in no published study has this putative mechanism been rigorously demonstrated. In fact, in no published study have the oligonucleotides been shown to bind to the sequences for which they were designed.

In our laboratory, we have designed oligonucleotides to bind to 5′ cap structures and reagents to specifically cleave the unique 5′ cap structure.[40] These studies demonstrate that 5′ cap targeted oligonucleotides were capable of inhibiting the binding of the translation initiation factor eIF-4a.[41]

2. *Inhibition of 3′ Polyadenylation*

In the 3′ untranslated region of pre-mRNA molecules are sequences that result in the post-transcriptional addition of long (hundreds of nucleotides) tracts of polyadenylate. Polyadenylation stabilizes mRNA and may play other roles in the intermediary metabolism of RNA species. Theoretically, interactions in the 3′ terminal region of pre-mRNA could inhibit polyadenylation and destabilize the RNA species. Although there are a number of oligonucleotides that interact in the 3′ untranslated region and display antisense activities, to date, no study has reported evidence for alterations in polyadenylation.[17]

C. Other Mechanisms

In addition to 5′ capping and 3′ adenylation, there are clearly other sequences in the 5′ and 3′ untranslated regions of mRNA that affect the stability of the molecules. Again, there are a number of antisense drugs that may work by these mechanisms.

Zamecnik and Stephenson reported that a 13-mer targeted to the untranslated 3′ and 5′ terminal sequences in Rous sarcoma viruses was active.[42] Oligonucleotides conjugated to an acridine derivative and targeted to a 3′ terminal sequence in type A influenza viruses were reported to be active against several RNA targets. Studies in our laboratories have shown that sequences in the 3′ untranslated region of RNA molecules are often the most sensitive.[43-45] For example, ISIS 1939, a 20-mer phosphorothioate that binds to and appears to disrupt a predicted stem loop structure in the 3′ untranslated region of the mRNA for ICAM, is a potent antisense inhibitor. However, inasmuch as a 2′ methoxy analog of ISIS 1939 was much less active, it is likely that, in addition to destabilization and cellular nucleolytic activity, activation of RNase H (see below) is also involved in the activity of ISIS 1939.[17]

D. Activation of RNase H

RNase H is a ubiquitous enzyme that degrades the RNA strand of an RNA-DNA duplex. It has been identified in organisms as diverse as viruses and human cells.[46] At least two classes of RNase H have been identified in eukaryotic cells. Multiple enzymes with RNase H activity have been observed in prokaryotes.[46]

Although RNase H is involved in DNA replication, it may play other roles in the cell and is found in the cytoplasm as well as the nucleus.[47] However, the concentration of the enzyme in the nucleus is thought to be greater, and some of the enzyme found in cytoplasmic preparations may be due to nuclear leakage.

RNase H activity is quite variable in cells. It is absent or minimal in rabbit reticulocytes but present in wheat germ extracts.[46,48] In HL-60 cells, for example, the level of activity in undifferentiated cells is greatest, relatively high in DMSO and vitamin D differentiated cells, and much lower in PMA-differentiated cells (Hoke, unpublished data).

The precise recognition elements for RNase H are not known; however, it has been shown that oligonucleotides with DNA-like properties as short as tetramers can activate RNase H.[49] Changes in the sugar influence RNase H activation as sugar modifications that result in RNA-like oligonucleotides, e.g., 2′ fluoro or 2′ methoxy do not appear to serve as substrates for RNase H.[50-51] Alterations in the orientation of the sugar to the base can also affect RNase H activation as α-oligonucleotides are unable to induce RNase H or may require parallel annealing.[52-53] Additionally, backbone modifications influence the ability of oligonucleotides to activate RNase H. Methylphosphonates do not activate RNase H.[54-55] In contrast, phosphorothioates are excellent substrates.[34,56-57] In addition, chimeric molecules have been studied as oligonucleotides that bind to RNA and activate RNase H.[58-59] For example, oligonucleotides comprised of wings of 2′ methoxy phosphonates and a 5-base gap of deoxyoligonucleotides bind to their target RNA and activate RNase H.[58-59] Furthermore, a single ribonucleotide in a sequence of deoxyribonucleotides was shown to be sufficient to serve as a substrate for RNase H when bound to its complementary deoxyoligonucleotide.[60]

That it is possible to take advantage of chimeric oligonucleotides designed to activate RNase H, have greater affinity for their RNA receptors, and to enhance specificity has also been demonstrated.[61-62] In a recent study, RNase H-mediated cleavage of target transcript was much more selective when deoxyoligonucleotides comprised of methylphosphonate deoxyoligonucleotide wings and phosphodiester gaps were compared to full phosphodiester oligonucleotides.[62]

Despite the information about RNase H and the demonstration that many oligonucleotides may activate RNase H in lysate and purified enzyme assays, relatively little is still known about the role of structural features in RNA targets in activating RNase H.[63-65] In fact, direct proof that RNase H activation is, in fact, the mechanism of action of oligonucleotides in cells is to a large extent lacking.

Recent studies in our laboratories provide additional, albeit indirect, insights into these questions. ISIS 1939 is a 20-mer phosphorothioate complementary to a sequence in the 3′ untranslated region of ICAM-1 RNA.[17] It inhibits ICAM production in human umbilical vein endothelial cells, and Northern blots demonstrate that ICAM-1 mRNA is rapidly degraded. A 2′ methoxy analog of ISIS 1939 displays higher affinity for the RNA than the phosphorothioate, is stable in cells, but inhibits ICAM-1 protein production much less potently than ISIS 1939. It is likely that ISIS 1939 destabilizes the RNA and activates RNase H. In contrast, ISIS 1570, an 18-mer phosphorothioate that is complementary to the translation initiation codon of the ICAM-1 message inhibited production of the protein, but it caused no degradation of the RNA. Thus, two oligonucleotides that are capable of activating RNase H had different effects depending on the site in the mRNA at which they bound.[17]

A more direct demonstration that RNase H is likely a key factor in the activity of many antisense oligonucleotides was provided by studies in which reverse-ligation polymerase chain reaction (PCR) was used to identify cleavage products from bcr-abl mRNA in cells treated with phosphorothioate oligonucleotides.[66]

Given the emerging role of chimeric oligonucleotides with modifications in the 3′ and 5′ wings designed to increase nuclease stability and to enhance affinity for the target RNA, and a DNA-type gap to serve as a substrate for RNase H, studies focused on understanding the effects of various modifications on the efficiency of the enzyme(s) are also of considerable importance. In one such study on *Escherichia coli* RNase H, we have recently reported that the enzyme displays minimal sequence specificity and is processive. When a chimeric oligonucleotide with 2′ modified sugars in the wings was hybridized to the RNA, the initial site of cleavage was the nucleotide adjacent to the methoxy-deoxy junction closest to the 3′ end of the RNA substrate. The initial rate of cleavage increased as the size of the DNA gap increased, and the efficiency of the enzyme was considerably less against an RNA target duplexed with a chimeric antisense oligonucleotide than a full DNA-type oligonucleotide.[67]

IV. CHARACTERISTICS OF PHOSPHOROTHIOATE OLIGODEOXYNUCLEOTIDES

A. Introduction

Of the first generation of oligonucleotide analogs, the class that has resulted in the broadest range of activities and about which the most is known, is the phosphorothioate class. Phosphorothioate oligonucleotides were first synthesized in 1969 when a poly rI-rC phosphorothioate was synthesized.[68] Their modification clearly achieves the objective of increased nuclease stability. In this class of oligonucleotides, one of the oxygen atoms in the phosphate group is replaced with a sulfur. The resulting compound is negatively charged, as is a chiral phosphodiester, but it is much more resistant to nucleases.[69]

B. Hybridization

The hybridization of phosphorothioate oligonucleotides to DNA and RNA has been thoroughly characterized.[1,70-71] The T_m of a phosphorothioate oligodeoxynucleotide for RNA is approximately 0.5°C less per nucleotide than for a corresponding phosphodiester oligodeoxynucleotide. This reduction in T_m per nucleotide is virtually independent of the number of phosphorothioate units substituted for phosphodiesters. However, sequence context has some influence as the ΔT_m can vary from –0.3 to 1°C depending on sequence. Compared to RNA and RNA duplex formation, a phosphorothioate oligodeoxynucleotide has a T_m approximately –0.2°C lower per unit.[4] This means that to be effective *in vitro*, phosphorothioate oligodeoxynucleotides must typically be 17-to 20-mer in length and that invasion of double-stranded regions in RNA is difficult.[6,36,61,72]

Association rates of phosphorothioate oligodeoxynucleotide to unstructured RNA targets are typically 10^6 to $10^7 M^{-1}S^{-1}$ independent of oligonucleotide length or sequence.[4,6] Association rates to structured RNA targets can vary from 10^2 to 10^8 $M^{-1}S^{-1}$ depending on the structure of the RNA, site of binding in the structure, and other factors.[4] In another words, association rates for oligonucleotides that display acceptable affinity constants are sufficient to support biological activity at therapeutically achievable concentrations.

The specificity of hybridization of phosphorothioate oligonucleotides is, in general, slightly greater than that of phosphodiester analogs. For example, a T-C mismatch results in a 7.7°C or 12.8°C reduction in T_m, respectively, for a phosphodiester or phosphorothioate oligodeoxynucleotide 18 nucleotides in length with the mismatch centered.[4] Thus, from this perspective, the phosphorothioate modification is quite attractive.

C. Interactions with Proteins

Phosphorothioate oligonucleotides bind to proteins. The interactions with proteins can be divided into nonspecific, sequence specific, and structure specific binding events, each of which may have different characteristics and effects. Nonspecific binding to a wide variety of proteins has been demonstrated. Exemplary of this type of binding is the interaction of phosphorothioate oligonucleotides with serum albumin. The affinity of such interactions is low, the kDa for albumin being approximately 200 μm.[73-74] Thus, its kDa is in a range similar to that of aspirin or penicillin. Furthermore, in this study, no competition between phosphorothioate oligonucleotides and several drugs that bind to bovine serum albumin was observed. In this study, binding and competition were determined in an assay in which electrospray mass spectrometry was used. In contrast, in a study in which an equilibrium dissociation constant was derived from an assay using albumin loaded on a CH-sephadex column, the Km ranged from 1 to 5×10^{-5} M for bovine serum albumin and 2 to 3×10^{-4} M for human serum albumin. Moreover, warfarin and indomethacin were reported to compete for binding to serum albumin.[75] Clearly, much more work is required before definitive conclusions can be drawn.

Phosphorothioate oligonucleotides can interact with nucleic acid-binding proteins, such as transcription factors and single-strand nucleic acid-binding proteins. However, very little is known about these binding events. Additionally, it has been reported that phosphorothioates bind to an 80-kDa membrane protein that was suggested to be involved in cellular uptake processes.[10] However, again, little is known about the affinities, sequence, or structural specificities of these putative interactions.

Phosphorothioates interact with nucleases and DNA polymerases. These compounds are slowly metabolized by both endo- and exonucleases and inhibit these enzymes.[67,70] The inhibition of these enzymes appears to be competitive and this may account for some early data suggesting that phosphorothioates are almost infinitely stable to nucleases. In these studies, the oligonucleotide-to-enzyme ratio was very high and, thus, the enzyme was inhibited. Phosphorothioates also bind to RNase H when in an RNA-DNA duplex, and the duplex serves as a substrate for RNase H.[76] At higher concentrations, presumably by binding as a single strand to RNase H, phosphorothioates inhibit the enzyme.[67,70] Again, the oligonucleotides appear to be competitive antagonists for the DNA-RNA substrate.

Phosphorothioates have been shown to be competitive inhibitors of DNA polymerase α and β with respect to the DNA template, and noncompetitive inhibitors of DNA polymerases γ and δ.[76] Despite this inhibition, several studies have suggested that phosphorothioates might serve as primers for polymerases and be extended.[56,67,77] In our laboratories, we have shown extensions of 2 to 3 nucleotides only. At present, a full explanation as to why no longer extensions are observed is not available.

Phosphorothioate oligonucleotides have been reported to be competitive inhibitors for HIV reverse transcriptase and to inhibit RT-associated RNase H activity.[78-79] They have been reported to bind to the cell surface protein, CD4, and to protein kinase C.[80] Various viral polymerases have also been shown to be inhibited by phosphorothioates.[56] Additionally, we have shown potent, nonsequence-specific inhibition of RNA splicing by phosphorothioates.[26]

Like other oligonucleotides, phosphorothioates can adopt a variety of secondary structures. As a general rule, self-complementary oligonucleotides are avoided, if possible, to avoid duplex formation between oligonucleotides. However, other structures that are less well understood can also form. For example, oligonucleotides containing runs of guanosines can form tetrameric structures called G-quartets, and these appear to interact with a number of proteins with relatively greater affinity than unstructured oligonucleotides.[3]

In conclusion, phosphorothioate oligonucleotides may interact with a wide range of proteins via several types of mechanisms. These interactions may influence the pharmacokinetic, pharmacologic, and toxicologic properties of these molecules. They may also complicate studies on the mechanism of action of these drugs.

D. Pharmacokinetic Properties

To study the pharmacokinetics of phosphorothioate oligonucleotides, a variety of labeling techniques have been used. In some cases, 3′ or 5′ ^{32}P-end-labeled or fluorescently labeled oligonucleotides have been used in *in vitro* or *in vivo* studies. These are probably less satisfactory than internally labeled compounds because terminal phosphates are rapidly removed by phosphatases, and fluorescently labeled oligonucleotides have physicochemical properties that differ from the unmodified oligonucleotides. Consequently, either uniformly ^{32}S- or base-labeled phosphorothioates are preferable for pharmacokinetic studies. In our laboratories, a tritium exchange method that labels a slowly exchanging proton at the C8 position in purines was developed and proved to be quite useful.[81] Very recently, a method that added radioactive methyl groups via *S*-adenosyl methionine has also been successfully used.[82] Finally, advances in extraction, separation, and detection methods have resulted in methods that provide excellent pharmacokinetic analyses without radiolabeling.[73]

1. *Nuclease Stability*

The principle metabolic pathway for oligonucleotides is cleavage via endo- and exonucleases. Phosphorothioate oligonucleotides, while quite stable to various nucleases, are competitive inhibitors of nucleases.[9,76,83-85] Consequently, the stability of phosphorothioate oligonucleotides to nucleases is probably slightly less than initially thought, as high concentrations (that inhibited nucleases) of oligonucleotides were employed in the early studies. Similarly, phosphorothioate oligonucleotides are degraded slowly by cells in tissue culture with a half-life of 12 to 24 h and are slowly metabolized in animals.[9,11,83] The pattern of metabolites suggests primarily exonuclease activity with perhaps modest contributions by endonucleases. However, a number of lines of evidence suggest that, in many cells and tissues, endonucleases play an important role in the metabolism of oligonucleotides. For example, 3′ and 5′ modified oligonucleotides with phosphodiester backbones have been shown to be relatively rapidly degraded in cells and after administration to animals.[13,86] Thus, strategies in which oligonucleotides are modified at only the 3′ and 5′ terminus as a means of enhancing stability have not proven to be successful.

2. In Vitro *Cellular Uptake*

Phosphorothioate oligonucleotides are taken up by a wide range of cells *in vitro*.[2,9,76,87,88] In fact, uptake of phosphorothioate oligonucleotides into a prokaryote, *Vibrio parahaemolyticus*, has been reported as has uptake into *Schistosoma mansoni*.[89-90] Uptake is time- and temperature-dependent. It is also influenced by cell type, cell culture conditions, media and sequence, and length of the oligonucleotide.[9] No obvious correlation has been identified between uptake and the lineage of cells, whether the cells are transformed or whether the cells are virally infected.[9] Nor are the factors that result in differences in uptake of different sequences of oligonucleotide understood. Although several studies have suggested that receptor-mediated endocytosis may be a significant mechanism of cellular uptake, these data are not yet compelling enough to conclude that receptor-mediated endocytosis accounts for a significant portion of the uptake in most cells.[10]

Numerous studies have shown that, once taken up, phosphorothioate oligonucleotides distribute broadly in most cells.[9,91] Again, however, significant differences in subcellular distribution between various types of cells have been noted.

Cationic lipids and other approaches have been used to enhance uptake of phosphorothioate oligonucleotides in cells that take up little oligonucleotide *in vitro*.[92-94] Again, however, there are substantial variations from cell type to cell type. Other approaches to enhanced intracellular uptake *in vitro* have included streptolysin D treatment of cells and the use of dextran sulfate and other liposome formulations as well as physical means such as microinjection.[16,66,95]

3. In Vivo *Pharmacokinetics*

Phosphorothioate oligonucleotides bind to serum albumin and α-2 macroglobulin. The apparent affinity for albumin is quite low (200 to 400 μM) and comparable to the low affinity binding observed for a number of drugs, e.g., aspirin and penicillin.[73-75] Serum protein binding, therefore, provides a repository for these drugs and prevents rapid renal excretion. As serum protein binding is saturable, at higher doses, intact oligomer may be found in urine.[77,96] Studies in our laboratory suggest that in rats, oligonucleotides administered intravenously (i.v.) at doses of 15 to 20 mg/kg saturate the serum protein binding capacity (Leeds, unpublished data).

Phosphorothioate oligonucleotides are rapidly and extensively absorbed after parenteral administration. For example, in rats, after an intradermal dose 3.6 mg/kg of ^{14}C-ISIS 2105, a 20-mer phosphorothioate, approximately 70% of the dose was absorbed within 4 h and total systemic bioavailability was in excess of 90%.[12] After intradermal injection in man, absorption of ISIS 2105 was similar to that observed in rats.[8] Subcutaneous (s.c.) administration to rats and monkeys results in somewhat lower bioavailability and greater distribution to lymph as would be expected (Leeds, unpublished observations).

Distribution of phosphorothioate oligonucleotides from blood after absorption or i.v. administration is extremely rapid. We have reported distribution half-lives of less than one hour, and similar data have been reported by others.[11-12,77,96] Blood and plasma clearance is multi-exponential with a terminal elimination half-life from 40 to 60 h in all species except man. In man, the terminal elimination half-life may be somewhat longer.[8]

Phosphorothioates distribute broadly to all peripheral tissues. Liver, kidneys, bone marrow, skeletal muscle, and skin accumulate the highest percentage of a dose, but other tissues display small quantities of drug.[11-12] No evidence of significant penetration of the blood-brain barrier has been reported. The rates of incorporation and clearance from tissues vary as a function of the organ studied, with liver accumulating drug most rapidly (20% of a dose within 1 to 2 h) and other tissues accumulating drug more slowly. Similarly, elimination of drug is more rapid from liver than from any other tissue; e.g., the terminal half-life from liver was 62 h and from renal medulla was 156 h. The distribution into the kidney has been studied more extensively and drug has been shown to be present in Bowman's capsule, the proximal convoluted tubule, the bush border membrane, and within renal tubular epithelial cells.[97] These data suggested that the oligonucleotides are filtered by the glomerulus, then reabsorbed by the proximal convoluted tubule epithelial cells.

Moreover, the authors suggested that reabsorption might be mediated by interactions with specific proteins in the bush border membranes.

At relatively low doses, clearance of phosphorothioate oligonucleotides is due primarily to metabolism.[11-12,96] Metabolism is mediated by exo- and endonucleases that result in shorter oligonucleotides and, ultimately, nucleosides that are degraded by normal metabolic pathways. Although no direct evidence of base excision or modification has been reported, these are theoretical possibilities that may occur. In one study, a larger molecular weight radioactive material was observed in urine, but not fully characterized.[77] Clearly, the potential for conjugation reactions and extension of oligonucleotides via these drugs serving as primers for polymerases must be explored in more detail. In a very thorough study, 20 nucleotide phosphodiester and phosphorothioate oligonucleotides were administered i.v. to mice at a dose of 6 mg/kg. The oligonucleotides were internally labeled with ^3H-CH_3 by methylation of an internal deoxycytidine residue using Hha1 methylase and S-[^3H] adenosyl methionine.[82] The observations for the phosphorothioate oligonucleotide were entirely consistent with those made in our studies. Additionally, in this paper, autoradiographic analyses showed drug in renal cortical cells.[82]

One study of prolonged infusions of a phosphorothioate oligonucleotide to human beings has been reported.[98] In this study, five patients with leukemia were given ten-day i.v. infusions at a dose of 0.05 mg/kg/h. Elimination half-lives reportedly varied from 5.9 to 14.7 days. Urinary recovery of radioactivity was reported to be 30 to 60% of the total dose, with 30% of the radioactivity being intact drug. Metabolites in urine included both higher and lower molecular weight compounds. In contrast, when GEM-91 (a 25-mer phosphorothioate oligodeoxynucleotide) was administered to humans as a 2-h i.v. infusion at a dose of 0.1 mg/kg, a peak plasma concentration of 295.8 mg/ml was observed at the cessation of the infusion. Plasma clearance of total radioactivity was biexponential with initial and terminal elimination half-lives of 0.18 and 2.7 h, respectively. However, degradation was extensive and intact drug pharmacokinetic models were not presented. Nearly 50% of the administered radioactivity was recovered in urine, but most of the radioactivity represented degradation products. In fact, no intact drug was found in the urine at any time.[99]

In a more recent study in which the level of intact drug was carefully evaluated using capillary gel electrophoresis, the pharmacokinetics of ISIS 2302, a 20-mer phosphorothioate oligodeoxynucleotide, after a 2-h infusion, were determined. Doses from 0.06 mg/kg to 2.0 mg/kg were studied, and the peak plasma concentrations were shown to increase linearly with dose, with the 2 mg/kg dose resulting in peak plasma concentrations of intact drug of approximately 9.5 μg/ml. Clearance from plasma, however, was dose-dependent, with the 2 mg/kg dose having a clearance of 1.28 ml $min^{-1}kg^{-1}$, while that of 0.5 mg/kg was 2.07 ml $min^{-1}kg^{-1}$. Essentially, no intact drug was found in urine.

Clearly, the two most recent studies differ from the initial report in several facets, but the most likely explanation is related to the evolution of assay methodology, not difference between compounds. Overall, the behavior of phosphorothioates in the plasma of humans appears to be similar to that in other species.

We have also performed oral bioavailability experiments in rodents treated with an H2 antagonist to avoid acid-mediated depurination or precipitation. In these studies, very limited (<5%) bioavailability was observed (Crooke, unpublished observations). However, it seems likely that the principal limiting factor in the oral bioavailability of phosphorothioates may be degradation in the gut rather than absorption. Studies using everted rat jejunum sacs demonstrated passive transport across the intestinal epithelium.[100] Further, studies using more stable 2′

methoxy phosphorothioate oligonucleotides showed a significant increase in oral bioavailability that appeared to be associated with the improved stability of the analogs.[101]

In summary, pharmacokinetic studies of several phosphorothioates demonstrate that they are well absorbed from parenteral sites, distribute broadly to all peripheral tissues, do not cross the blood-brain barrier, and are eliminated primarily by slow metabolism. In short, once a day or every other day systemic dosing should be feasible. Although the similarities between oligonucleotides of different sequences are far greater than the differences, additional studies are required before determining whether there are subtle effects of sequence on the pharmacokinetic profile of this class of drugs.

E. Pharmacological Properties

1. *Molecular Pharmacology*

Antisense oligonucleotides are designed to bind to RNA targets via Watson-Crick hybridization. As RNA can adopt a variety of secondary structures via Watson-Crick hybridization, one useful way to think of antisense oligonucleotides is as competitive antagonists for self-complementary regions of the target RNA. Obviously, creating oligonucleotides with the highest affinity per nucleotide unit is pharmacologically important, and a comparison of the affinity of the oligonucleotide to a complementary RNA oligonucleotide is the most sensible comparison. In this context, phosphorothioate oligodeoxynucleotides are relatively competitively disadvantaged as the affinity per nucleotide unit of oligomer is less than that of RNA folding back on itself (>-2.0°C T_m per unit).[102] This results in a requirement of at least 15 to 17 nucleotides in order to have sufficient affinity to produce biological activity.[72]

Although multiple mechanisms by which an oligonucleotide may terminate the activity of an RNA species to which it binds are possible, examples of biological activity have been reported for only three oligonucleotides. Antisense oligonucleotides have been reported to inhibit RNA splicing, to inhibit translation of mRNA, and to induce degradation of RNA by RNase H.[17,22,27] Without question, the mechanism that has resulted in the most potent compounds and is best understood is RNase H activation. To serve as a substrate for RNase H, a duplex between RNA and a "DNA-like" oligonucleotide is required. Specifically, a sugar moiety in the oligonucleotide that induces a duplex conformation equivalent to that of a DNA-RNA duplex and a charged phosphate are required.[103] Thus, phosphorothioate oligodeoxynucleotides are expected to induce RNase H-mediated cleavage of the RNA when bound. As will be discussed later, many chemical approaches that enhance the affinity of an oligonucleotide for RNA result in duplexes that are no longer substrates for RNase H.

Selection of sites at which optimal antisense activity may be induced in an RNA molecule is complex, dependent on the terminating mechanism involved and is influenced by the chemical class of the oligonucleotide. Each RNA appears to display unique patterns of sites of sensitivity. Within the phosphorothioate oligodeoxynucleotide chemical class, studies in our laboratory have shown antisense activity can vary from undetectable to 100% by shifting an oligonucleotide by just a few bases in the RNA target.[17,70,104] Although significant progress has been made in developing general rules that help define potentially optimal sites in RNA species, to a large extent this remains an empirical process that must be performed for each RNA target and every new chemical class of oligonucleotides.

Phosphorothioates have also been shown to have effects inconsistent with the antisense mechanism for which they were designed. Some of these effects are due to sequence and structure specific, as well as nonspecific, interactions with proteins. These effects are particularly prominent in *in vitro* tests for antiviral activity as often high concentrations of cells, viruses, and oligonucleotides are coincubated.[15,105] HIV is particularly problematic as many oligonucleotides bind to the gp120 protein of the virus.[3] However, the potential for confusion arising from the misinterpretation of an activity as being due to an antisense mechanism when, in fact, it is due to non-antisense effects is certainly not limited to antiviral or just *in vitro* tests.[106-108] Again, these data simply urge caution and argue for careful dose-response curves, direct analyses of target protein or RNA, and inclusion of appropriate controls before drawing conclusions concerning the mechanisms of action of oligonucleotide-based drugs. In addition to protein interactions, other factors such as overrepresented sequences of RNA and unusual structures that may be adopted by oligonucleotides can contribute to unexpected results.[3]

Given the variability in cellular uptake of oligonucleotides, the variability in potency as a function of binding site in an RNA target, and potential non-antisense activities of oligonucleotides, careful evaluation of dose-response curves and clear demonstration of the antisense mechanism are required before drawing conclusions from *in vitro* experiments. Nevertheless, numerous well-controlled studies have been reported in which antisense activity was conclusively demonstrated. As many of these studies have been reviewed previously, suffice it to say that antisense effects of phosphorothioate oligodeoxynucleotides against a variety of targets are well documented.[1,56,70-71,109-110]

2. In Vivo *Pharmacological Activities*

A relatively large number of reports of *in vivo* activities of phosphorothioate oligonucleotides have now appeared documenting activities both after local and systemic administration (Table 1).[16] However, only for a few of these reports have sufficient studies been performed to draw relatively firm conclusions concerning the mechanism of action. Consequently, I will review in some detail only a few reports that provide sufficient data to support a relatively firm conclusion with regard to mechanism of action. Local effects have been reported for phosphorothioate and methylphosphonate oligonucleotides. A phosphorothioate oligonucleotide designed to inhibit c-myb production and applied locally was shown to inhibit intimal accumulation in the rat carotid artery.[111] In this study, a Northern blot showed a significant reduction in c-myb RNA in animals treated with the antisense compound, but there was no effect by a control oligonucleotide. In a recent study, the effects of the oligonucleotide were suggested to be due to a non-antisense mechanism.[107] However, only one dose level was studied, thus much remains to be done before definitive conclusions are possible.

Similar effects were reported for phosphorothioate oligodeoxynucleotides designed to inhibit cyclin-dependent kinases (CDC-2 and CDK-2). Again, the antisense oligonucleotide inhibited intimal thickening and cyclin-dependent kinase activity, while a control oligonucleotide had no effect.[112] Additionally, local administration of a phosphorothioate oligonucleotide designed to inhibit N-myc resulted in reduction in N-myc expression and slower growth of a subcutaneously transplanted human tumor in nude mice.[113]

Antisense oligonucleotides administered intraventricularly have been reported to induce a variety of effects in the central nervous system. Intraventricular injection of antisense oligonucleotides to neuropeptide-Y-Y1 receptors reduced the density of

TABLE 1

Reported Activity of Antisense Oligonucleotides in Animal Models

Target	Route	Species	Ref.
Cardiovascular models:			
c-*myb*	Topically	Rat	111
cdc2 Kinase	Topically	Rat	174
PCNA	Topically	Rat	174
cdc2 Kinase	Topically	Rat	112
CDK2	Topically	Rat	112
Cyclin B1	Topically	Rat	175
PCNA	Topically	Rat	176
Angiotensin 1 receptor	Intracerebral	Rat	177
Angiotensinogen	Intracerebral	Rat	178
c-*fos*	Intracerebral	Rat	179
Inflammatory models:			
Type 1 IL-1 receptor	Intradermal	Mouse	122
ICAM-1	Intravenous	Mouse	180
ICAM-1	Intravenous	Mouse	181
ICAM-1	Intravenous	Mouse	182
ICAM-1	Intravenous	Mouse	183
ICAM-1	Intravenous	Mouse	184
Cancer models:			
N-*myc*	Subcutaneous	Mouse	113
NF-kB p65	Intraperitoneal	Mouse	123
c-*myb*	Subcutaneous	Mouse	185
p120 Nucleolar antigen	Intraperitoneal	Mouse	186
NK-kB p65	Subcutaneous	Mouse	124
Protein kinase C-α	Intraperitoneal	Mouse	18
c-*myb*	Subcutaneous	Mouse	20
Ha-*ras*	Intratumor	Mouse	187
BCR-ABL	Intravenous	Mouse	19
PTHrP	Intraventricular	Rat	188
c-raf Kinase	Intravenous	Mouse	126
Protein kinase C-α	Intravenous	Mouse	125
Protein kinase C-α	Intravenous	Mouse	189
Neurological models:			
c-*fos*	Intracerebral	Rat	190
SNAP-25	Intracerebral	Chicken	121
Kinesin heavy chain	Intravitreal	Rabbit	191
Arginine vasopressin	Intracerebral	Rat	192
c-*fos*	Intracerebral	Rat	193
Progesterone receptor	Intracerebral	Rat	194
Dopamine D_2 receptor	Intracerebral	Rat	195
Y-Y1 receptor	Intracerebral	Rat	114
Neuropeptide Y	Intracerebral	Rat	196
κ-Opioid receptor	Intracerebral	Rat	197
IGF-1	Intracerebral	Rat	198
κ-Opioid receptor	Intracerebral	Rat	197
c-*fos*	Intraspinal	Rat	199
c-*fos*	Intracerebral	Rat	200
c-*fos*	Intraspinal	Rat	201
NMDA receptor	Intracerebral	Rat	202
CREB	Intracerebral	Rat	203
Delta-opioid receptor	Intracerebral	Mice	204

TABLE 1 (CONTINUED)

Reported Activity of Antisense Oligonucleotides in Animal Models

Target	Route	Species	Ref.
Progesterone receptor	Intracerebral	Rat	205
GAD65	Intracerebral	Rat	206
GAD67	Intracerebral	Rat	206
AT1-angiotensin receptor	Intracerebral	Rat	207
Tryptophan hydroxylase	Intracerebral	Mouse	120
AT1-angiotensin receptor	Intracerebral	Rat	119
CRH_1-corticotropin-releasing hormone receptor	Intracerebral	Rat	208
opioid receptor	Intracerebral	Rat	209
opioid receptor	Intracerebral	Mouse	210
Oxytocin	Intracerebral	Rat	211
Oxytocin	Intracerebral	Rat	212
Substance P receptor	Intracerebral	Rat	213
Tyrosine hydroxylase	Intracerebral	Rat	214
c-*jun*	Intracerebral	Rat	215
D_1 dopamine receptor	Intracerebral	Mouse	118
D_2 dopamine receptor	Intracerebral	Mouse	116
D_2 dopamine receptor	Intracerebral	Mouse	115
D_2 dopamine receptor	Intracerebral	Mouse	117
Viral models:			
HSV-1		Mouse	22
Tick-born encephalitis		Mouse	216
Duck hepatitis virus	Intravenous	Duck	217

the receptors and resulted in behavioral signs of anxiety.[114] Similarly, an antisense oligonucleotide designed to bind to NMDA-R1 receptor channel RNA inhibited the synthesis of these channels and reduced the volume of focal ischemia produced by occlusion of the middle cerebral artery in rats.[114]

In a series of well-controlled studies, antisense oligonucleotides administered intraventricularly selectively inhibited dopamine type 2 receptor expression, dopamine type 2 receptor RNA levels, and behavioral effects in animals with chemical lesions. Controls included randomized oligonucleotides and the observation that no effects were observed on dopamine type 1 receptor or RNA levels.[115-117] This laboratory also reported the selective reduction of dopamine type 1 receptor and RNA levels with the appropriate oligonucleotide.[118]

Similar observations were reported in studies on AT-1 angiotensin receptors and tryptophan hydroxylase. In studies in rats, direct observations of AT-1 and AT-2 receptor densities in various sites in the brain after administration of different doses of phosphorothioate antisense, sense, and scrambled oligonucleotides were reported.[119] Again, in rats, intraventricular administration of phosphorothioate antisense oligonucleotide resulted in a decrease in tryptophan hydroxylase levels in the brain, while a scrambled control did not.[120]

Injection of antisense oligonucleotides to synaptosomal-associated protein-25 into the vitreous body of rat embryos reduced the expression of the protein and inhibited neurite elongation by rat cortical neurons.[121]

In addition to local and regional effects of antisense oligonucleotides, a growing number of well-controlled studies have demonstrated systemic effects of phosphorothioate oligodeoxynucleotides. Expression of interleukin-1 (IL-1) in mice was inhibited by systemic administration of antisense oligonucleotides.[122] Oligonucleotides to the NF-κB p65 subunit administered intraperitoneally (i.p.) at 40 mg/kg every three days slowed tumor growth in mice transgenic for the human T-cell leukemia viruses.[123] Similar results with other antisense oligonucleotides were shown in another *in vivo* tumor model after either prolonged s.c. infusion or intermittent s.c. injection.[124]

Several recent reports further extend the studies of phosphorothioate oligonucleotides as antitumor agents in mice. In one study, a phosphorothioate oligonucleotide directed to inhibition of the bcr-abl oncogene was administered at a dose of 1 mg/day for nine days i.v. to immunodeficient mice injected with human leukemic cells. The drug was shown to inhibit the development of leukemic colonies in the mice and to selectively reduce bcr-abl RNA levels in peripheral blood lymphocytes, spleen, bone marrow, liver, lungs, and brain.[19] However, it is possible that the effects on the RNA levels were secondary to effects on the growth of various cell types. In the second study, a phosphorothioate oligonucleotide antisense to the proto-oncogene myb, inhibited the growth of human melanoma in mice. Again, myb mRNA levels appeared to be selectively reduced.[20]

A number of studies from our laboratories that directly examined target RNA levels, target protein levels, and pharmacological effects using a wide range of control oligonucleotides, and examination of the effects on closely related isotypes have been completed. Single and chronic daily administration of a phosphorothioate oligonucleotide designed to inhibit mouse protein kinase C-α, (PKC-α), selectively inhibited expression of PKC-α RNA in mouse liver without effects on any other isotype. The effects lasted at least 24 h after a dose, and a clear dose-response curve was observed, with a dose of 10 to 15 mg/kg i.p. reducing PKC-α RNA levels in liver by 50% 24 h after a dose.[18]

A phosphorothioate oligonucleotide designed to inhibit human PKC-α expression selectively inhibited expression of PKC-α RNA and PKC-α protein in human tumor cell lines implanted s.c. in nude mice after i.v. administration.[125] In these studies, effects on RNA and protein levels were highly specific and observed at doses lower than 6 mg/kg/day, and antitumor effects were detected at doses as low as 0.6 mg/kg/day. A large number of control oligonucleotides failed to show activity.

In a similar series of studies, Monia et al.[126-127] demonstrated highly specific loss of human *c-raf* kinase RNA in human tumor xenografts and antitumor activity that correlated with the loss of RNA. Moreover, a series of control oligonucleotides with 1 to 7 mismatches showed decreasing potency *in vitro* and precisely the same rank order potencies *in vivo*.

Finally, a single injection of a phosphorothioate oligonucleotide designed to inhibit c-AMP-dependent protein kinase type 1 was reported to selectively reduce RNA and protein levels in human tumor xenografts and to reduce tumor growth.[128]

Thus, there is a growing body of evidence that phosphorothioate oligonucleotides can induce potent systemic and local effects *in vivo*. More importantly, there are now a number of studies with sufficient controls and direct observation of target RNA and protein levels to suggest highly specific effects that are difficult to explain via any mechanism other than antisense. As would be expected, the potency of these effects varies depending on the target, the organ, and the endpoint measured as well as the route of administration and the time after a dose when the effect is measured.

In conclusion, although it is of obvious importance to interpret *in vivo* activity data cautiously, and it is clearly necessary to include a range of controls and to evaluate effects on target RNA and protein levels and control RNA and protein levels directly, it is difficult to argue with the conclusion today that some effects have been observed in animals that are most likely primarily due to an antisense mechanism.

Additionally, in studies on patients with CMV-induced retinitis, local injections of ISIS 2922 have resulted in impressive efficacy, though it is obviously impossible to prove the mechanism of action is antisense in these studies.[129]

F. Toxicological Properties

1. *In Vitro*

In our laboratory, we have evaluated the toxicities of scores of phosphorothioate oligodeoxynucleotides in a significant number of cell lines in tissue culture. As a general rule, no significant cytotoxicity is induced at concentrations below 100 μ*M* oligonucleotide. Additionally, with a few exceptions, no significant effect on macromolecular synthesis is observed at concentrations below 100 μ*M*.[87,91]

Polynucleotides and other polyanions have been shown to cause release of cytokines.[130] Also, bacterial DNA species have been reported to be mitogenic for lymphocytes *in vitro*.[131] Furthermore, oligodeoxynucleotides (30 to 45 nucleotides in length) were reported to induce interferons and enhance natural killer (NK) cell activity.[132] In the latter study, the oligonucleotides that displayed NK-stimulating activity contained specific palindromic sequences and tended to be guanosine rich. Collectively, these observations indicate that nucleic acids may have broad immunostimulatory activity.

It has been shown that phosphorothioate oligonucleotides stimulate B-lymphocyte proliferation in a mouse splenocyte preparation (analogous to bacterial DNA), and the response may underlie the observations of lymphoid hyperplasia in the spleen and lymph nodes of rodents caused by repeated administration of these compounds (see below).[133] We also have evidence of enhanced cytokine release by immunocompetent cells when exposed to phosphorothioates *in vitro*.[134] In this study, both human keratinocytes and an *in vitro* model of human skin released IL-1-a when treated with 250 μ*M* to 1 m*M* of phosphorothioate oligonucleotides. The effects seemed to be dependent on the phosphorothioate backbone and independent of sequence or 2′ modification. In a study in which murine B lymphocytes were treated with phosphodiester oligonucleotides, B-cell activation was induced by oligonucleotides with unmethylated CpG dinucleotides.[135] This has been extrapolated to suggest that the CpG motif may be required for immune stimulation of oligonucleotide analogs such as phosphorothioates. This clearly is not the case with regard to release of IL-1-a from keratinocytes;[134] nor is it the case with regard to *in vivo* immune stimulation (see below).

2. *Genotoxicity*

As with any new chemical class of therapeutic agents, concerns about genotoxicity cannot be dismissed as little *in vitro* testing has been performed and no data from long-term studies of oligonucleotides are available. Clearly, given the limitations in our understanding about the basic mechanisms that might be involved, empirical data must be generated. We have performed mutagenicity studies on two phosphorothioate oligonucleotides, ISIS 2105 and ISIS 2922, and found them to be nonmutagenic at all concentrations studied.[8]

Two mechanisms of genotoxicity that may be unique to oligonucleotides have been considered. One possibility is that an oligonucleotide analog could be integrated into the genome and produce mutagenic events. Although integration of an oligonucleotide into the genome is conceivable, it is extremely rare. For most viruses, viral DNA integration is itself a rare event and, of course, viruses have evolved specialized enzyme-mediated mechanisms to achieve integration. Moreover, preliminary studies in our laboratory have shown that phosphorothioate oligodeoxynucleotides are generally poor substrates for DNA polymerases, and it is unlikely that enzymes such as integrases, gyrases, and topoisomerases (that have obligate DNA cleavage as intermediate steps in their enzymatic processes) will accept these compounds as substrates. Consequently, it would seem that the risk of genotoxicity due to genomic integration is no greater and probably less than that of other potential mechanisms, for example, alteration of the activity of growth factors, cytokine release, nonspecific effects on membranes that might trigger arachidonic acid release, or inappropriate intracellular signaling. Presumably, new analogs that deviate significantly more from natural DNA would be even less likely to be integrated.

A second concern that has been raised about possible genotoxicity is the risk that oligonucleotides might be degraded to toxic or carcinogenic metabolites. However, metabolism of phosphorothioate oligodeoxynucleotides by base excision would release normal bases, which presumably would be nongenotoxic. Similarly, oxidation of the phosphorothioate backbone to the natural phosphodiester structure would also yield nonmutagenic (and probably nontoxic) metabolites. Finally, it is possible that phosphorothioate bonds could be hydrolyzed slowly, releasing nucleoside phosphorothioates that presumably would be rapidly oxidized to natural (nontoxic) nucleoside phosphates. However, oligonucleotides with modified bases and/or backbones may pose different risks.

3. *In Vivo*

The acute LD_{50} in mice of all phosphorothioate oligonucleotides tested to date is in excess of 500 mg/kg (Kornbrust, unpublished observations). In rodents, we have had the opportunity to evaluate the acute and chronic toxicities of multiple phosphorothioate oligonucleotides administered by multiple routes.[136-137] The consistent dose-limiting toxicity was immune stimulation manifested by lymphoid hyperplasia, splenomegaly, and a multi-organ monocellular infiltrate. These effects occurred only with chronic dosing at doses >20 mg/kg and were dose dependent. The liver and kidney were the organs most prominently affected by monocellular infiltrates. All of these effects appeared to be reversible, and chronic intradermal administration appeared to be the most toxic route, probably because of high local concentrations of the drugs, resulting in local cytokine release and initiation of a cytokine cascade. There were no obvious effects of sequence. At doses of 100 mg/kg and greater, minor increases in liver enzyme levels and mild thrombocytopenia were also observed.

In monkeys, however, the toxicological profile of phosphorothioate oligonucleotides is quite different. The most prominent dose-limiting side effect is sporadic reductions in blood pressure associated with bradycardia. When these events are observed, they are often associated with activation of C-5 complement and they are dose-related and peak plasma concentration-related. This appears to be related to the activation of the alternative pathway.[138] All phosphorothioate oligonucleotides tested to date appear to induce these effects, though there may be slight variations in potency as a function of sequence and/or length.[139-141]

A second prominent toxicologic effect in the monkey is the prolongation of activated partial thromboplastin time. At higher doses, evidence of clotting abnormalities is observed. Again, these effects are dose- and peak plasma concentration-dependent.[140-141] Although no evidence of sequence dependence has been observed, there appears to be a linear correlation between number of phosphorothioate linkages and potency between 18 to 25 nucleotides (Nicklin, P., unpublished observations). The mechanisms responsible for these effects are likely very complex, but preliminary data suggest that direct interactions with thrombin may be at least partially responsible for the effects observed.[142]

In man, again the toxicological profile differs somewhat. When ISIS 2922 is administered intravitreally to patients with CMV retinitis, the most common adverse event is anterior chamber inflammation which is easily managed with steroids. A relatively rare and dose-related adverse event is morphological changes in the retina associated with loss in peripheral vision.[129]

ISIS 2105, a 20-mer phosphorothioate designed to inhibit the replication of human papilloma viruses that cause genital warts, was administered intradermally at doses as high as 3 mg per wart weekly for three weeks. Essentially no toxicities have been observed, including, remarkably, a complete absence of local inflammation (Grillone, L., unpublished results).

Every other day administration of 2-h i.v. infusions of ISIS 2302, at doses as high as 2 mg/kg, resulted in no significant toxicities including no evidence of immune stimulation and no hypotension. A slight subclinical increase in APTT was observed at the 2 mg/kg dose.[143]

G. Therapeutic Index

In Figure 2, an attempt to put the toxicities and their dose-response relationships in a therapeutic context is shown. This is particularly important as considerable confusion has arisen concerning the potential utility of phosphorothioate oligonucleotides for selected therapeutic purposes deriving from unsophisticated interpretation of toxicological data. As can be readily seen, the immune stimulation induced by these compounds appears to be particularly prominent in rodents and unlikely to be dose limiting in man; nor have we, to date, observed hypotensive events in humans. Thus, this toxicity appears to occur at lower doses in monkeys than man and certainly is not dose limiting in man.

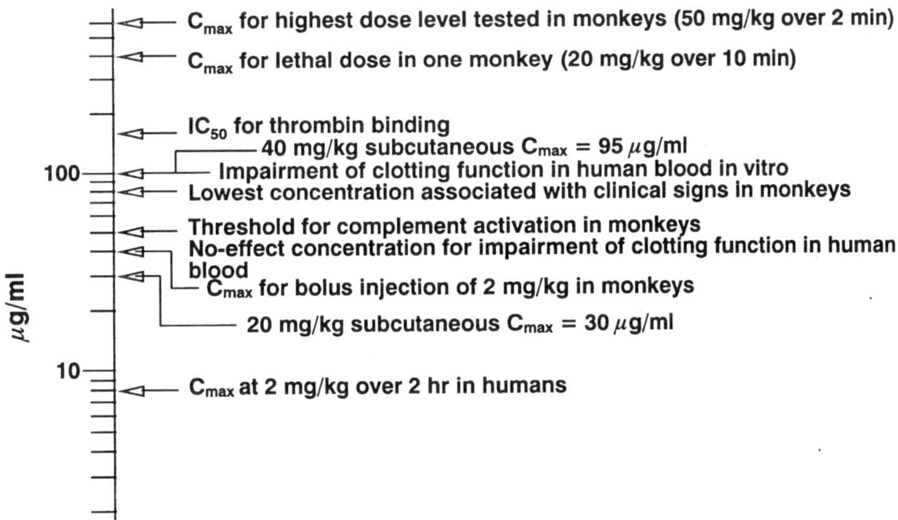

FIGURE 2
Plasma concentrations of ISIS 2302 at which various activities are observed. These concentrations are determined by extracting plasma and analyzing by capillary gel electrophoresis and represent intact ISIS 2302.

Based on our experience to date, we believe that the dose-limiting toxicity in man will be clotting abnormalities, and this will be associated with peak plasma concentrations well in excess of 10 μg/ml. In animals, pharmacological activities have been observed with i.v. bolus doses from 0.006 mg/kg to 10 to 15 mg/kg depending on the target, the endpoint, the organ studied, and the time after a dose when the effect is measured. Thus, it would appear that phosphorothioate oligonucleotides have a therapeutic index that supports their evaluation for a number of therapeutic indications.

H. Conclusions

Phosphorothioate oligonucleotides have perhaps outperformed many expectations. They display attractive parenteral pharmacokinetic properties. They have produced potent systemic effects in a number of animal models and, in many experiments, the antisense mechanism has been directly demonstrated as the hoped for selectivity. Further, these compounds appear to display satisfactory therapeutic indices for many indications.

Nevertheless, phosphorothioates clearly have significant limits (Table 2). Pharmacodynamically, they have relatively low affinity per nucleotide unit. This means that longer oligonucleotides are required for biological activity and that invasion of many RNA structures may not be possible. At higher concentrations, these compounds inhibit RNase H as well. Thus, the higher end of the pharmacologic dose-response curve is lost. Pharmacokinetically, phosphorothioates do not cross the blood-brain barrier, are not significantly orally bioavailable, and may display dose-dependent pharmacokinetics. Toxicologically, clearly the release of cytokines, activation of complement, and interference with clotting will pose dose limits if they are encountered in the clinic.

TABLE 2

Phosphorothioate Oligonucleotides

Limits
Pharmacodynamic
Low affinity per nucleotide unit
Inhibition of RNase H at high concentrations
Pharmacokinetic
Limited bioavailability
Limited blood-brain barrier penetration
Dose-dependent pharmacokinetics
Possible drug-drug interactions
Toxicologic
Release of cytokines
Complement associated effects on blood pressure?
Clotting effects

As several clinical trials are in progress with phosphorothioates, and others will be initiated shortly, we shall soon have more definitive information about the activities, toxicities, and value of this class of antisense drugs in human beings.

V. THE MEDICINAL CHEMISTRY OF OLIGONUCLEOTIDES

A. Introduction

The core of any rational drug discovery program is medicinal chemistry. Although the synthesis of modified nucleic acids has been a subject of interest for some time, the intense focus on the medicinal chemistry of oligonucleotides dates perhaps to no more than five years prior to this chapter. Consequently, the scope of medicinal chemistry has recently expanded enormously, but the biological data to support conclusions about synthetic strategies are only beginning to emerge.

Modifications in the base, sugar, and phosphate moieties of oligonucleotides have been reported. The subjects of medicinal chemical programs include approaches to create enhanced affinity and more selective affinity for RNA or duplex structures, the ability to cleave nucleic acid targets, enhanced nuclease stability, cellular uptake and distribution, and *in vivo* tissue distribution, metabolism, and clearance.

B. Heterocycle Modifications

1. *Pyrimidine Modifications*

A relatively large number of modified pyrimidines have been synthesized and are now incorporated into oligonucleotides and evaluated. The principle sites of modification are C-2, C-4, C-5, and C-6. These and other nucleoside analogs have recently been thoroughly reviewed.[144] Consequently, a very brief summary of the analogs that displayed interesting properties is incorporated here.

Inasmuch as the C-2 position is involved in Watson-Crick hybridization, C-2-modified pyrimidine containing oligonucleotides has shown unattractive hybridization properties. An oligonucleotide containing 2-thiothymidine was found to hybridize well to DNA and, in fact, even better to RNA (ΔT_m 1.5°C/modification; Swayze et al., unpublished results).

In contrast, several modifications in the 4 position that have interesting properties have been reported. 4-thiopyrimidines have been incorporated into oligonucleotides with no significant negative effect on hybridization.[145] A bicyclic and an N4-methoxy analog of cytosine were shown to hybridize with both purine bases in DNA with T_ms approximately equal to natural base pairs.[146] Additionally, a fluorescent base has been incorporated into oligonucleotides and shown to enhance DNA-DNA duplex stability.[147]

A large number of modifications at the C-5 position have also been reported including halogenated nucleosides. Although the stability of duplexes may be enhanced by incorporating 5-halogenated nucleosides, the occasional mispairing with G and the potential that the oligonucleotide might degrade and release toxic nucleoside analogs cause concern.[144]

Furthermore, oligonucleotides containing 5-propynylpyrimidine modifications have been shown to enhance the duplex stability (ΔT_m 1.6°C/modification[105]) and support the RNase H activity. The 5-heteroarylpyrimidines were also shown to influence the stability of duplexes.[105,148] A more dramatic influence was reported for the tricyclic 2′ deoxycytidine analogs, exhibiting an enhancement of 2 to 5°C/modification depending on the positioning of the modified bases.[149] It is believed that the enhanced binding properties of these analogs are due to extended stacking and increased hydrophobic interactions.

In general, as expected, modifications in the C-6 position of pyrimidines are highly duplex destabilizing.[150] Oligonucleotides containing 6-aza pyrimidines have been shown to reduce T_m by 1 to 2°C/modification, but to enhance the nuclease stability of oligonucleotides and to support RNase H-induced degradation of RNA targets.[144]

2. *Purine Modifications*

Although numerous purine analogs have been synthesized, when incorporated into oligonucleotides they usually result in destabilization of duplexes. However, there are a few exceptions where a purine modification had a stabilizing effect. A brief summary of some of these analogs is discussed below.

Generally, N-1 modifications of purine moiety have resulted in destabilization of the duplex.[157] Similarly, C-2 modifications have usually resulted in destabilization. However, 2-6-diaminopurine has been reported to enhance hybridization by approximately 1°C/modification when paired with T.[152] Of the 3-position substituted bases reported to date, only the 3-deaza adenosine analog has been shown to have no negative effective on hybridization.

Modifications at the C-6 and C-7 positions have likewise resulted in only a few interesting bases from the point of view of hybridization. Inosine has been shown to have little effect on duplex stability, but because it can pair and stack with all four normal DNA bases, it behaves as a universal base and creates an ambiguous position in an oligonucleotide.[153] Incorporation of 7-deaza inosine into oligonucleotides was destabilizing, and this was considered to be due to its relatively hydrophobic nature.[154] 7-Deaza guanine was similarly destabilizing, but when 8-aza-7-deaza guanine was incorporated into oligonucleotides, it enhanced hybridizations.[155] Thus, on occasion, introduction of more than one modification in a nucleobase may compensate for destabilizing effects of some modifications. Interestingly, a 7-iodo 7-deazaguanine residue was recently incorporated into oligonucleotides and shown to enhance the binding affinity dramatically (ΔT_m 10.0°C/modification compared to 7-deazaguanine).[156] The increase in T_m value was attributed to (1) the hydrophobic nature of the modification, (2) increased stacking interaction, and (3) favorable pKa of the base.

In contrast, some C-8 substituted bases have yielded improved nuclease resistance when incorporated in oligonucleotides, but they seem to be somewhat destabilizing.[144]

3. *Oligonucleotide Conjugates*

Although conjugation of various functionalities to oligonucleotides has been reported to achieve a number of important objectives, the data supporting some of the claims are limited and generalizations are not possible based on the data presently available.

a. Nuclease Stability

Numerous 3′ modifications have been reported to enhance the stability of oligonucleotides in serum.[157] Both neutral and charged substituents have been reported to stabilize oligonucleotides in serum and, as a general rule, the stability of a conjugated oligonucleotide tends to be greater as bulkier substituents are added. Inasmuch as the principal nuclease in serum is a 3′ exonuclease, it is not surprising that 5′ modifications have resulted in significantly less stabilization. Internal modifications of base, sugar and backbone have also been reported to enhance nuclease stability at or near the modified nucleoside.[157] In a recent study, thiono triester (adamantyl, cholesteryl and others) modified oligonucleotides have shown improved nuclease stability, cellular association, and binding affinity.[158]

The demonstration that modifications may induce nuclease stability sufficient to enhance activity in cells in tissue culture and in animals has proven to be much more complicated because of the presence of 5′ exonucleases and endonucleases. In our laboratory, 3′ modifications and internal point modifications have not provided sufficient nuclease stability to demonstrate pharmacological activity in cells.[83] In fact, even a 5 nucleotide long phosphodiester gap in the middle of a phosphorothioate oligonucleotide resulted in sufficient loss of nuclease resistance to cause complete loss of pharmacological activity.[72]

In mice, neither a 5′ cholesterol nor 5′ C-18 amine conjugate altered the metabolic rate of a phosphorothioate oligodeoxynucleotide in liver, kidneys or plasma.[73] Furthermore, blocking the 3′ and 5′ termini of a phosphodiester oligonucleotide did not markedly enhance the nuclease stability of the parent compound in mice.[13] However, 3′ modification of a phosphorothioate oligonucleotide was reported to enhance its stability in mice relative to the parent phosphorothioate.[159] Moreover, a phosphorothioate oligonucleotide with a 3′ hairpin loop was reported to be more stable in rats than its parent.[158] Thus, 3′ modifications may enhance the stability of the relatively stable phosphorothioates sufficiently to be of value.

b. Enhanced Cellular Uptake

Although oligonucleotides have been shown to be taken up by a number of cell lines in tissue culture, with perhaps the most compelling data relating to phosphorothioate oligonucleotides, a clear objective has been to improve cellular uptake of oligonucleotides.[2,8] Inasmuch as the mechanisms of cellular uptake of oligonucleotides are still very poorly understood, the medicinal chemistry approaches have been largely empirical and based on many unproven assumptions.

Because phosphodiester and phosphorothioate oligonucleotides are water soluble, the conjugation of lipophilic substituents to enhance membrane permeability has been a subject of considerable interest. Unfortunately, studies in this area have not been systematic and, at present, there is precious little information about the changes in physicochemical properties of oligonucleotides actually effected by specific lipid conjugates. Phospholipids, cholesterol and cholesterol derivatives, cholic acid, and simple alkyl chains have been conjugated to oligonucleotides at various sites in the oligonucleotide. The effects of these modifications on cellular uptake have been assessed using fluorescent, or radiolabeled, oligonucleotides or by measuring pharmacological activities. From the perspective of medicinal chemistry, very few systematic studies have been performed. The activities of short alkyl chains, adamantine, daunomycin, fluorescein, cholesterol, and porphyrin conjugated oligonucleotides were compared in one study.[160] A cholesterol modification was reported to be more effective at enhancing uptake than the other substituents. It also seems likely that the effects of various conjugates on cellular uptake may be affected by the cell type and target studied. For example, we have studied cholic acid conjugates of phosphorothioate deoxyoligonucleotides or phosphorothioate 2′ methoxy oligonucleotides and observed enhanced activity against HIV and no effect on the activity of ICAM directed oligonucleotides.

Additionally, polycationic substitutions and various groups designed to bind to cellular carrier systems have been synthesized. Although many compounds have been synthesized, the data reported to date are insufficient to draw firm conclusions about the value of such approaches or structure-activity relationships.[157]

c. RNA Cleaving Groups

Oligonucleotide conjugates were recently reported to act as artificial ribonucleases, albeit in low efficiencies.[161] Conjugation of chemically reactive groups such as alkylating agents, photo-induced azides, prophine, and psoralene have been utilized extensively to effect a cross-linking of oligonucleotide and the target RNA. In principle, this treatment may lead to translation arrest. In addition, lanthanides and complexes thereof have been reported to cleave RNA via a hydrolytic pathway. Recently, a novel europium complex was covalently linked to an oligonucleotide and shown to cleave 88% of the complementary RNA at physiological pH.[162]

d. In Vivo *Effects*

To date, relatively few studies have been reported *in vivo*. The properties of a 5′ cholesterol and 5′ C-18 amine conjugates of a 20-mer phosphorothioate oligodeoxynucleotide have been determined in mice. Both compounds increased the fraction of an i.v. bolus dose found in the liver. The cholesterol conjugate, in fact, resulted in more than 80% of the dose accumulating in the liver. Neither conjugate enhanced stability in plasma, liver, or kidneys.[73] Interestingly, the only significant change in the toxicity profile was a slight increase in effects on serum transaminases and histopathological changes indicative of slight liver toxicity associated with the cholesterol conjugate.[163] A 5′ cholesterol phosphorothioate conjugate was also recently reported to have a longer elimination half-life, to be more potent, and to induce greater liver toxicity in rats.[164]

4. Sugar Modifications

The focus of second generation oligonucleotide modifications has centered on the sugar moiety. In oligonucleotides, the pentofuranose sugar ring occupies a contral connecting manifold that also positions the nucleobases for effective stacking. Recently, a symposium series has been published on the carbohydrate modifications in antisense research which covers this topic in great detail.[165] Therefore, the content of the following discussion is restricted to a summary of the main events in this area.

A growing number of oligonucleotides in which the pentofuranose ring is modified or replaced have been reported.[166] Uniform modifications at the 2′ position have been shown to enhance hybridization to RNA, and in some cases, to enhance nuclease resistance.[166] Chimeric oligonucleotides containing 2′ deoxyoligonucleotide gaps with 2′ modified wings have been shown to be more potent than parent molecules.[61]

Other sugar modifications include α-oligonucleotides, carbocyclic oligonucleotides, and hexapyranosyl oligonucleotides.[166] Of these, α-oligonucleotides have been most extensively studied. They hybridize in parallel fashion to single-stranded DNA and RNA and are nuclease resistant. All these oligonucleotides support RNase H and, as can be seen, a direct correlation between affinity and potency exists.

A growing number of oligonucleotides in which the C-2′ position of the sugar ring is modified have been reported.[157,161] These modifications include lipophilic alkyl groups, intercalators, amphipathic amino-alkyl tethers, positively charged polyamines, highly electronegative fluoro or fluoro alkyl moieties, and sterically bulky methylthio derivatives. The beneficial effects of a C-2′ substitution on the antisense oligonucleotide cellular uptake, nuclease resistance, and binding affinity have been well documented in the literature. In addition, excellent review articles have appeared in the last few years on the synthesis and properties of C-2′ modified oligonucleotides.[161,167-169]

Other modifications of the sugar moiety have also been studied, including other sites as well as more substantial modifications. However, much less is known about the antisense effects of these modifications.[16]

2′ Methoxy-substituted phosphorothioate oligonucleotides have recently been reported to be more stable in mice than their parent compounds and to display enhanced oral bioavailability.[158,101] The analogs displayed tissue distribution similar to that of the parent phosphorothioate.

Similarly, we have compared the pharmacokinetics of 2′ propoxy modified phosphodiester and phosphorothioate deoxynucleotides.[73] As expected, the 2′ propoxy modification increased lipophilicity and nuclease resistance. In fact, in mice the 2′ propoxy phosphorothioate was too stable in liver or kidney to measure an elimination half-life.

Interestingly, the 2′ propoxy phosphodiester was much less stable than the parent phosphorothioate in all organs except the kidney in which the 2′ propoxy phosphodiester was remarkably stable. The 2′ propoxy phosphodiester did not bind to albumin significantly, while the affinity of the phosphorothioate for albumin was enhanced. The only difference in toxicity between the analogs was a slight increase in renal toxicity associated with the 2′ propoxy phosphodiester analog.[163]

Incorporation of the 2′ methoxyethyoxy group into oligonucleotides increased the T_m by 1.1°C/modification when hybridized to the complement RNA. In a similar manner, several other 2′ *O*-alkoxy modifications have been reported to enhance the affinity.[170] The increase in affinity with these modifications was attributed to (1) the favorable gauche effect of side chain and (2) additional solvation of the alkoxy substituent in water.

More substantial carbohydrate modifications have also been studied. Hexose-containing oligonucleotides were created and found to have very low affinity for RNA.[171] Also, the 4′ oxygen has been replaced with sulfur. Although a single substitution of a 4′ thio modified nucleoside resulted in destabilization of a duplex, incorporation of two 4′ thio modified nucleosides increased the affinity of the duplex.[172] Finally, bicyclic sugars have been synthesized with the hope that preorganization into more rigid structures would enhance hybridization. Several of these modifications have been reported to enhance hybridization.[165]

5. *Backbone Modifications*

Substantial progress in creating new backbones for oligonucleotides that replace the phosphate or the sugar-phosphate unit has been made. The objectives of these programs are to improve hybridization by removing the negative charge, enhance stability, and potentially improve pharmacokinetics.

For a review of the backbone modifications reported to date, please see References 9, 16, and 165. Suffice it to say that numerous modifications have been made that replace phosphate, retain hybridization, alter charge, and enhance stability. Because these modifications are now being evaluated *in vitro* and *in vivo*, a preliminary assessment should be possible shortly.

Replacement of the entire sugar-phosphate unit has also been accomplished, and the oligonucleotides produced have displayed very interesting characteristics. PNA oligonucleotides have been shown to bind to single-stranded DNA and RNA with extraordinary affinity and high sequence specificity. They have been shown to be able to invade some double-stranded nucleic acid structures. PNA oligonucleotides can form triple-stranded structures with DNA or RNA.

PNA oligonucleotides were shown to be able to act as antisense and transcriptional inhibitors when microinjected in cells.[173] PNA oligonucleotides appear to be quite stable to nucleases and peptidases as well.

In summary, then, in the past five years enormous advances in the medicinal chemistry of oligonucleotides has been reported. Modifications at nearly every position in oligonucleotides have been attempted and numerous potentially interesting analogs have been identified. Although it is far too early to determine which of the modifications may be most useful for particular purposes, it is clear that a wealth of new chemicals is available for systematic evaluation and that these studies should provide important insights into the SAR of oligonucleotide analogs.

VI. CONCLUSIONS

Although many more questions about antisense remain to be answered than are answered, progress has continued to be gratifying. Clearly, as more is learned, we will be in the position to perform progressively more sophisticated studies and to understand more of the factors that determine whether an oligonucleotide actually works via an antisense mechanism. We should also have the opportunity to learn a great deal more about this class of drugs as additional studies are completed in humans.

ACKNOWLEDGMENT

The author wishes to thank Colleen Matzinger for excellent typographic and administrative assistance.

ABBREVIATIONS

PNA, peptide nucleic acid; mRNA, messenger RNA; Ha-*ras*, Harvey *ras*; IL, interleukin; TAR, transactivator response element; ICAM, intercellular adhesion molecule; PKC, protein kinase C; HIV, human immune deficiency virus; NK, natural killer; CMV, cytomegalovirus; HPV, human papilloma virus; HSV, herpes simplex virus; and PTHrP, parathyroid hormone-related peptide.

REFERENCES

1. Crooke, S.T. and Lebleu, B. (Eds.), *Antisense Research and Applications,* CRC Press, Boca Raton, FL, 1993.
2. Crooke, R.M. *In vitro* toxicology and pharmacokinetics of antisense oligonucleotides, *Anti-Cancer Drug Des.,* 6, 609, 1991.
3. Wyatt, J.R., Vickers, T.A., Roberson, J.L. et al., Combinatorially selected guanosine-quartet structure is a potent inhibitor of human immunodeficiency virus envelop-mediated cell fusion, *Proc. Natl. Acad. Sci. U.S.A.,* 91, 1356, 1994.
4. Freier, S.M., Hybridization: Considerations affecting antisense drugs, in *Antisense Research and Applications,* Crooke, S.T. and Lebleu, B., Eds., CRC Press, Boca Raton, FL, 1993, 67.
5. Ecker, D.J. Strategies for invasion of RNA secondary structure, in *Antisense Research and Applications,* Crooke, S.T. and Lebleu, B., Eds., CRC Press, Boca Raton, FL, 1993, 387.

6. Lima, W.F., Monia, B.P., Ecker, D.J. et al., Implication of RNA structure on antisense oligonucleotide hybridization kinetics, *Biochemistry*, 31, 12055, 1992.
7. Ecker, D.J., Vickers, T.A., Bruice, T.W. et al., Pseudo-half knot formation with RNA, *Science*, 257, 958, 1992.
8. Crooke, S.T., Grillone, L.R., Tendolkar, A. et al., A pharmacokinetic evaluation of ^{14}C labeled afovirsen sodium in genital wart patients, *J. Pharmacol. Exp. Ther.*, 56, 641, 1994.
9. Crooke, R.M., Graham, M.J., Cooke, M.E. et al., *In vitro* pharmacokinetics of phosphorothioate antisense oligonucleotides, *J. Pharmacol. Toxicol.*, 275, 462, 1995.
10. Loke, S.L., Stein, C.A., Zhang, X.H. et al., Characterization of oligonucleotide transport into living cells, *Proc. Natl. Acad. Sci. U.S.A.*, 86, 3474, 1989.
11. Cossum, P.A., Sasmor, H., Dellinger, D. et al., Disposition of the ^{14}C-labeled phosphorothioate oligonucleotide ISIS 2105 after intravenous administration to rats, *J. Pharmacol. Exp. Ther.*, 267, 1181, 1993.
12. Cossum, P.A., Truong, L., Owens, S.R. et al., Pharmacokinetics of a ^{14}C labeled phosphorothioate oligonucleotides, ISIS 2105, after intradermal administration to rats, *J. Pharm. Exp. Ther.*, 269, 89, 1994.
13. Sands, H., Gorey-Feret, L.J., Ho, S.P. et al., Biodistribution and metabolism of internally ^{3}H-labeled oligonucleotides. II. 3′, 5′-blocked oligonucleotides, *Mol. Pharmacol.*, 47, 636, 1995.
14. Cowsert, L. Antiviral activities of oligonucleotides, in *Antisense Research and Applications*, CRC Press, Boca Raton, FL, 1993, 521.
15. Azad, R.F., Driver, V.B., Tanaka, K. et al., Antiviral activity of a phosphorothioate oligonucleotide complementary to RNA of the human cytomegalovirus major immediate-early region, *Antimicrob. Agents Chemother.*, 37, 1945, 1993.
16. Crooke, S.T., *Therapeutic Applications of Oligonucleotides*, R.G. Landes Co., Austin, TX, 1995.
17. Chiang, M.Y., Chan, H., Zounes, M.A. et al., Antisense oligonucleotides inhibit ICAM-1 expression by two distinct mechanisms, *J. Biol. Chem.*, 266, 18162, 1991.
18. Dean, N.M. and McKay, R., Inhibition of PKC-a expression in mice after systemic administration of phosphorothioate antisense oligonucleotides, *Proc. Natl. Acad. Sci. U.S.A.*, 91, 11762, 1994.
19. Skorski, T., Nieborowska-Skorska, M., Nicolaides, N.C. et al., Suppression of Ph^1 leukemia cell growth in mice by BCR-ABL antisense oligodeoxynucleotide, *Proc. Natl. Acad. Sci. U.S.A.*, 91, 4504, 1994.
20. Hijya, N., Zhang, J., Ratajczak, M.Z. et al., Biological and therapeutic significance of MYB expression in human melanoma, *Proc. Natl. Acad. Sci. U.S.A.*, 91, 4499, 1994.
21. McManaway, M.E., Neckers, L.M., Loke, S.L. et al., Tumour-specific inhibition of lymphoma growth by an antisense oligodeoxynucleotide, *Lancet*, 335, 808, 1990.
22. Kulka, M., Smith, C., Aurelian, L. et al., Site specificity of the inhibitory effects of oligo(nucleoside methylphosphonates) complementary to the acceptor splice junction of herpes simplex virus type 1 immediately early mRNA, *Proc. Natl. Acad. Sci. U.S.A.*, 86, 6868, 1989.
23. Zamecnik, P.C., Goodchild, J., Taguchi, Y. et al., Inhibition of replication and expression of human T-cell lymphotropic virus type III in cultured cells by exogenous synthetic oligonucleotides complementary to viral RNA, *Proc. Natl. Acad. Sci. U.S.A.*, 83, 4143, 1986.
24. Smith, C.C., Aurelian, L., Reddy, M.P. et al., Antiviral effect of an oligo(nucleoside methylphosphonate) complementary to the splice junction of herpes simplex virus type 1 immediate early pre-mRNAs 4 and 5, *Proc. Natl. Acad. Sci. U.S.A.*, 83, 2787, 1986.
25. Dominski, Z. and Kole, R., Restoration of correct splicing in thalassemic pre-mRNA by antisense oligonucleotides, *Proc. Natl. Acad. Sci. U.S.A.*, 90, 8673, 1993.
26. Hodges, D. and Crooke, S.T., Inhibition of wild-type and mutated luciferase-adenovirus pre-mRNAs by antisense oligonucleotides, *Mol. Pharmacol.*, 48, 905, 1995.
27. Agrawal, S., Goodchild, J., Civeira, M.P. et al., Oligodeoxynucleoside phosphoramidates and phosphorothioates as inhibitors of human immunodeficiency virus, *Proc. Natl. Acad. Sci. U.S.A.*, 85, 7079, 1988.
28. Lemaitre, M., Bayard, B., and Lebleu, B., Specific antiviral activity of a poly (L-lysine)-conjugated oligodeoxyribonucleotide sequence complementary to vesicular stomatitis virus N-protein mRNA initiation site, *Proc. Natl. Acad. Sci. U.S.A.*, 84, 648, 1987.
29. Rosolen, A., Whitesell, L., Olegalo, M. et al., Antisense inhibition of single copy N-myc expression results in decreased cell growth without reduction of c-myc protein in a neuroepithelioma cell line, *Cancer Res.*, 50, 6316, 1990.
30. Vasanthakumar, G. and Ahmed, N.K., Modulation of drug resistance in a daunorubicin resistant subline with oligonucleoside methylphosphonates, *Cancer Commun.*, 1, 225, 1989.
31. Sburlati, A.R., Manrow, R.E., and Berger, S.L., Prothymosin a antisense oligomers inhibit myeloma cell division, *Proc. Natl. Acad. Sci. U.S.A.*, 88, 253, 1991.

32. Zheng, H., Sahai, B.M., Kilgannon, P. et al., Specific inhibition of cell-surface T-cell receptor expression by antisense oligodeoxynucleotides and its effect on the production of an antigen-specific regulatory T-cell factor, *Proc. Natl. Acad. Sci. U.S.A.*, 86, 3758, 1989.
33. Maier, J.A.M., Voulalas, P., Roeder, D. et al., Extension of the life-span of human endothelial cells by an interleukin-1a antisense oligomer, *Science*, 249, 1570, 1990.
34. Mirabelli, C.K., Bennett, C.F., Anderson, K. et al., *In vitro* and *in vivo* pharmacologic activities of antisense oligonucleotides, Anti-Cancer Drug Des., 6, 647, 1991.
35. Cowsert, L.M., Fox, M.C., Zon, G. et al., *In vitro* evaluation of phosphorothioate oligonucleotides targeted to the E_2 mRNA of papillomavirus: Potential treatment of genital warts, *Antimicrob. Agents Chemother.*, 37, 171, 1993.
36. Vickers, T., Baker, B.F., Cook, P.D. et al., Inhibition of HIV-LTR gene expression by oligonucleotides targeted to the TAR element, *Nucleic Acids Res.,*, 19, 3359, 1991.
37. Saxena, S.K. and Ackerman, E.J., Microinjected oligonucleotides complementary to the a-sarcin loop of 28 S RNA abolish protein synthesis in *Xenopus* oocytes, *J. Biol. Chem.,*, 265, 3263, 1990.
38. Walker, K., Elela, S.A., and Nazar, R.N., Inhibition of protein synthesis by anti-5.8 S rRNA oligodeoxyribonucleotides, *J. Biol. Chem.*, 265, 2428, 1990.
39. Westerman, P., Gross, B., and Hoinkis, G., Inhibition of expression of SV40 virus large T-antigen by antisense oligodeoxyribonucleotides, *Biomed. Biochim. Acta*, 48, 85, 1989.
40. Baker, B. Decapitation of a 5′ capped oligoribonucleotide by ortho-Phenanthroline:Cu(II), *J. Am. Chem. Soc.*, 115, 3378, 1993.
41. Baker, B.F., Miraglia, L., and Hagedorn, C.H., Modulation of eurkaryotic initiation factor-4E binding to 5′ capped oligoribonucleotides by modified antisense oligonucleotides, *J. Biol. Chem.*, 267, 11495, 1992.
42. Zamecnik, P.C. and Stephenson, M.L., Inhibition of Rous sarcoma virus replication and cell transformation by a specific oligodeoxynucleotides, *Proc. Natl. Acad. Sci. U.S.A.*, 75, 280, 1978.
43. Zerial, A., Thuong, N.T., and Helene, C., Selective inhibition of the cytopathic effect of type A influenza viruses by oligodeoxynucleotides covalently linked to an intercalating agent, *Nucleic Acids Res.*, 15, 9909, 1987.
44. Thuong, N.T., Asseline, U., and Monteney-Garestier, T., Oligodeoxynucleotides covalently linked to intercalating and reactive substances: Synthesis, characterization and physicochemical studies, *Oligodeoxynucleotides: Antisense Inhibitors of Gene Expression*, Cohen, J.S., Ed., CRC Press, Boca Raton, FL, 1989, 25.
45. Helene, C. and Toulme, J.J., Control of gene expression by oligonucleotides covalently linked to intercalating agents and nucleic acid-cleaving reagents, *Oligodeoxynucleotides: Antisense Inhibitors of Gene Expression*, Cohen, J.S., Ed., CRC Press, Boca Raton, FL, 1989, 137.
46. Crouch, R.J. and Dirksen, M.-L., Ribonucleases H., *Nucleases*, Linn, S.M. and Roberts, R.J., Eds., Cold Spring Harbor Laboratory, Cold Spring Harbor, NY, 1985, 211.
47. Crum, C., Johnson, J.D., Nelson, A. et al., Complementary oligodeoxynucleotide mediated inhibition of tobacco mosaic virus RNA translation *in vitro*, *Nucleic Acids Res.*, 16, 4569, 1988.
48. Haeuptle, M.T., Frank, R., and Dobberstein, B., Translation arrest by oligodeoxynucleotides complementary to mRNA coding sequences yields polypeptides of predetermined length, *Nucleic Acids Res.*, 14, 1427, 1986.
49. Doris-Keller, H., Site specific enzymatic cleavage of RNA, *Nucleic Acid Res.*, 7, 179, 1979.
50. Kawasaki, A.M., Casper, M.D., Freier, S.M. et al., Uniformly modified 2′-deoxy-2′fluoro phosphorothioate oligonucleotides as nuclease resistant antisense compounds with high affinity and specificity for RNA targets, *J. Med. Chem.*, 36, 831, 1993.
51. Sproat, B.S., Lamond, A.L., Beijer, B. et al., Highly efficient chemical synthesis of 2′-*O*-methyloligoribonucleotides and tetrabiotinylated derivatives; novel probes that are resistant to degradation by RNA or DNA specific nucleases, *Nucleic Acids Res.*, 17, 3373, 1989.
52. Morvan, F., Rayner, B., and Imbach, J.-L., α-Oligonucleotides: A unique class of modified chimeric nucleic acids, *Anti-Cancer Drug Des.*, 6, 521, 1991.
53. Gagnor, C., Rayner, B., Leonetti, J.-P. et al., α-DNA IX. Parallel annealing of α-anomeric oligodeoxyribonucleotides to natural mRNA is required for interference in RNase H mediated hydrolysis and reverse transcription, *Nucleic Acids Res.*, 17, 5107, 1989.
54. Maher, J.L., III, Wold, B., and Dervan, P.G., Inhibition of DNA binding properties by oligonucleotide-directed triple helix formation, *Science*, 245, 725, 1989.
55. Miller, P.S. Non-ionic antisense oligonucleotides, *Oligodeoxynucleotides: Antisense Inhibitors of Gene Expression*, Cohen, J.S., Ed., CRC Press, Boca Raton, FL, 1989, 79.
56. Stein, C.A. and Cheng, Y.-C., Antisense oligonucleotides as therapeutic agents. Is the bullet really magic?, *Science*, 261, 1004, 1993.
57. Cazenave, C., Stein, C.A., Loreau, N. et al., Comparative inhibition of rabbit globin mRNA translation by modified antisense oligodeoxynucleotides, *Nucleic Acids Res.*, 17, 4255, 1989.

58. Quartin, R., Brakel, C., and Wetmur, J., Number and distribution of methylphosphonate linkages in oligodeoxynucleotides affect exo- and endonuclease sensitivity and ability to form RNase H substrates, *Nucleic Acids Res.*, 17, 7253, 1989.
59. Furdon, P., Dominski, Z., and Kole, R., RNase H cleavage of RNA hybridized to oligonucleotides containing methylphosphonate, phosphorothioate and phosphodiester bonds, *Nucleic Acids Res.*, 17, 9193, 1989.
60. Eder, P.S. and Walder, J.A., Ribonuclease H from K562 human erythroleukemia cells, *J. Biol. Chem.*, 206, 6472, 1991.
61. Monia, B.P., Lesnik, E.A., Gonzalez, C. et al., Evaluation of 2′ modified oligonucleotides containing 2′-deoxy gaps as antisense inhibitors of gene expression, *J. Biol. Chem.*, 268, 1993.
62. Giles, R.V. and Tidd, D.M., Increased specificity for antisense oligodeoxynucleotide targeting of RNA cleavage of RNase H using chimeric methylphosphorodiester structures, *Nucleic Acids Res.*, 20, 763, 1992.
63. Walder, R.Y. and Walder, J.A., Role of RNase H in hybrid-arrested translation by antisense oligonucleotides, *Proc. Natl. Acad. Sci. U.S.A.*, 85, 5011, 1988.
64. Minshull, J. and Hunt, T., The use of single-stranded DNA and RNase H to promote quantitative hybrid arrest of translation of mRNA/DNA hybrids in reticulocyte lysate cell-free translations, *Nucleic Acids Res.*, 14, 6433, 1986.
65. Gagnor, C., Bertrand, J., Thenet, S. et al., Alpha-DNA VI: Comparative study of alpha- and beta-anomeric oligodeoxyribonucleotides in hybridization to mRNA and in cell free translation inhibition, *Nucleic Acids Res.*, 15, 10419, 1987.
66. Giles, R.V., Spiller, D.G., and Tidd, D.M., Detection of ribonuclease H-generated mRNA fragments in human leukemia cells following reversible membrane permeabilization in the presence of antisense oligodeoxynucleotides, *Antisense Res. Dev.*, 5, 23, 1995.
67. Crooke, S.T., Lemonidis, K.M., Neilson, L., et al., Kinetic characteristics of *E. coli* RNase H1: Cleavage of various antisense oligonucleotide-RNA duplexes, *Biochem. J.*, 312, 599, 1995.
68. DeClercq, E., Eckstein, F., and Merigan, T.C., Interferon induction increased through chemical modification of a synthetic polyribonucleotide, *Science*, 165, 1137, 1969.
69. Cohen, J.S., Phosphorothioate oligodeoxynucleotides, *Antisense Research and Applications*, Crooke, S.T. and Lebleu, B., Eds., CRC Press, Boca Raton, FL, 1993, 205.
70. Crooke, S.T., Therapeutic applications of oligonucleotides, *Annu. Rev. Pharmacol. Toxicol.*, 32, 329, 1992.
71. Crooke, S.T., Progress toward oligonucleotide therapeutics: Pharmacodynamic properties, *FASEB J.*, 7, 533, 1993.
72. Monia, B.P., Johnston, J.F., Ecker, D.J. et al., Selective inhibition of mutant Ha-ras mRNA expression by antisense oligonucleotides, *J. Biol. Chem.*, 267, 19954, 1992.
73. Crooke, S.T., Graham, M.J., Zuckerman, J.E. et al., Pharmacokinetic properties of several novel oligonucleotide analogs in mice, *J. Pharmacol. Exp. Ther.*, 277(2), 923, 1996.
74. Joos, R.W. and Hall, W.H., Determination of binding constants of serum albumin for penicillin, *J. Pharmacol. Exp. Ther.*, 166, 113, 1969.
75. Srinivasan, S.K., Tewary, H.K., and Iversen, P.L., Characterization of binding sites, extent of binding and drug interactions of oligonucleotides with albumin, *Antisense Res. Dev.*, 5, 131, 1995.
76. Gao, W.-Y., Han, F.-S., Storm, C. et al., Phosphorothioate oligonucleotides are inhibitors of human DNA polymerases and RNase H: Implications for antisense technology, *Mol. Pharmacol.*, 41, 223, 1991.
77. Agrawal, S., Temsamani, J., and Tang, J.Y., Pharmacokinetics, biodistribution and stability of oligodeoxynucleotide phosphorothioates in mice, *Proc. Natl. Acad. Sci. U.S.A.*, 88, 7595, 1991.
78. Majumdar, C., Stein, C.A., Cohen, J.S. et al., Stepwise mechanism of HIV reverse transcriptase: primer function of phosphorothioate oligodeoxynucleotide, *Biochemistry*, 28, 1340, 1989.
79. Cheng, Y.-C., Gao, W., and Han, F., Against human immunodeficiency virus and herpes viruses, *Nucleosides Nucleotides*, 10, 155, 1991.
80. Stein, C.A., Neckers, L.M., Nair, B.C. et al., Phosphorothioate oligodeoxycytidine interferes with binding of HIV-1 with gp120 to CD4, *J. AIDS*, 4, 686, 1991.
81. Graham, M.J., Freier, S.M., Crooke, R.M. et al., Tritium labeling of antisense oligonucleotides by exchange with tritiated water, *Nucleic Acids Res.*, 21, 3737, 1993.
82. Sands, H., Gorey-Feret, L.J., Cocuzza, A.J. et al., Biodistribution and metabolism of internally ^{3}H-labeled oligonucleotides. I. Comparison of a phosphodiester and a phosphorothioate, *Mol. Pharmacol.*, 45, 932, 1994.
83. Hoke, G.D., Draper, K., Freier, S.M. et al., Effects of phosphorothioate capping on antisense oligonucleotide stability, hybridization and antiviral efficacy versus herpes simplex virus infection, *Nucleic Acids Res.*, 19, 5743, 1991.

84. Wickstrom, E. Oligodeoxynucleotide stability in subcellular extracts and culture media, *J. Biochem. Biophys. Methods*, 13, 97, 1986.
85. Campbell, J.M., Bacon, T.A., and Wickstrom, E., Oligodeoxynucleoside phosphorothioate stability in subcellular extracts, culture media, sera and cerebrospinal fluid, *J. Biochem. Biophys. Methods*, 20, 259, 1990.
86. Miyao, T., Takakura, Y., Akiyama, T. et al., Stability and pharmacokinetic characteristics of oligonucleotides modified at terminal linkages in mice, *Antisense Res. Dev.*, 5, 115, 1995.
87. Crooke, R.M., *In vitro* and *in vivo* toxicology of first generation analogs, in *Antisense Research and Applications*, Crooke, S.T. and Lebleu, B., Eds., CRC Press, Boca Raton, FL, 1993b, 471.
88. Neckers, L.M., Cellular internalization of oligodeoxynucleotides, *Antisense Research and Applications*, Crooke, S.T. and Lebleu, B., Eds., CRC Press, Boca Raton, FL, 1993, 451.
89. Chrissey, L.A., Walz, S.E., Pazirandeh, M. et al., Internalization of oligodeoxyribonucleotides by *Vibrio parahaemolyticus*, *Antisense Res. Dev.*, 3, 367, 1993.
90. Tao, L.-F., Marz, K.A., Wongwit, W. et al., Uptake, intracellular distribution, and stability of oligodeoxynucleotide phosphorothioate by *Schistosoma mansoni*, *Antisense Res. Dev.*, 5, 123, 1995.
91. Crooke, R.M., Cellular uptake, distribution and metabolism of phosphorothioate, phosphorodiester and methylphosphonate oligonucleotides, *Antisense Research and Applications*, Crooke, S.T. and Lebleu, B., Eds., CRC Press, Boca Raton, FL, 1993a, 427.
92. Bennett, C.F., Chiang, M.-Y., Chan, H. et al., Use of cationic lipids to enhance the biological activity of antisense oligonucleotides, *J. Liposome Res.*, 3, 85, 1993.
93. Bennett, C.F., Chiang, M.-Y., Chan, H. et al., Cationic lipids enhance cellular uptake and activity of phosphorothioate antisense oligonucleotides, *Mol. Pharmacol.*, 41, 1023, 1992.
94. Quattrone, A., Papucci, L., Schiavone, et al., Intracellular enhancement of intact antisense oligonucleotide steady-state levels by cationic lipids, *Anti-Cancer Drug Des.*, 9, 549, 1994.
95. Wang, S., Lee, R.J., Cauchon, G. et al., Delivery of antisense oligodeoxyribonucleotides against the human epidermal growth factor receptor into cultured KB cells with liposomes conjugated to folate via polyethylene glycol, *Proc. Natl. Acad. Sci. U.S.A.*, 92, 3318, 1995.
96. Iversen, P., *In vivo* studies with phosphorothioate oligonucleotides: Pharmacokinetic prologue, *Anti-Cancer Drug Des.*, 6, 531, 1991.
97. Rappaport, J., Hanss, B., Kopp, J.B. et al., Transport of phosphorothioate oligonucleotides in kidney: Implications for molecular therapy, *Kidney Int.*, 47, 1462, 1995.
98. Bayever, E., Iversen, P.L., Bishop, M.R. et al., Systemic administration of a phosphorothioate oligonucleotide with a sequence complementary to p53 for acute myelogenous leukemia and myelodysplastic syndrome: Initial results of a phase 1 trial, *Antisense Research Dev.*, 3, 383, 1993.
99. Zhang, R., Yan, J., Shahinian, H. et al., Pharmacokinetics of an anti-human immunodeficiency virus antisense oligodeoxynucleotide phosphorothioate (GEM 91) in HIV-infected subjects, *Clin. Pharmacol. Ther.*, 58, 44, 1995a.
100. Hughes, J.A., Avrutskaya, A.V., Brouwer, K.L.R. et al., Radiolabeling of methylphosphonate and phosphorothioate oligonucleotides and evaluation of their transport in everted rat jejunum sacs, *Pharm. Res.*, 12, 817, 1995.
101. Agrawal, S., Zhang, X., Lu, Z. et al., Absorption, tissue distribution and *in vivo* stability in rats of a hybrid antisense oligonucleotide following oral administration, *Biochem. Pharmacol.*, 50, 571, 1995.
102. Cook, P.D., Medicinal chemistry strategies for antisense research, *Antisense Research and Applications*, Crooke, S.T. and Lebleu, B., Eds., CRC Press, Boca Raton, FL, 1993, 303.
103. Mirabelli, C.K. and Crooke, S.T., Antisense oligonucleotides in the context of modern molecular drug discovery and development, in *Antisense Research and Applications*, Crooke, S.T. and Lebleu, B., Eds., CRC Press, Boca Raton, FL, 1993, 7.
104. Bennett, C.F. and Crooke, S.T., Oligonucleotide-based inhibitors of cytokine expression and function, in *Pharmacological Modulation of Cytokines*, Henderson, B. and Bodner, M. W., Eds., CRC Press, Boca Raton, FL, 1996, 171.
105. Wagner, R.W., Matteucci, M.D., Lewis, J.G. et al., Antisense gene inhibition by oligonucleotides containing C-5 propyne pyrimidines, *Science*, 260, 1510, 1993.
106. Barton, C.M. and Lemoine, N.R., Antisense oligonucleotides directed against p53 have antiproliferative effects unrelated to effects on p53 expression, *Br. J. Cancer*, 71, 429, 1995.
107. Burgess, T.L., Fisher, E.F., Ross, S.L. et al., The antiproliferative activity of c-myb and c-myc antisense oligonucleotides in smooth muscle cells is caused by a nonantisense mechanism, *Proc. Natl. Acad. Sci. U.S.A.*, 92, 4051, 1995.
108. Hertl, M., Neckers, L.M., and Katz, S.I., Inhibition of interferon-y-induced intercellular adhesion molecule-1 expression on human keratinocytes by phosphorothioate antisense oligodeoxynucleotides is the consequence of antisense-specific and antisense-non-specific effects, *J. Invest. Dermatol.*, 104, 813, 1995.

109. Crooke, S.T., Oligonucleotide therapeutics, *Burger's Medicinal Chemistry and Drug Discovery, Vol. 1, 5th ed.*, Wolff, M.E., Ed., J. Wiley & Sons, 1995, 863.
110. Nagel, K.M., Holstad, S.G., and Isenberg, K.E., Oligonucleotide pharmacotherapy. An antigene strategy, *Pharmacotherapy*, 13, 177, 1993.
111. Simons, M., Edelman, E.R., DeKeyser, J.-L. et al., Antisense c-myb oligonucleotides inhibit intimal arterial smooth muscle cell accumulation *in vivo*, *Nature*, 359, 67, 1992.
112. Abe, J., Zhou, W., Taguchi, J. et al., Suppression of neointimal smooth muscle cell accumulation *in vivo* by antisense CDC2 and CDK2 oligonucleotides in rat carotid artery, *Biochem. Biophys. Res. Commun.*, 198, 16, 1994.
113. Whitesell, L., Rosolen, A., and Neckers, L.M., *In vivo* modulation of N-myc expression by continuous perfusion with an antisense oligonucleotide, *Antisense Res. Dev.*, 1, 343, 1991.
114. Wahlestedt, C., Pich, E.M., Koob, G.F. et al., Modulation of anxiety and neuropeptide Y-Y1 receptors by antisense oligodeoxynucleotides, *Science*, 259, 528, 1993.
115. Weiss, B., Zhou, L.-W., Zhang, S.-P. et al., Antisense oligodeoxynucleotide inhibits D_2 dopamine receptor-mediated behavior and D_2 messenger RNA, *Neuroscience*, 55, 607, 1993.
116. Zhou, L.-W., Zhang, S.-P., Qin, Z.-H. et al., *In vivo* administration of an oligodeoxynucleotide antisense to the D_2 dopamine receptor messenger RNA inhibits D_2 dopamine receptor-mediated behavior and the expression of D_2 dopamine receptors in mouse striatum, *J. Pharmacol. Exp. Ther.*, 268, 1015, 1994.
117. Qin, Z.-H., Zhou, L.-W., Zhang, S.-P. et al., D_2 dopamine receptor antisense oligodeoxynucleotide inhibits the synthesis of a functional pool of D_2 dopamine receptors, *Mol. Pharmacol.*, 48, 730, 1995.
118. Zhang, S.-P., Zhou, L.-W., and Weiss, B., Oligodeoxynucleotide antisense to the D_1 dopamine receptor mRNA inhibits D_1 dopamine receptor-mediated behaviors in normal mice and in mice lesioned with 6-hydroxydopamine, *J. Pharmacol. Exp. Ther.*, 271, 1462, 1994.
119. Ambuhl, P., Gyurko, R., and Phillips, M.I., A decrease in angiotensin receptor binding in rat brain nuclei by antisense oligonucleotides to the angiotensin AT_1 receptor, *Reg. Peptides*, 59, 171, 1995.
120. McCarthy, M.M., Nielsen, D.A., and Goldman, D., Antisense oligonucleotide inhibition of tryptophan hydroxylase activity in mouse brain, *Reg. Peptides*, 59, 163, 1995.
121. Osen-Sand, A., Catsicas, M., Staple, J.K. et al., Inhibition of axonal growth by SNAP-25 antisense oligonucleotides *in vitro* and *in vivo*, *Nature*, 364, 445, 1993.
122. Burch, R.M. and Mahan, L.C., Oligonucleotides antisense to the interleukin 1 receptor mRNA block the effects of interleukin 1 in cultured murine and human fibroblasts and in mice, *J. Clin. Invest.*, 88, 1190, 1991.
123. Kitajima, I., Shinohara, T., Bilakovics, J. et al., Ablation of transplanted HTLV-1 tax-transformed tumors in mice by antisense inhibition of NF-kB, *Science*, 258, 1792, 1992.
124. Higgins, K.A., Perez, J.R., Coleman, T.A. et al., Antisense inhibition of the p65 subunit of NF-kB blocks tumorigenicity and causes tumor regression, *Proc. Natl. Acad. Sci. U.S.A.*, 90, 9901, 1993.
125. Dean, N.M., McKay, R., Miraglia, L. et al., Inhibition of growth of human tumor cell lines in nude mice by an antisense oligonucleotide inhibitor of PKC-a expression, *Cancer Res.*, 56(15), 3499, 1996.
126. Monia, B.P., Johnston, J.F., Geiger, T. et al., Antitumor activity of a phosphorothioate antisense oligodeoxynucleotide targeted against C-*raf* kinase, *Nature Med.*, 2(6), 668, 1996.
127. Monia, B.P., Johnston, J.F., Sasmor, H. et al., Nuclease resistance and antisense activity of modified oligonucleotides targeted to Ha-*ras*, *J. Biol. Chem.*, 271(24), 14533, 1996.
128. Nesterova, M. and Cho-Chung, Y.S., A single injection protein kinase a-directed antisense treatment to inhibit tumor growth, *Nature Med.*, 1, 528, 1995.
129. Hutcherson, S.L., Palestine, A.G., Cantrill, H.L. et al., Antisense oligonucleotide safety and efficacy for CMV retinitis in AIDS patients, *35th Intl. Conf. on Antimicrobial Agents and Chemotherapy*, 1995, 204.
130. Colby, C., The induction of interferon by natural and synthetic polynucleotides, *Prog. Nucleic Acid Res. Mol. Biol.*, 11, 1, 1971.
131. Messina, J.P., Gilkeson, G.S., and Pisetsky, D.S., Stimulation of *in vitro* murine lymphocyte proliferation by bacterial DNA, *J. Immunol.*, 147, 1759, 1991.
132. Kuramoto, E., Yano, O., Kimura, Y. et al., Oligonucleotide sequences required for natural killer cell activation, *Jpn. J. Cancer Res.*, 83, 1128, 1992.
133. Psietsky, D.S. and Reich, C.F., Stimulation of murine lymphocyte proliferation by a phosphorothioate oligonucleotide with antisense activity for herpes simplex virus, *Life Sci.*, 54, 101, 1993.
134. Crooke, R.M., Crooke, S.T., Graham, M.J. et al., Effect of antisense oligonucleotides on cytokine release from human keratinocytes in an *in vitro* model of skin, *Toxicol. Appl. Pharmacol.*, 140, 85, 1996.
135. Krieg, A.M., Yi, A.-K., Matson, S. et al., CpG motifs in bacterial DNA trigger direct B-cell activation, *Nature*, 374, 546, 1995.

136. Henry, S.P., Orr, J.L., Bruner, R.H. et al., Comparison of the toxicities of ISIS 1082 and ISIS 2105, phosphorothioate oligonucleotides, following subacute intradermal administration in Sprague-Dawley rats, *Toxicology*, in press.
137. Henry, S.P., Taylor, J., Midgley, L. et al., Evaluation of the toxicity of ISIS 2302, a phosphorothioate oligonucleotides: in a 4-week study in CD-1 mice, *Fundam. Appl. Toxicol.*, submitted.
138. Henry, S.P., Giclas, P., Leeds, J. et al., Activation of the alternative pathway of complement by a phosphorothioate oligonucleotide: Potential mechanism of action, in preparation.
139. Cornish, K.G., Iversen, P., Smith, L. et al., Cardiovascular effects of a phosphorothioate oligonucleotide with sequence antisense to p53 in the conscious rhesus monkey, *Pharmacol. Res. Commun.*, 3, 239, 1993.
140. Galbraith, W.M., Hobson, W.C., Giclas, P.C. et al., Complement activation and hemodynamic changes following intravenous administration of phosphorothioate oligonucleotides in the monkey, *Antisense Res. Dev.*, 4, 201, 1994.
141. Henry, S.P., Bolte, H., Auletta, C. et al., Evaluation of the toxicity of ISIS 2302, a phosphorothioate oligonucleotide: 2) 4-week study in cynomolgus monkeys, *Fundam. Appl. Toxicol.*, submitted.
142. Henry, S.P., Novotny, W., Leeds, J. et al., Inhibition of clotting parameters by a phosphorothioate oligonucleotide, in preparation.
143. Glover, J.M., Leeds, J.M., Mant, T.G.K. et al., Phase I safety and pharmacokinetic profile of an ICAM-1 antisense oligonucleotide (ISIS 2302), in preparation.
144. Sanghvi, Y.S., Heterocyclic base modifications in nucleic acids and their applications in antisense oligonucleotides, *Antisense Research and Applications*, Crooke, S.T. and Lebleu, B., Eds., CRC Press, Boca Raton, FL, 1993, 273.
145. Nikiforov, T.T. and Connolly, B.A., The synthesis of oligodeoxynucleotides containing 4-thiothymidine residues, *Tetahedron Lett.*, 32, 3851, 1991.
146. Lin, K.T.P. and Brown, D.M., Synthesis and duplex stability of oligonucleotides containing cytosine-thymine analogues, *Nucleic Acids Res.*, 17, 10373, 1989.
147. Inoue, H. and Ohtsuka, E., Synthesis and hybridization of dodecadeoxyribonucleotides containing a fluorescent pyridopyrimidine deoxynucleoside, *Nucleic Acids Res.*, 13, 7119, 1985.
148. Gutierrez, A.J., Terhorst, T.J., Matteucci, M.D. et al., 5-Heteroaryl-2′-deoxyuridine analogs. Synthesis and incorporation into high-affinity oligonucleotides, *J. Am. Chem. Soc.*, 116, 5540, 1994.
149. Lin, K.-Y., Jone, R.J., and Matteucci, M., Tricyclic-2′-deoxycytidine analogs: Syntheses and incorporation into oligodeoxynucleotides which have enhanced binding to complementary RNA, *J. Am. Chem. Soc.*, 117, 3873, 1995.
150. Sanghvi, Y.S., Hoke, G.D., Freier, S.M. et al., Antisense oligonucleotides: Synthesis and biological evaluation of oligodeoxynucleotides containing modified pyrimidines, *Nucleic Acids Res.*, 21, 3197, 1993.
151. Hagenberg, L., Gassen, H.G., and Matthaei, H., Synthesis and coding properties of poly (c^1A), poly (c^3A), poly (c^7A) and poly (h^6A), *Biochem. Biophys. Res. Commun.*, 50, 1104, 1973.
152. Sproat, B.S., Iribarren, A.M. et al., New synthetic routes to synthons suitable for 2′-O-allyloligoribonucleotide assembly, *Nucleic Acids Res.*, 19, 733, 1991.
153. Martin, F.H., Castro, M.M., Aboul-ela, F. et al., Base pairing involving deoxyinosine: Implications for probe design, *Nucleic Acids Res.*, 13, 8927, 1985.
154. Santa Lucia, J., Kierzek, R., and Turner, D.H., Functional group substitutions as probes of hydrogen bonding between GA mismatches in RNA internal loops, *J. Am. Chem. Soc.*, 113, 4314, 1991.
155. Seela, F., Kaiser, K., and Bindig, U., 2′-deoxy-β D-ribofuranosides of N^6-methylated 7-dazaadenine and 8-aza-7-deazaadenine: Solid phase synthesis of oligodeoxyribonucleotides and properties of self-complementary duplexes, *Helv. Chim. Acta*, 72, 868, 1989.
156. Seela, F., Ramzaeva, N., and Chen, Y., Oligonucleotide duplex stability controlled by the 7-substituents of 7-deazaguanine bases, *Bioorg. Med. Chem. Lett.*, Vol. 5, 3049, 1995.
157. Manoharan, M., Designer antisense oligonucleotides: Conjugation chemistry and functionality placement. *Antisense Research and Therapeutics*, Crooke, S.T. and Lebleu, B., Eds., CRC Press, Boca Raton, FL, 1993, 303.
158. Zhang, R., Lu, Z., Zhang, X. et al., *In vivo* stability and disposition of a self-stabilized oligodeoxynucleotide phosphorothioate in rats, *Clin. Chem.*, 41, 836, 1995b.
159. Temsamani, J., Tang, J.-Y., Padmapriya, A. et al., Pharmacokinetics, biodistribution and stability of capped oligodeoxynucleotide phosphorothioates in mice, *Antisense Res. Dev.*, 3, 277, 1993.
160. Boutorine, A., Huet, C., Saison, T. et al., Cell penetration studies of oligonucleotides derivatized with cholesterol and porphyrins, *Conf. on Nucleic Acid Therapeutics*, 60 (Abstr.), 1991.
161. DeMesmaeker, A., Haner, R., Martin, P. et al., Antisense oligonucleotides, *Acc. Chem. Res.*, 28, 366, 1995.
162. Hall, J., Husken, D., Pieles, U. et al., Efficient sequence-specific cleavage of RNA using novel europium complexes conjugated to oligonucleotides, *Chem. Biol.*, 1, 185, 1994.

163. Henry, S.P., Zuckerman, J.E., Rojko, J. et al., Toxicologic properties of several novel oligonucleotide analogs in mice, *J. Pharmacol. Exp. Ther.*, submitted.
164. Desjardins, J., Mata, J., Brown, T. et al., Cholesteryl-conjugated phosphorothioate oligodeoxynucleotides modulate CYP2B1 expression *in vivo*, *J. Drug Targeting*, 2, 477, 1995.
165. Sanghvi, Y.S. and Cook, P.D., Eds., *Carbohydrate Modifications in Antisense Research*, American Chemial Society, Washington, D.C., 1994.
166. Breslauer, K.J., Frank, R., Blocker, H. et al., Predicting DNA duplex stability from base sequence, *Proc. Natl. Acad. Sci. U.S.A.*, 83, 8746, 1986.
167. Lamond, A.I. and Sproat, B.S., Antisense oligonucleotides made of 2′-O-alkyl RNA: Their properties and applications in RNA biochemistry, *FEBS Lett.*, 325, 123, 1993.
168. Sproat, B.S. and Lamond, A.I., 2′-O-alkyloligoribonucleotides, *Antisense Research and Applications*, Crooke, S.T. and Lebleu, B., Eds., CRC Press, Boca Raton, FL, 1993, 351.
169. Parmentier, G., Schmitt, G., Dolle, F. et al., A convergent synthesis of 2′-*O*-methyl uridine, *Tetrahedron*, 50, 5361, 1994.
170. Martin, P., New access to 2′-O-alkylated ribonucleosides and properties of 2′-*O*-alkylated oligoribonucleotides, *Helv. Chim. Acta*, 78, 486, 1995.
171. Pitsch, S., Krishnamurthy, R., Bolli, M. et al., Pyranosyl-RNA ("p-RNA"): Base-pairing selectivity and potential to replicate, *Helv. Chim. Acta.*, 78, 1621, 1995.
172. Bellon, L., Leydier, C., Barascut, J.-L., et al., 4′-Thio RNA: A novel class of sugar-modified β-RNA, *Carbohydrate Modifications in Antisense Research*, Sanghvi, Y.S. and Cook, P.D., Eds., American Chemical Society, Washington, D.C., 1994, 68.
173. Hanvey, J.C., Peffer, N.J., Bisi, J.E. et al., Antisense and antigene properties of peptide nucleic acids, *Science*, 258, 1481, 1992.
174. Morishita R., Gibbons, G.H., Ellison, K.E. et al., Single intraluminal delivery of antisense cdc2 kinase and proliferating-cell nuclear antigen oligonucleotides results in chronic inhibition of neointimal hyperplasia, *Proc. Natl. Acad. Sci. U.S.A.*, 90, 8474, 1993.
175. Morishita R., Gibbons, G.H., Kaneda, Y. et al., Pharmacokinetics of antisense oligodeoxyribonucleotides (cyclin B_1 and CDC-2 kinase) in the vessel wall *in vivo*: Enhanced therapeutic utility for restenosis by HVJ-liposome delivery, *Gene*, 149, 13, 1994.
176. Simons, M., Edelman, E.R., and Rosenberg, R.D., Antisense proliferating cell nuclear antigen oligonucleotides inhibit intimal hyperplasia in a rat carotid artery injury model, *J. Clin. Invest.*, 9, 2351, 1994.
177. Gyurko, F., Wielbo, D., and Phillips, M.I., Antisense inhibition of AT_1 receptor mRNA and angiotensinogen mRNA in the brain of spontaneously hypertensive rats reduces hypertension of neurogenic origin, *Regulatory Peptide*, 49, 167, 1993.
178. Phillips, M.I., Wielbo, D., and Gyurko, R., Antisense inhibition of hypertension: A new strategy for renin-angiotensin candidate genes, *Kidney Int.*, 46, 1554, 1994.
179. Suzuki, S., Pilowsky, P., Minson, J. et al., *c-fos* antisense in rostral ventral medulla reduces arterial blood pressure, *J. Physiol.*, R1418, 1994.
180. Stepkowski, S.M., Tu, Y., Condon, T.P. et al., Blocking of heart allograft rejection by intercellular adhesion molecule-1 antisense oligonucleotides alone or in combination with other immunosuppresive modalities, *J. Immunol.*, 10, 5336, 1994.
181. Kumasaka, T., Quinlan, W.M., Doyle, N.A. et al., The role of ICAM-1 in endotoxin-induced pneumonia evaluated using ICAM-1 antisense oligonucleotides, anti-ICAM-1 monoclonal antibodies and ICAM-1 mutant mice, *J. Clin. Invest.*, in press.
182. Katz, S.M., Browne, B., Pham, T. et al., Efficacy of ICAM-1 antisen se oligonucleotide in pancreatic islet transplantation, Transplant Proc., in press.
183. Stepkowski, S.M., Tu, Y., Condon, T.P. et al., Induction of transplantation tolerance by treatment with ICAM-1 antisense oligonucleotides and anti-LFA-1 monoclonal antibodies, *Tranplant Proc.*, 27, 113, 1995.
184. Bennett, C.F., Kornbrust, D., Henry, S. et al., An ICAM-1 antisense oligonucleotide, ISIS 3082, prevents and reverses dextran sulfate sodium-induced colitis in mice, submitted.
185. Ratajczak, M.Z., Kant, J.A., Luger, S.M. et al., *In vivo* treatment of human leukemia in a *scid* mouse model with *c-myb* antisense oligodeoxynucleotides, *Proc. Natl. Acad. Sci. U.S.A.*, 89, 11823, 1992.
186. Perlaky, L., Saijo, Y., Busch. R.K. et al., Growth inhibition of human tumor cell lines by antisense oligonucleotides designed to inhibit p120 expression, *Anti-Cancer Drug Des.*, 8, 3, 1993.
187. Schwab, G., Chavany C., Duroux, I. et al., Antisense oligonucleotides adsorbed to polyalkylcyanoacrylate nanoparticles specifically inhibit mutated Ha-*ras* mediated cell proliferation and tumorigenicity in nude mice, *Proc. Natl. Acad. Sci. U.S.A.*, 91, 10460, 1994.
188. Akino, K., Ohtsuru, A., Yano, H. et al., Antisense inhibition of parathyroid hormone-related peptide gene expression reduces malignant pituitary tumor progression and metastases in the rat, *Cancer Res.*, 56, 77, 1996.

189. Yazaki, T., Ahmad, S., Chahlavi, A. et al., Treatment of glioblastoma U-87 by systemic administration of an antisense protein kinase C-α phosphorothioate oligodeoxynucleotide, submitted.
190. Chiasson, B.J., Hooper, M.L., Murphy, P.R. et al., Antisense oligonucleotide eliminates *in vivo* expression of c-*fos* in mammalian brain, *Eur. J. Pharmacol.*, 227, 451-1992.
191. Amaratunga, A., Morin, P.J., Kosik, K.S. et al., Inhibition of kinesin synthesis and rapid anterograde anxonal transport *in vivo* by an antisense oligonucleotide, *J. Biol. Chem.*, 268, 17427, 1993.
192. Flanagan, L.M., McCarthy, M.M., Brooks, P.J., Pfaff, D.W., and McEwen, B.S., Arginine vasopressin levels after daily infusions of antisense oligonucleotides into the supraoptic nucleus, *Ann. NY Acad. Sci.*, 689, 520, 1993.
193. Heilig, M., Engel, J.A., and Soderpalm. B., C-*fos* antisense in the nucleus accumbens blocks the locomotor stimulant action of cocaine, *Eur. J. Pharmacol.*, 236, 339, 1993.
194. Pollio, G., Xue, P., Zanisi, M. et al., Antisense oligonucleotide blocks progesterone-induced lordosis behavior in ovariectomized rats, *Mol. Brain Res.*, 19, 135, 1993.
195. Zhang M. and Creese, I., Antisense oligodeoxynucleotide reduces brain dopamine D_2 receptors: Behavioral correlates, *Neurosci. Lett.*, 161, 223, 4947, 1993.
196. Akabayashi, A., Wahlestedt, C., Alexander, J.T. et al., Specific inhibition of endogenous neuropeptide Y synthesis in arcuate nucleus by antisense oligonucleotides suppresses feeding behavior and insulin secretion, *Mol. Brain Res.*, 21, 55, 1994.
197. Adams, J.U., Chen, X.H., deRiel, J.K. et al., *In vivo* treatment with antisense oligodeoxynucleotide to kappa-opioid receptors inhibited kappa-agonist-induced analgesia in rats, *Regul. Pept.*, 54, 1, 1994.
198. Castro-Alamancos, M.A. and Torres-Aleman, I., Learning of the conditioned eye-blink response is impaired by an antisense insulin-like growth factor I oligonucleotide, *Proc. Natl. Acad. Sci. U.S.A.*, 91, 10203, 1994.
199. Gillardon, F., Beck, H., Uhlmann, E. et al., Inhibition of c-*fos* protein expression in rat spinal cord by antisense oligodeoxynucleotide superfusion, *Eur. J. Neurosci.*, 6, 880, 1994.
200. Hooper, M.L., Chiasson, B.J., and Robertson, H.A., Infusion into the brain of an antisense oligonucleotide to the immediate-early gene c-*fos* suppresses production of *fos* and produces a behavioral effect, *Neuroscience*, 63, 917, 1994.
201. Woodburn, V.L., Hunter, J.C., Durieux, C., Poat, J.A., and Hughes, J., The effect of c-*fos* antisense in the formalin-paw test, *Regul. Pept.*, 54, 327, 1994.
202. Kindy, M.S. NMDA receptor inhibition using antisense oligonucleotides prevents delayed neuronal death in gerbil hippocampus following cerebral ischemia, *Neurosci. Res. Commun.*, 14, 175, 1994.
203. Konradi, C., Cole, R.L., Heckers, S. et al., Amphetamine regulates gene expression in rat striatum via transcription factor CREB, *J. Neurosci.*, 14, 5623, 1994.
204. Lai, J., Bilsky, E.J., Rothman, R.B. et al., Treatment with antisense oligodeoxynucleotide to the opioid-∂ receptor selectively inhibits ∂_2-agonist antinociception, *Neuroreport*, 5, 1049, 1994.
205. Mani, S.K., Blaustein, J.D., Allen, J.M.C. et al., Inhibition of rat sexual behavior by antisense oligonculeotides to the progesterone receptor, *Endocrinology*, 135, 1994.
206. McCarthy, M.M., Masters, D.B., Rimvall, K. et al., Intracerebral administration of antisense oligodeoxynucleotides to GAD_{65} and GAD_{67} mRNAs modulate reproductive behavior in the female rat, *Brain Res.*, 636, 209, 1994.
207. Sakai, R.R., Ma, L.Y., He, P.F. et al., Intracerebroventricular administration of angiotensin type 1 (AT_1) receptor antisense oligonucleotide attenuate thirst in the rat, *Regul. Pept.*, 59, 183, 1995.
208. Liebsch, G., Landgraf, R., Gerstberger, R. et al., Chronic infusion of a CRH_1 receptor antisense oligodeoxynucleotide into the central nucleus of the amygdala reduced anxiety-related behavior in socially defeated rats, *Regul. Pept.*, 59, 229, 1995.
209. Cha, X.Y., Xu, H., Ni, Q. et al., Opioid peptide receptor studies. 4. Antisense oligodeoxynucleotide to the ∂-opioid receptor delineates opioid receptor subtypes, *Regul. Pept.*, 59, 247, 1995.
210. Mizoguchi, H., Narita, M., Nagase, H. et al., Antisense oligodeoxynucleotide to a ∂-opioid receptor blocks the antinociception induced by cold water swimming, *Regul. Pept.*, 59, 255, 1995.
211. Morris, M., Barrett, C., and Callahan, M.F., Oxytocin antisense reduces salt intake in the baroreceptor-denervated rat, *Regul. Pept.*, 59, 261, 1995.
212. Neumann, I., Porter, D.W.F., Landgraf, R. et al., Rapid effect on suckling of an oxytocin antisense oligonucleotide administered into rat supraoptc nucleus, *Am. Phys. Soc.*, R852, 1994.
213. Ogo, H., Hirai, Y., Miki, S. et al., Modulation of substance P/neurokinin-1 receptor in human astrocytoma cells by antisense oligodeoxynucleotides, *Gen. Pharmacol.*, 25, 1131, 1994.
214. Skutella, T., Probst, J.C., Jirikowski, G.F. et al., Ventral tegmental area (VTA) injections of tyrosine hydroxylase phosphorothioate antisense oligonucleotide suppress operant behavior in rats, *Neurosci. Lett.*, 167, 55, 1994.
215. Tischmeyer, W., Grimm, R., Schicknick, H. et al., Sequence-specific impairment of learning by c-*jun* antisense oligonucleotides, *Neuroreport*, 5, 1501, 1994.

216. Vlassov, V.V., Inhibition of tick-borne viral encephalitis expression using covalently linked oligonucleotide analogs. Meeting on *Oligodeoxynucleotides as Antisense Inhibitors of Gene Expression: Therapeutic Implications,* Rockville, MD, June 18-21, 1989.

217. Offensperger, W.-B., Offensperger, S., Walter, E. et al., *In vivo* inhibition of duck hepatitis B virus replication and gene expression by phosphorothioate modified antisense oligodeoxynucleotides, *EMBO J.*, 12, 1257, 1993.

Chapter 3

Pharmacokinetics of Phosphorothioate Oligonucleotides and Their Novel Analogs

Sudhir Agrawal and Ruiwen Zhang

CONTENTS

0-8493-8552-0/97/$0.00+$.50

Antisense oligonucleotides and their analogs have been used to modulate the expression of both foreign and cellular genes and their effectiveness as novel therapeutic agents is currently being studied.[1] To be an effective therapeutic agent, an antisense oligonucleotide should have a favorable pharmacokinetic profile, tissue disposition, and *in vivo* stability. Oligonucleotides containing phosphodiester linkages have a plasma half-life of less than five minutes in mice,[2] rabbits,[3] and monkeys.[4] To increase the stability against nucleases, several oligonucleotide analogs with various backbone (internucleotide linkages) modifications have been synthesized.[5] Phosphorothioate oligodeoxynucleotides (PS-oligos) in which one of the nonbridged oxygens is replaced with sulfur are more stable against nucleases than are their phosphodiester counterparts.[5,6] PS-oligos are studied extensively in *in vitro* and *in vivo* models, and their pharmacokinetics and pharmacodynamics are being evaluated in clinical trials.[6,7] In this chapter, we will summarize our recent work on the pharmacokinetics of a PS-oligo and its three novel analogs following intravenous (i.v.) dosing in rats to illustrate the role of chemical modifications on the improvement of pharmacokinetics of antisense oligonucleotides. Initial studies examining oral bioavailability of antisense oligonucleotides also will be reviewed.

I. EXPERIMENTAL PROTOCOLS

A. Oligonucleotides

A 25-mer PS-oligo and its three novel analogs (Figure 1) have been compared for their *in vivo* stability, pharmacokinetics, tissue disposition, and elimination. PS-oligo (Oligo **1**; Gemai™) is targeted to the initiation codon of HIV-1 and is presently in phase II clinical trials.[8-10] Oligo **2** is a self- stabilized oligo with a hairpin loop at the 3′ end. The presence of the hairpin loop domain at the 3′ end provides greater stability against nuclease degradation by keeping the 3′ end involved in hydrogen bonding, but the hairpin domain gets destablized in the presence of a complementary RNA target.[11,12] Oligo **3** is a "hybrid" oligo, in which four contiguous deoxynucleosides at both the 3′ and 5′ ends are replaced with 2′-*O*-methylribonucleotides.[13-15] In general, 2′-*O*- methylribonucleotide phosphorothioates are more resistant to nucleases and placement of these linkages in Oligo **3** further increases its *in vivo* stability. Oligo **4** is a chimeric oligo in which four phosphorothioate linkages are replaced with four methylphosphonate linkages.[16,17] Methylphosphonate linkages are nonionic and very resistant to nucleolytic degradation, and placement of these linkages at the 3′ and 5′ ends should protect the PS-oligo from degradation *in vivo*. All oligos used in the *in vivo* studies are labeled with ^{35}S at the sites shown in Figure 1.

B. Animals and Procedures

Male Sprague-Dawley rats (110 ± 10 g, Harlan Laboratories, Indianapolis, IN) were used for the pharmacokinetic studies.[4,14,15,17] Generally, 30 animals were used for each oligo. Following administration of a single i.v. dose of 30 mg/kg of oligo into the tail vein, three animals were euthanized at time points 5, 30, and 60 min and 3, 6, 12, 24, 48, 120, and 240 h. Blood from each animal was collected in heparinized tubes and the plasma was separated by centrifugation. All tissues/organs were homogenized, mixed with tissue solubilizer, and the total radioactivity was counted. The total excreted urine and feces were collected from each animal at various time points and the radioactivity was counted.

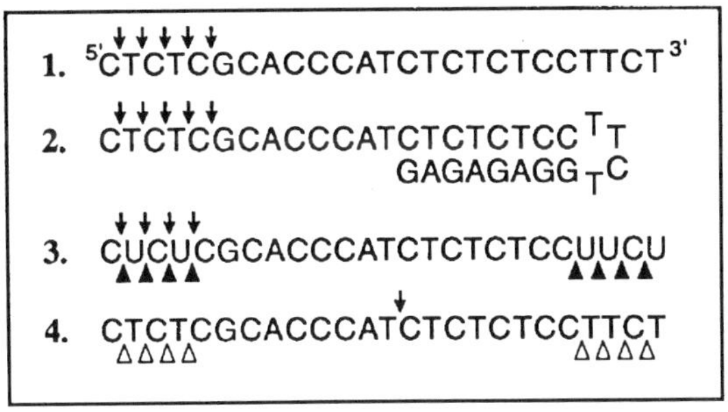

↓ = ^{35}S-labeled site

▲ = 2'-O-methylribonucleoside phosphorothioate

Δ = methylphosphonate internucleotide linkages

FIGURE 1
Structure of oligos. Oligo **1** is a phosphorothioate, Oligo **2** is a phosphorothioate which has a hairpin loop region at the 3′ end; Oligo **3** is a phosphorothioate, which contains four 2′-*O*-methylnucleotides at both the 3′ and 5′ ends, and Oligo **4** is a phosphorothioate, which contains contiguous four methylphosphonate linkages at both the 3′ and 5′ ends. The sites of ^{35}S-labeling are shown by arrows.

From plasma, tissue homogenates, and excreted urine and feces, the oligos were extracted for further analysis by polyacrylamide gel electrophoresis (PAGE)[4,14,15,17] and high performance liquid chromatography (HPLC)[14,15,17] to establish the integrity of the radioactivity and its association with the oligos or their metabolites.

II. PHARMACOKINETIC ANALYSIS

To understand the therapeutic potential, the mechanism of action and/or any side effects of an oligo, one needs to understand: (1) what is the maximum plasma concentration (C_{max}), rate of adsorption and elimination (half-lives), mean residue time (MRT), the area under the curve (AUC), and the *in vivo* stability of the oligo; (2) from the plasma compartment, where is the oligo distributed — whether to all tissues, or specifically to certain organs, and what is the stability in each tissue/organ; (3) what percentage of the administered dose of the oligonucleotide is distributed to each tissue at various times; and (4) what percentage of the administered dose is excreted by different elimination pathways (e.g., urine and feces) and what is the integrity of the oligo. In the present study, pharmacokinetic parameters were estimated using computer-mediated programs.[14,17]

A. Plasma Clearance

Figure 2 illustrates the comparative plasma concentration time courses of four radiolabeled oligos following i.v. bolus administration. The concentrations were expressed as the oligo equivalents in µg/ml of plasma based on the radioactivity levels. The pharmacokinetic parameters of all four oligos are listed in Table 1. Oligos **1** and **2** have similar values of $T_{1/2}\alpha$, $t_{1/2}\beta$ and the other parameters studied, whereas Oligos **3** and **4** have a $T_{1/2}\alpha$ shorter than that of Oligos **1** and **2**, suggesting a rapid distribution of Oligos **3** and **4**. Furthermore, Oligos **3** and **4** have a longer elimination half-life ($t_{1/2}\beta$), indicating that these two oligos are retained in the body for a longer period.

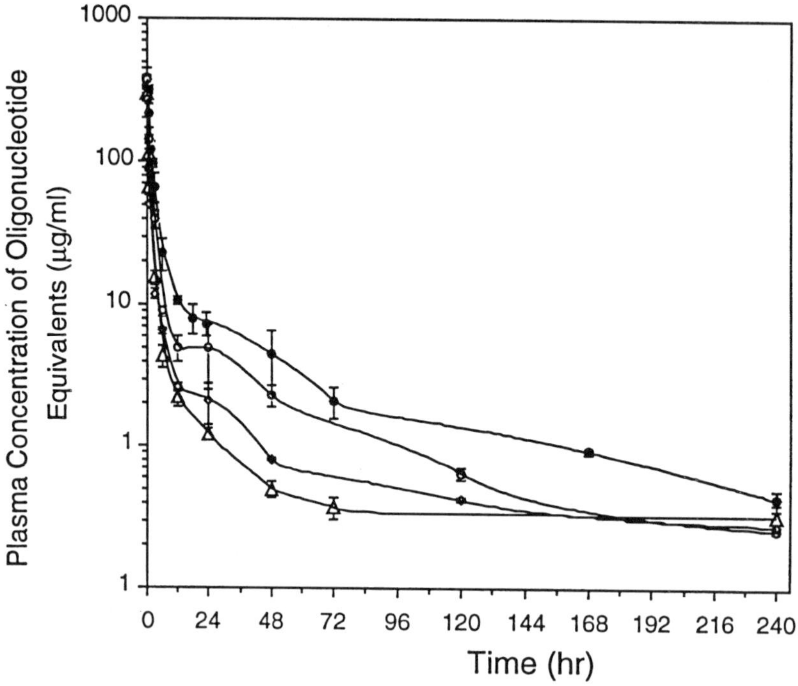

FIGURE 2
Plasma concentration-time curves of Oligo **1** (•), Oligo **2** (○), Oligo **3** (Δ), and Oligo **4** (◊). The concentrations were based on the quantitation of radioactivity. Pharmacokinetic analyses of plasma clearance (Table 1) indicate that there are differences among the four oligos.

TABLE 1
Plasma Pharmacokinetic Parameters of Oligonucleotides

Oligonucleotide number	C_{max} (µg/ml)	$T_{1/2}\alpha$ (h)	$T_{1/2}\beta$ (h)	AUC (µg/ml · h)	MRT (h)	CL (ml/kg/h)
Oligo **1**	418.4	0.95	47.57	1432.51	42.59	20.94
Oligo **2**	343.2	0.54	41.44	1039.10	45.2	28.90
Oligo **3**	339.73	0.34	52.02	704.09	57.53	42.61
Oligo **4**	301.15	0.38	52.29	584.96	54.93	51.29

A longer retention period for Oligos **3** and **4** is also shown by a longer MRT for Oligos **3** and **4**. Oligos and their metabolites from the plasma were analyzed by gel electrophoresis and HPLC following standard phenol extraction and protein kinase K digestion. Analysis of Oligo **1** showed that the presence of the intact oligo could be detected up to 12 to 24 h, along with the degraded forms of the oligo. HPLC analysis revealed a similar profile to that observed on gel electrophoresis. Representative HPLC profiles are presented in Figure 3. The other three oligos, **2**, **3**, and **4**, showed significantly greater *in vivo* stability and a majority of the radioactivity was associated with the intact oligos. Based on the radioactivity levels, less than one percent of the administered dose of any of the four oligos was present in the plasma compartment at 3 to 6 h post-dosing (Figure 4, Panel A for each oligo), suggesting that the plasma compartment may not be the best to illustrate the pharmacokinetic characteristics of oligos.

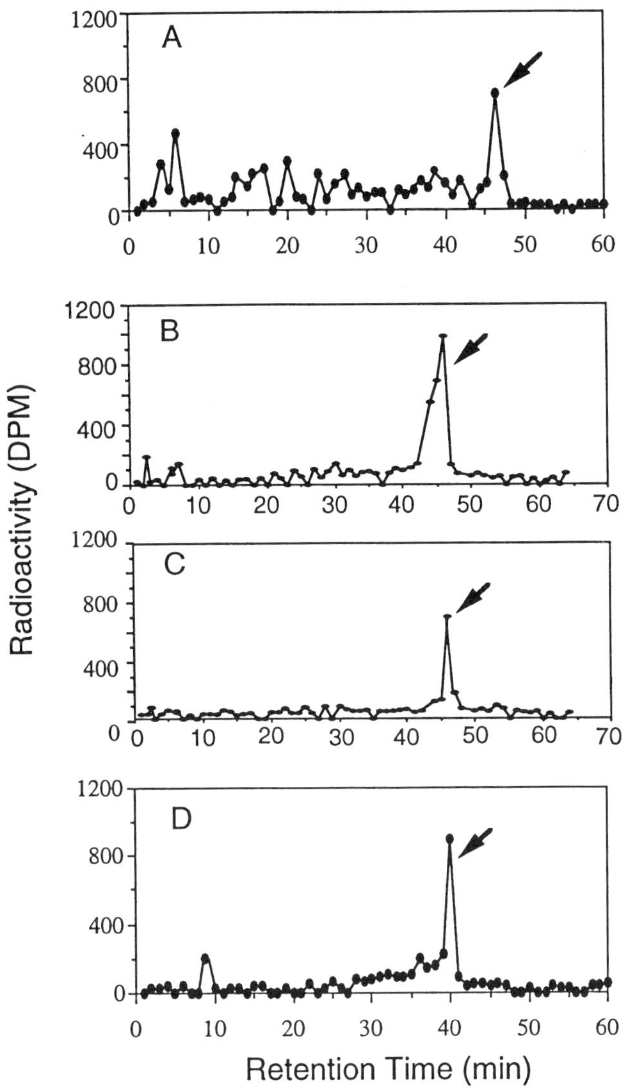

FIGURE 3
Stability of oligos in plasma. HPLC profiles of extracted radioactivity are from plasma samples at 3 h following i.v. administration of either Oligo **1** (A), Oligo **2** (B), Oligo **3** (C), or Oligo **4** (D). Significant degradation of Oligo **1** was observed, but the other three oligos were shown to have greater *in vivo* stability. Arrows indicate the position of intact oligo.

B. Elimination through Urine and Feces

The major pathway of elimination of oligos from the body is through urinary excretion, although some oligos are eliminated in feces. Figure 4, Panels C shows the cumulative excretion of oligos in urine based on the radioactivity level during the 240-h period following administration. Oligos **1** and **2** were excreted to approximately 65% over a period of 240 h; Oligos **3** and **4** were excreted in urine to only 42 to 44 percent in the same time period. Analysis of the extracted radioactivity in the cases of Oligos **1** and **2** showed the presence of degraded forms of the oligos; in the cases of Oligos **3** and **4**, the excreted radioactivities were associated with the intact oligos (up to 24 h), as well as the degraded forms of the oligos. The elimination

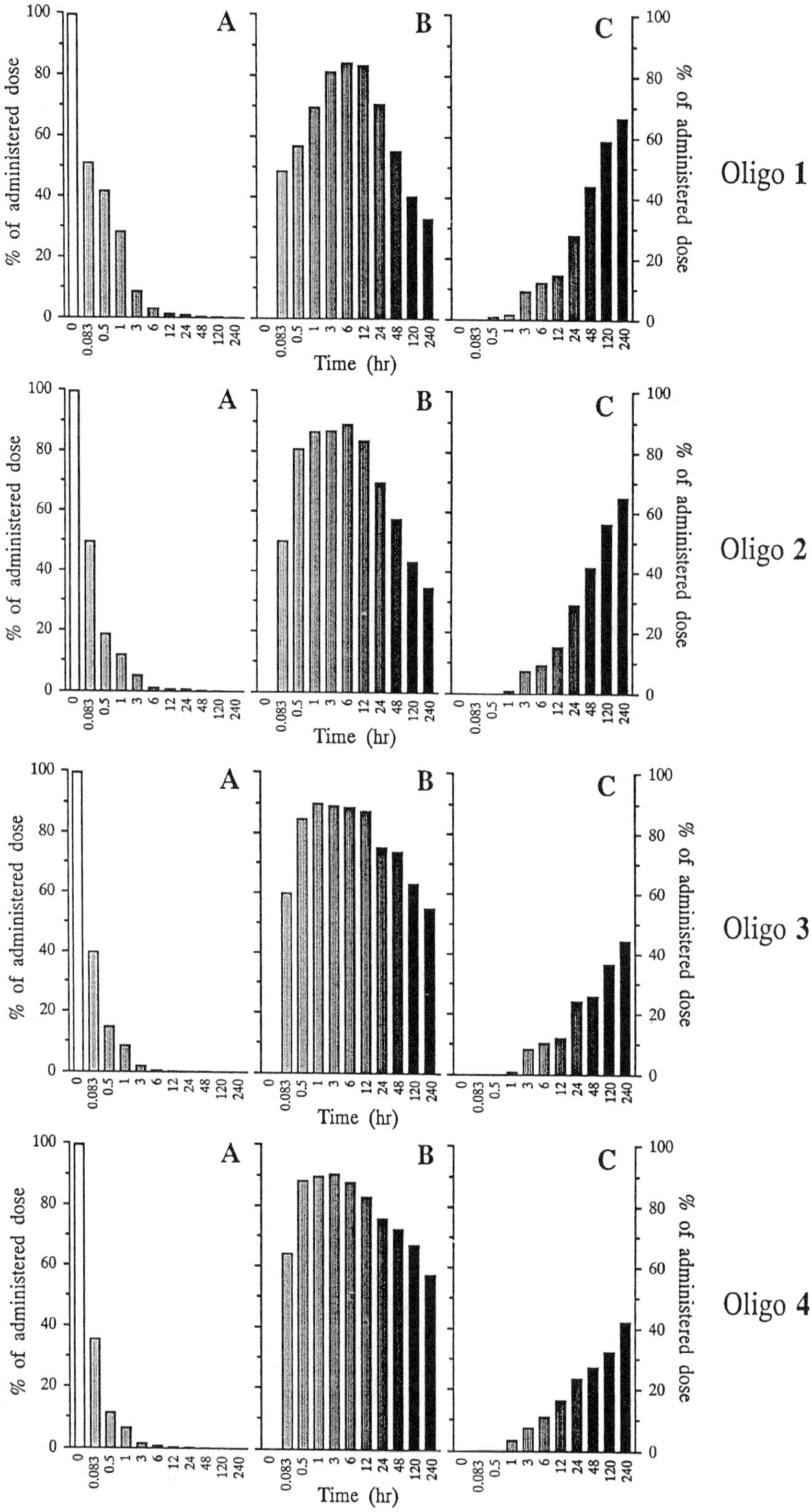
% of administered dose
Time (hr)
A
B
C
0
0.083
0.5
1
3
6
12
24
48
120
240
0
20
40
60
80
100
Oligo 1
Oligo 2
Oligo 3
Oligo 4

FIGURE 4

of the oligos in feces represents only 5 to 10% of the administered dose. No significant differences were observed among the four oligos. The radioactivity in the feces was associated with degradative products.

C. Tissue Distribution

Following i.v. administration, oligos were cleared from the plasma compartment and distributed to various tissues. Radioactivity was detected within five minutes of administration in the kidneys, liver, bone marrow, spleen, lymph nodes, pancreas, thyroid, adrenals, lungs, heart, and fat, and a small amount was detected in the brain.[4,14,18] Radioactivity was also detected in the gastrointestinal tissues, including the stomach and small and large intestines, and the contents of stomach and small and large intestines, suggesting an enterohepatic circulation of the oligos (and their metabolites). Figure 4, Panels B shows the combined tissue accumulation of the oligos at various time points following i.v. administration. A large percent of the administered oligos (based on radioactivity levels) was present in tissues and was slowly eliminated over a period of 240 h (Figure 4, Panels C).

Oligos **1** and **2** showed very similar profiles of tissue accumulation and elimination over the 240-h period after administration. About 12% of the administered dose was present in the liver at 12 h and was eliminated thereafter with time (Figure 5). At 240 h after administration, about 2.3% of Oligo **1** (based on radioactivity levels) was still present in the liver (Figure 5). Oligo **2** had a distribution profile similar to that of Oligo **1**. The liver disposition of Oligos **3** and **4** was different from that of Oligos **1** and **2**; the concentration increased with time following administration and peaked to about 10% at 12 to 24 h. The elimination of radioactivity for Oligos **3** and **4** was slower than that for Oligos **1** and **2**; at 240 h post-dosing, about 5 to 7% of the radioactivity was still present in the liver (Figure 5). Analysis by PAGE of the extracted radioactivity from liver homogenates showed that, in the cases of Oligos **2**, **3** and **4**, at up to 48 h post-dosing a majority of the radioactivity was associated with the intact oligo along with some metabolites, whereas in the case of Oligo **1**, more metabolites were observed (Figure 6).

In general, the disposition of the oligos in the kidneys showed a profile similar to that in the liver. The concentrations of Oligos **1** and **2** reached a peak (6 to 8% of the administered dose) at 12 h post-dosing and a slow elimination was observed (Figure 5). In the case of Oligos **3** and **4**, peak concentrations of the oligos were reached at a later time (24 to 48 h), and the elimination was much slower than that observed for Oligos **1** and **2**. HPLC analysis of the extracted oligos from kidney homogenates showed that the majority of radioactivity was associated with the intact oligos for Oligos **2**, **3**, and **4**, whereas for Oligo **1**, the radioactivity was associated with both the intact oligo and its degradative metabolites (Figure 7). A lower percentage of oligo disposition and elimination was observed in the spleen (Figure 5). Interestingly, compared to the other oligos, Oligo **1**, evidenced a higher spleen concentration at an early stage, but no difference was observed thereafter.

FIGURE 4
Distribution in plasma (A) and tissues (B) and elimination in urine (C) of Oligo **1**, Oligo **2**, Oligo **3**, and Oligo **4**. Following i.v. administration, all oligos had similar plasma clearance and by 6-h post-dosing, the majority of the oligos were eliminated from the plasma. The oligos significantly accumulated in the vaious tissues tested. Elimination of oligos from the tissues was different for Oligos **1** and **2**, as compared to Oligos **3** and **4**, which are significantly more stable and have a slower elimination, suggesting that elimination from the tissues is mainly related to metabolism. Elimination in urine was time-dependent. Up to 65% of the administered dose was eliminated in urine for Oligos **1** and **2**, whereas only about 40% of the administered dose was eliminated for Oligos **3** and **4**.

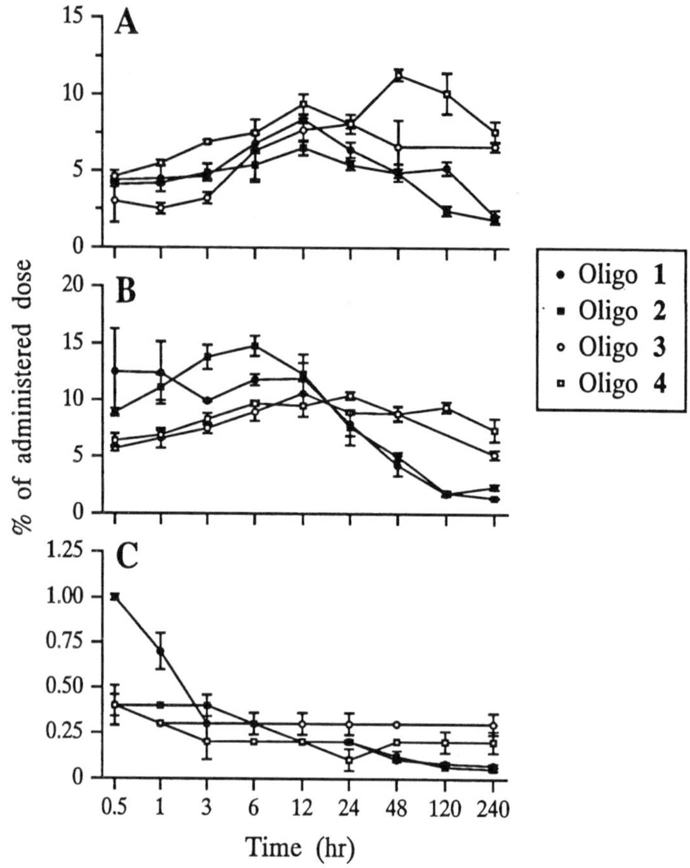

FIGURE 5
Comparative distribution of Oligo **1** (-•-), Oligo **2** (-▪-), Oligo **3** (-○-), and Oligo **4** (-□-) in kidneys (A), liver (B), and spleen (C). In general, very similar profiles of distribution were observed for all four oligos. Oligos **3** and **4** were retained in the tissues to a greater extent and for a longer time than Oligos **1** and **2**.

In summary, the pharmacokinetic study of the four oligos establishes the following points:

1. Following i.v. administration, oligos are rapidly cleared from the plasma compartment and distributed to various tissues. The $t_{1/2}\alpha$ is shorter than 60 min and $t_{1/2}\beta$ is longer than 24 h.
2. The major route of elimination of the oligos from the body is in urine, with minor elimination in the feces.
3. The rate of elimination in urine depends on the *in vivo* stability and the nature of the oligo and its metabolites. Oligos with increased *in vivo* stability are eliminated slowly.
4. Following administration, oligos are distributed to the majority of organs. The highest concentrations of oligos are observed in the kidneys and the liver.
5. The metabolism of oligos in various tissues is time and structure-dependent.
6. Low radioactivity levels in the brain suggest that the oligos do not cross the blood-brain barrier efficiently.
7. The degradation of PS-oligos *in vivo* is primarily from the 3′ end. The *in vivo* stability of oligo can be increased by protecting the 3′ end by (1) capping, (2) incorporating

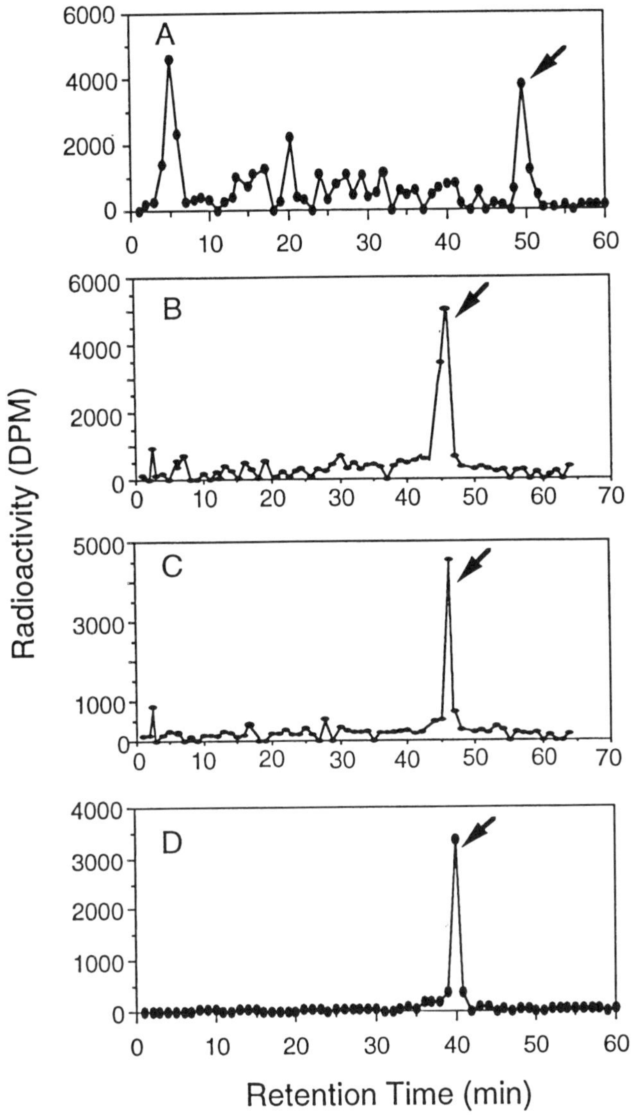

FIGURE 6
Stability of oligos in the kidneys. HPLC profiles show the composition of extracted radioactivity from kidney homogenates at 12 h following i.v. administration of either Oligo **1** (A), Oligo **2** (B), Oligo **3** (C), or Oligo **4** (D). Arrows indicate the position of intact oligo.

nuclease-resistant segments of oligos (e.g., 2′-*O*-methylribonucleosides or methylphosphonate linkages); or (3) creating a hairpin loop region.

8. The presence of radioactivity in the gastrointestinal tract and its contents suggest an enterohepatic circulation of oligos (and their metabolites).

III. ORAL ADMINISTRATION OF OLIGONUCLEOTIDES

Following i.v. administration of all four oligos to rats, we observed high radioactivity levels in gastrointestinal tissues and their contents. Analysis of the extracted radioactivity by HPLC and gel electrophoresis confirmed that the radioactivity was

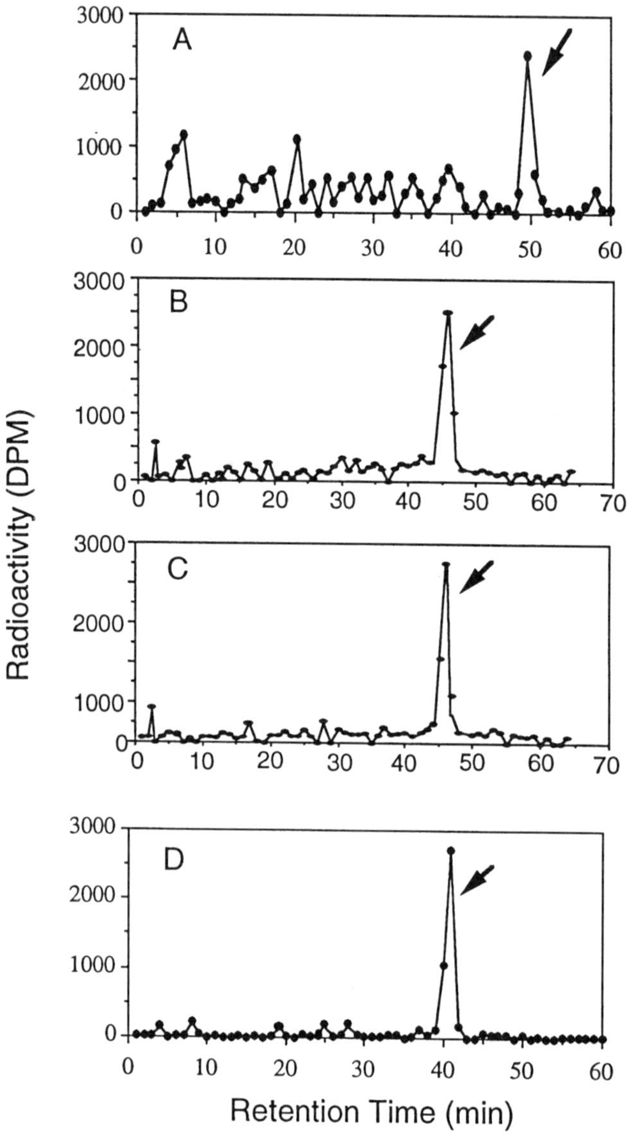

FIGURE 7
Stability of oligos in the liver. HPLC profiles show the composition of extracted radioactivity from liver homogenates at 12 h following i.v. administration of either Oligo **1** (A), Oligo **2** (B), Oligo **3** (C), or Oligo **4** (D). Arrows indicate the position of intact oligo.

associated with both intact and degraded oligos. In the case of Oligos **3** and **4**, more intact oligos were observed than with Oligos **1** and **2**. However, the oligo-associated radioactivity was not eliminated in feces in significant amounts, suggesting that there may be an enterohepatic circulation and reabsorption of the oligos from the intestinal tract, and, therefore, it may be possible to deliver oligos by oral administration.

This indication led us to determine the oral bioavailability of oligos. In earlier studies using Oligo **1**, following oral gavage in rats, we observed that the oligo was stable in stomach contents, but was extensively degraded in small intestinal contents. The mobility of the bands on gel electrophoresis suggested that degradation of Oligo **1** is primarily by exonucleases; a continuous ladder of bands of the degraded products was observed. To overcome digestion by nucleases, we studied the stability of

Oligo **3**,[15] which is significantly more stable *in vivo* following i.v. administration than Oligo **1**.[14] Following oral gavage, Oligo **3**, which was recovered from the stomach contents was not degraded at up to 3 h; minimal degradation was observed in the small intestinal contents (Figure 8). The degradation pattern of Oligo **3** suggests that the segment of oligo containing 2′-*O*-methylribonucleoside was removed by nuclease to generate 19-, 18-, and 17-mer (Figure 8). Intact Oligo **3** could be detected at up to 12 h in contents of the small intestine. Analysis by gel electrophoresis of the radioactivity excreted in feces showed the presence of both intact and degraded forms of Oligo **3**.

After establishing that Oligo **3** remains stable in the contents of stomach, small intestine and large intestine following oral gavage in rats, we measured the absorption of radioactivity from the gastrointestinal tract into the body. To measure the total absorption of Oligo **3**, animals (3 rats per group) were euthanized at 6 and 12 h after oral administration, and the gastrointestinal tract was then removed. The radioactivity in the gastrointestinal tract, feces, urine, plasma, and the remainder of the body was determined separately. The total recovery of the radioactivity was determined to be 95% ± 6%. The percentage of the absorbed Oligo **3**-derived radioactivity was determined using the following calculations:

$$\frac{[\text{Total radioactivity in the remainder of the body and plasma} + \text{total radioactivity in urine}]}{\text{Total radioactivity in the gastrointestinal tract, feces, plasma, and the remainder of the body}}$$

The total absorption of Oligo **3** was determined to be about 10% over 6 h and about 25% over 12 h based on radioactivity levels. Following absorption, the radioactivity was distributed to various organs with the same pattern as seen after i.v. administration. HPLC analysis of the extracted Oligo **3**-associated radioactivity from various tissues showed the presence of both the intact and degraded forms. Figure 9 shows the HPLC analysis of the extracted radioactivity from contents of the small intestine, the portal venous plasma, the liver, and the systemic plasma.

Within one hour after oral gavage radioactivity was detected in urine. The mean cumulative excretion of radioactivity in urine was determined to be 2.5% of the administered dose over 24 h and 3.8% over 48 h after administration (Figure 10). The majority of the radioactivity in the urine was associated with the degradation products of Oligo **3**. At the early time points, however, traces of intact oligo were also detected (Figure 10). After the studies with Oligo **3**, the oral bioavailability of Oligo **4** was further examined. Using a similar experimental protocol, we demonstrated that, following oral administration, Oligo **4** had increased stability in the gastrointestinal tract and increased absorption rate compared to the other oligos.

In summary, these studies establish the following points:

1. PS-oligo (Oligo **1**), when administered orally, remained stable in stomach contents, but was degraded in the intestinal contents.
2. PS-oligos, protected at both the 3′ and the 5′ ends with nuclease-resistant linkages, had increased *in vivo* stability in the stomach, the small intestine, and the contents of the large intestine.
3. Although the detailed mechanisms for oral absorption of oligos have not yet been defined, the detection of intact oligos in the portal venous plasma suggests that oligos may be transported across the intestinal walls.
4. Following absorption from the intestinal tract, oligos are distributed via systemic circulation to various tissues. Major metabolism of the absorbed oligos may occur in the liver.

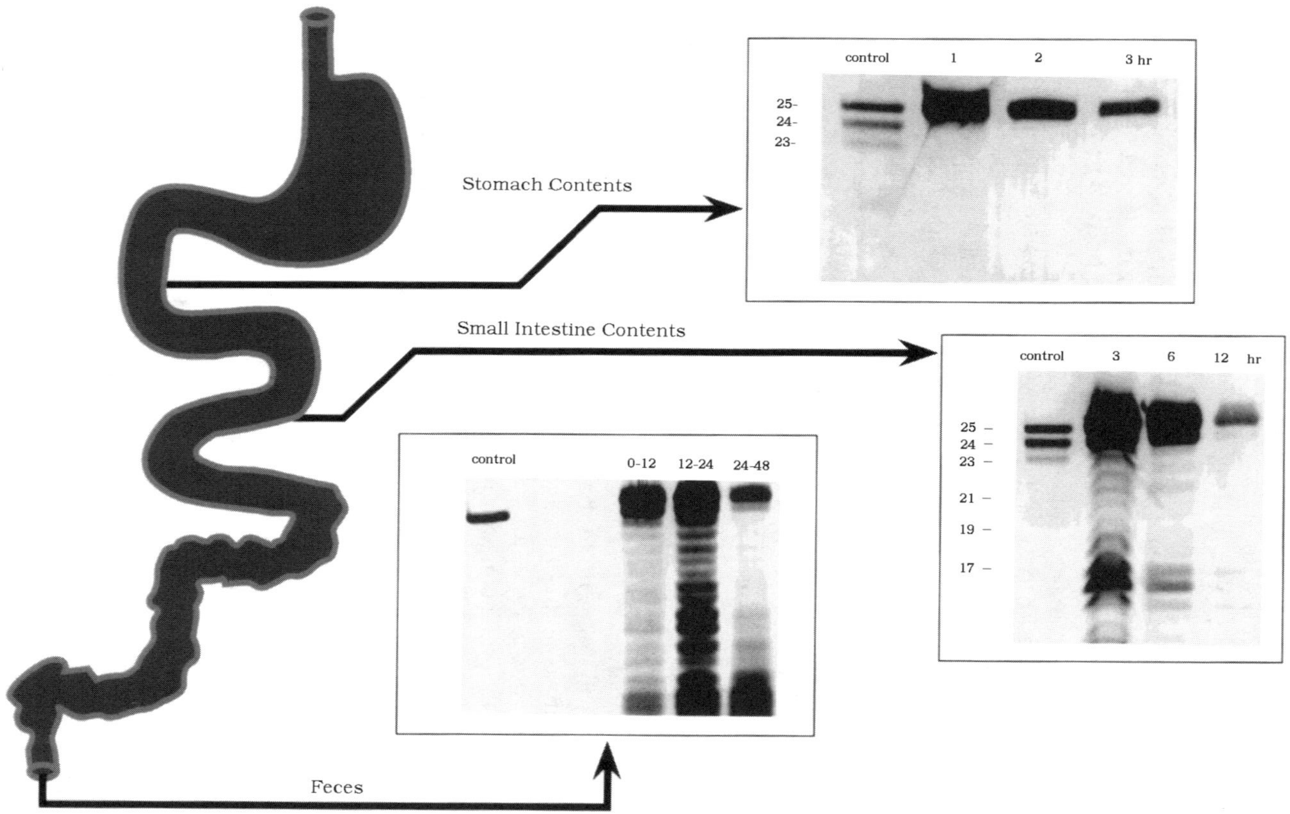

FIGURE 8
Stability of Oligo **3** in the stomach and small intestine contents and feces following oral gavage in rats at the indicated time points. The gastrointestinal contents were removed, and radioactivity was extracted and analyzed using PAGE. Radioactivity extracted from the stomach contents was associated with the intact oligo; however, radioactivity extracted from contents of the small intestine showed the presence of both intact and degraded forms. The presence of intact oligo along with degraded forms was also detected in feces. Control oligo in stomach contents and small intestine contents in a mixture of Oligo **3** and its shorter length (24, 33 etc.) which were not removed following labeling, and serves here as markers for degradation product.

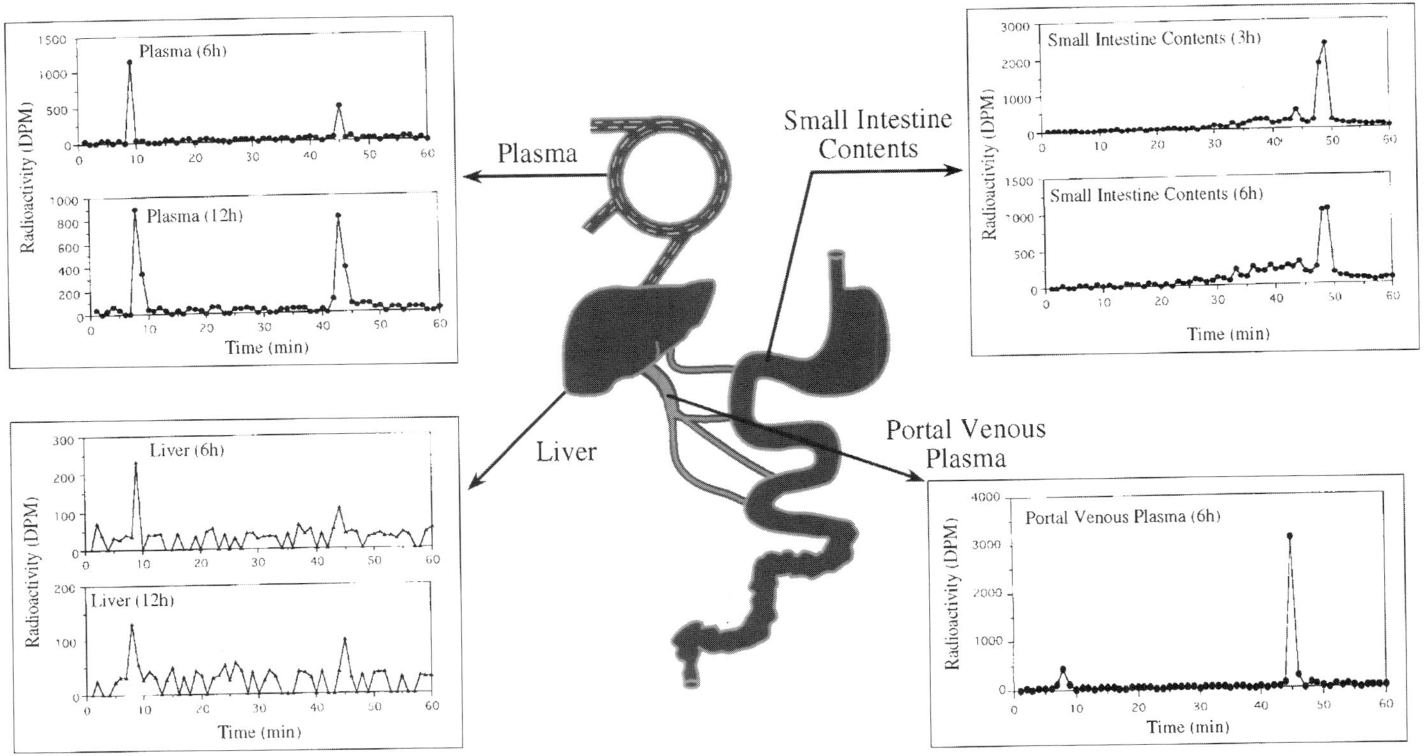

FIGURE 9
Analysis of the extracted radioactivity from the stomach and small intestine contents, portal venous plasma, liver, and systemic plasma using HPLC. Radioactivity extracted from stomach and small intestine contents and portal venous plasma was associated mainly with the intact oligo, whereas, radioactivity extracted from the liver homogenate and plasma was associated with both the intact and degraded forms of the oligo.

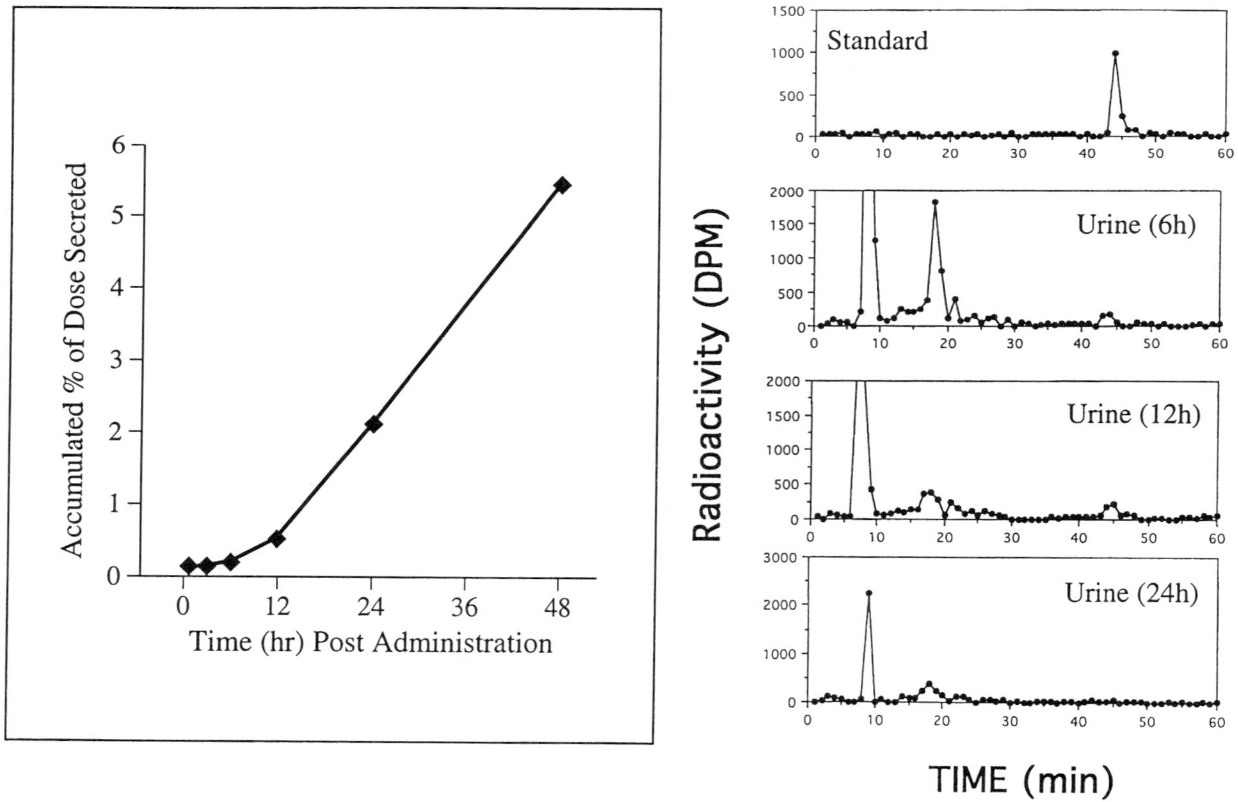

FIGURE 10
Urinary excretion of Oligo **3** following oral administration. Left panel shows the cumulative urinary excretion and the right panel shows the HPLC analysis of the extracted radioactivity at 6, 12, and 24 h post oral dosing.

5. Novel formulation of oligos or the use of carriers may further increase the stability of oligos in the stomach, the small intestine, the contents of the large intestine, and in the liver, and, therefore, may increase the oral bioavailability of the oligos.
6. Reduction in the charge of oligo (e.g., Oligo **4**) further increases the absorption of oligos following oral administration.

IV. DISCUSSION

In the past four years many reports have appeared describing the pharmacokinetics of various antisense oligos (Table 2). Oligos with varying lengths and base compositions have been studied in mice,[2,18-22] rats,[4,6,14,15,23-28] rabbits, monkeys,[4,29] and now in humans.[10,30,31] The majority of these studies were carried out using radiolabeled oligos, e.g., [^{35}S], [^{3}H] and [^{14}C]. Various routes of administration of oligos, e.g., i.v., intraperitoneal (i.p.), subcutaneous (s.c.), and intradermal (i.d.), have been employed (Table 2). Quantitation of the oligos in plasma, tissue homogenates, urine, and feces have been carried out by measuring radioactivity levels or, in some studies, using HPLC following extraction of an unlabeled oligo from plasma and urine.

In all cases, following i.v. administration or absorption from the site of administration (i.p., s.c., or i.d.), PS-oligos are rapidly cleared from the plasma. The half-life of distribution ($t_{1/2}\alpha$) is less than one h and the half-life of elimination ($t_{1/2}\beta$) is in the range of 40 to 60 h, based on radioactivity levels. The C_{max} achieved following s.c., i.p., and i.d. administration is significantly lower than that achieved following i.v. administration. For all PS-oligos studied, they are retained in most tissues examined, with the highest concentrations found in the kidneys and liver. Analysis of the extracted radioactivity from tissue homogenates indicated that the intact oligos were detectable up to 24 h post-dosing, but the majority of the radioactivity was associated with degraded forms of oligos. The degree of urinary elimination of the oligos varies significantly from study to study. These variations may result from differences in radiolabeling, administered doses and routes, and oligo sequence. Studies carried out in both our laboratories and in others, with [^{35}S]-labeled or [^{3}H]-labeled oligos, demonstrate that urinary excretion is the major pathway of elimination of oligos. Studies carried out with [^{14}C]-labeled oligos show that the major pathway of elimination is in expired air.[23,24]

In general, plasma pharmacokinetic analysis is based on the plasma concentration-time profiles, using various computer-aided programs. Therefore, interpretation of pharmacokinetic parameters should consider several important factors including but not limited to: (1) experimental procedure, e.g., sample size, sampling times, observation period; (2) analytical methods, e.g., sensitivity, lowest limits of detection; (3) chemical form of the monitored drug, i.e., total drug vs. free drug; parent drug vs. metabolites; and (4) programs for pharmacokinetic analysis, e.g., linear vs. non-linear; different simulation methods. It should be noted that the assumption for the use of plasma pharmacokinetic parameters to describe the fate of a given drug in the body is that the change of drug concentration and chemical forms will *represent* the changes in the whole body. This assumption may not always be correct due to the lower portion of oligos (<1% of the administered dose) in the plasma compartment and the limits of sensitivity of analytical methods used in quantitation of the oligo concentrations in plasma and tissues. In addition, the composition of oligo-associated radioactivity in plasma vs. tissues may vary significantly at various times. For example, in the later stage of experiment (24 h or later), minimal intact oligos were detected in the plasma sample, but the radioactivity in

TABLE 2

List of Pharmacokinetic Studies

Oligonucleotide details	Label	Dose and mode administration	$t_{1/2}$ (min)	$t_{1/2}\beta$	Ref.
In Mice:					
20-Mer, phosphorothioate	^{35}S-labeled	i) A 30 mg/kg single bolus i.v. injection (tail vein) ii) Same dose i.p.			18
20-Mer, end-capped phosphorothioate	^{35}S-labeled	30 mg/kg i.v.			19
20-Mer, phosphodiester and phosphorothioate	^{3}H-labeled	A single 6 mg/kg i.v. injection			2
20-Mer, phosphorothioate	Unlabeled	30 mg/kg			
In Rats:					
20-Mer, phosphorothioate	All thymidines were ^{14}C-labeled	3.6 mg/kg i.v. dose	24	Up to 51 h	23
20-Mer, phosphorothioate	^{14}C-labeled	Intradermal injection of 3.7 mg/kg dose	30	52.8 h	24
25-Mer, phosphorothioate	^{35}S-labeled	30 mg/kg single bolus i.v. injection	57.0	47.57 h	25
33-Mer, self-stabilized phosphorothioate	^{35}S-labeled	30 mg/kg single bolus i.v. injection	32.4	41.44 h	26
20-Mer, hybrid 2′O-methyl RNA phosphorothioate/ phosphorothioate oligo	^{35}S-labeled	30 mg/kg oral dose via gavage			15
i) Unmodified ii) 5′ Cholesterol modified-phosphorothioate	^{35}S-labeled	Up to 1 mg/kg i.p. dose	N.D.	23.2 h	27
i) 18-Mer, biotinylated phosphorothioate ii) Complexed with streptavidin-linked rat transferrin receptor antibody (OX26)	Internal ^{3}H-label on oligo-nucleotide	Up to 50 μg/200 μl injected via cannulated left femoral vein and animals sacrificed after 2 h	2.06		28
In Monkeys:					
15-Mer, phosphodiester	HPLC of unlabeled oligomer	Either constant i.v. infusion with up to 0.5 mg/kg/min or by bolus administration of up to 22.5 mg/kg	1.4	5.4	29
25-Mer, phosphodiester	Phosphodiester unlabeled	30 mg/kg i.v. administration			4
25-Mer, PS-oligonucleotide	^{35}S-labeled	1 and 5 mg/kg i.v.	36-60	42-56 h	
In Humans					
20-Mer, phosphorothioate	Unlabeled	i.v. Infusion			30
20-Mer, phosphorothioate	^{14}C-labeled at 2 position of all thymines	Intradermally			31
25-Mer, phosphorothioate	Internally ^{35}S-labeled	A 2-h i.v.infusion of 0.1 mg/kg	10.8	26.71 h	10

tissues was mainly associated with the intact oligos. Therefore, in the case of antisense oligos, precautions should be taken in interpreting plasma pharmacokinetic parameters.

As discussed above, it is generally accepted that PS-oligos and their modified analogs have a short distribution half-life ($t_{1/2}\alpha$) and a prolonged elimination half-life ($t_{1/2}\beta$). The short $t_{1/2}\alpha$ indicates a rapid clearance of the oligos from plasma, mainly distributed to various tissues. In the initial phase of distribution, the oligos are mainly distributed to highly perfused tissues like the liver, kidneys, and spleen. The prolonged elimination half-life ($t_{1/2}\beta$) indicates: (1) potential redistribution of oligos among tissues; (2) potential enterohepatic circulation; and (3) a slow clearance of oligos from the body. It should be noted that the major elimination of oligo-associated radioactivity is through urine, indicating that renal functions may have an impact on the clearance of oligos. In addition, several specific issues should be addressed as follows.

A. Structure and Stability of Oligos

In general, the plasma pharmacokinetics of oligos is not associated with the length and primary sequence of the oligos, but associated with the modification of the backbone and specific segments at the 3′ and/or 5′ end. We and others have demonstrated that these modifications increase the *in vivo* stability of the oligos and, therefore, increase tissue uptake and decrease total elimination, as indicated by the shorter $t_{1/2}\alpha$ and longer $t_{1/2}\beta$ compared to the PS-oligos. These observations are opening the door for future developments using different medicinal chemistry to modify the pharmacokinetics of antisense oligos.

B. Tissue Distribution

Apparently, oligos are well taken up by various tissues except for the brain, and tissue accumulation is related to the stability of oligos. These results suggest that specific delivery means may not be necessary. Qualitatively, no significant differences were observed between PS-oligos and modified analogs. However, quantitatively, significantly higher accumulation of modified oligos was seen in the liver and kidneys, compared to PS-oligos. Further analysis by HPLC and PAGE indicate that the majority of the radioactivity in these tissues was associated with the intact oligos, suggesting that: (1) metabolites with shorter lengths than that of the administered oligos are cleared out more rapidly that the intact oligos; (2) the kidneys have an important role in the retention of intact oligos and clearance of the metabolites; and (3) a lower plasma concentration may be also responsible for lower clearance of oligos. The selective clearance of intact oligos vs. their metabolites may have a significant impact on their antisense therapeutic effects, as well as on reducing any side effects that metabolites might have.

C. Protein Binding

Traditionally, in pharmacokinetic studies, total plasma drug concentrations are used to describe the distribution and elimination of studied drugs as well as their metabolites. However, for many drugs, the therapeutic and toxic effects correlate better with the concentration of diffusible, unbound drug than with the total drug concentration. Thus, it is very important to evaluate the plasma- or serum-protein binding of the drugs for proper pharmacokinetic studies and in routine clinical monitoring of drugs. Our previous studies[32] have provided a comprehensive analysis of the plasma- and serum-protein binding of a PS-oligo (Oligo **1**) and its modified analogs, a hybrid oligonucleotide (Oligo **3**) and a chimeric oligonucleotide (Oligo **4**) (Figure 1). Assays for protein-binding properties were conducted *in vitro* with plasma and serum from humans, rabbits, rats, and guinea pigs at various concentrations. In general, extensive protein binding of these oligonucleotides was dependent on the class and the concentration of oligo and on the species. Extensive protein-binding of the three oligos was observed, and the process seemed to be saturable. For example, the percentage of bound Oligo **1** to human plasma remained unchanged (94 to 91%) at concentrations ranging from 0.1 to 10 μg/ml, decreased at higher concentrations with 87% at 50 μg/ml, 77% at 200 μg/ml, and 62% at 500 μg/ml. Similar patterns were observed with Oligos **3** and **4** in human plasma. The extent of binding of oligos was a function of their concentration in plasma and serum. However, for the other three species, the percentage of Oligo **1** bound to plasma remained unchanged (>90) at concentrations from 0.1 to 200 μg/ml and decreased at higher concentrations (500 μg/ml) with the exception of guinea pigs, in which a significant decrease was seen only at 1000 μg/ml.

Although concentration-dependent protein binding was seen for all three oligos that were tested, quantitation analyses indicated that there were significant differences among the three oligos. In human plasma, the binding ratios observed were in the order of Oligo **3** > Oligo **1** > Oligo **4**. A similar pattern was seen in rat plasma but not in plasma from rabbits or guinea pigs. Significant differences in the protein binding of the oligo to plasma- and serum-proteins were observed among the four species tested in the present study. Generally, the percentage of oligo bound to plasma- and serum-proteins was in the rank order of guinea pigs > rabbits > rats > humans. In the guinea pig, nearly 95% or more of the three classes of oligos were bound to the plasma- and serum-proteins at all concentrations tested up to 500 μg/ml.

The mechanisms responsible for the differences in the plasma- and serum-protein binding between humans and experimental animals were not determined in the present study, but may be related to species-specific differences in the total levels and composition of the proteins. Further studies are needed. However, precautions should be employed when predicting drug doses for human studies based on animal data, since higher free drug concentrations in plasma are expected for humans in comparison with experimental animals at comparable total drug concentrations. The capacity for protein binding of the PS-oligo and its modified analogs was determined in the present study. However, further studies are needed to identify the specific proteins in the plasma or serum. In terms of the affinity of plasma-protein binding, our previous studies have shown that the affinity of PS-oligos for the protein in human blood is in the rank order of γ-globulins > fibrinogen > albumins, whereas for the hybrid oligo it is in the rank order of fibrinogen > γ-globulins > albumins.

D. Enterohepatic Circulation

We have demonstrated that the oligos and their metabolites are extensively subjected to biliary excretion following i.v. or oral administration.[33] Higher accumulation of oligo-associated radioactivity was observed in the intestinal tract and contents but limited fecal excretion of radioactivity was found. These results suggest an extensive enterohepatic circulation of oligos and their metabolites, which may have an important role in pharmacokinetics, therapeutic effects, and possible side effects of the oligos. Our computer modeling studies also support this hypothesis.[34] Further characterization of enterohepatic circulation of antisense oligos is underway in our laboratories, including the transport of oligos and their metabolites across the gastrointestinal wall, first-pass effect of the liver on the metabolism of the oligos, chemical forms of oligos at each site of the enterohepatic circulation (liver, bile, intestine, lumen, portal blood), and the impact on systemic circulation.

E. Therapeutic Effects vs. Side Effects

Obviously, to increase the therapeutic effects, it is desirable to increase the retention time of intact oligos in the body by means of increasing *in vivo* stability and decreasing clearance of the intact oligos. However, accumulation of oligos in the body may raise some concerns in terms of toxicity to specific organs. In addition, significant accumulation of oligos in certain tissues may also increase the risk of toxicity which may, in turn, increase further due to individual differences in the disease status and the organ functions. For example, significant accumulation of oligos in the kidneys in patients with renal disorders may have greater impact on host toxicity than in patients with normal renal function.

V. CONCLUSIONS

The understanding of pharmacokinetics, tissue disposition, *in vivo* stability, and elimination of antisense oligos is an important parameter in assessing the effectiveness (and potential side effects) as therapeutic agents. The pharmacokinetic profile also provides the basis for establishing a dosing regimen which is optimal with respect to efficacy and safety in humans.

It is clear from the studies with PS-oligos of varying length and base composition that following i.v. administration, PS-oligos are cleared rapidly from the plasma compartment. The same is true if PS-oligos are administered i.p., s.c., or i.d. Based on radioactivity levels, PS-oligos in plasma show long elimination half-lives; however, the majority of the radioactivity is associated with degraded forms of the PS-oligos.

PS-oligos are cleared from the plasma compartment but are retained in tissues for an extended time. The kidneys, liver, bone marrow, and spleen accumulate higher levels of PS-oligos compared to other tissues. The stability of PS-oligos following administration is tissue- and time-dependent. PS-oligos are degraded primarily from the 3′ end, and up to 24 h, the presence of intact oligos is detectable. Elimination of PS-oligos in urine is slow and the majority of the excreted PS-oligos are in degraded forms, suggesting that metabolism (degradation) is the key factor in determining the rate of elimination of the oligos.

The side effects which have been observed following administration of PS-oligos in mice and rats include thrombocytopenia, elevation of liver enzymes (AST and ALT), splenomegaly, hyperplasia of organ-associated reticuloendothelial cells, etc. In monkeys, the side effects also include complement activation (CH_{50}) and prolongation of the partial thromboplastin time (aPTT) and certain hemodynamic changes. Side effects such as CH_{50} and prolongation of aPTT are related to the plasma concentrations of oligos and can be minimized by keeping lower peak plasma concentrations by administering the oligos by slow infusion or s.c. injection. The other side effects are dependent on dosage and frequency of administration. It is not well established yet whether these side effects are due to PS-oligos or their metabolites, or due to the polyanionic nature of PS-oligos. In support of the latter possibility is evidence showing that the majority of these side effects have been observed with dextran sulfate, which is also polyanionic in nature.

The effectiveness of PS-oligos can be improved by increasing their *in vivo* stability thereby: (1) providing longer duration of action; (2) generating less metabolites and; (3) requiring less frequent administration. The three chemical modifications of PS-oligos described in this chapter provide a basis for further understanding the pharmacokinetics of antisense oligos. In all three cases, *in vivo* stability of the oligos has been improved and may allow less frequent dosing and improve the safety profile. Future studies are needed to further understand: (1) the mechanisms of cellular uptake, transport, and retention of oligos in various types of cells/tissues including the gastrointestinal tract; (2) the impact of pharmacokinetics of intact oligos and their metabolites on their *in vivo* therapeutic effectiveness and side effects; (3) metabolic pathways of oligos at cellular and molecular levels; and (4) potential species-specific differences in pharmacokinetics and their relation to therapeutic and toxic effects in order to extrapolate data from animal studies to humans.

REFERENCES

1. Zamecnik, P.C., History of antisense oligonucleotides, *Antisense Therapeutics*, Agrawal, S., Ed., Humana Press, Totowa, NJ, 1996, 1–12.
2. Sands, H., Gorey-Feret, L.J., and Cocuzza, A.J., Biodistribution and metabolism of internally ^{3}H-labeled oligonucleotides. I. Comparison of a phosphodiester and a phosphorothioate, *Mol. Pharmacol.*, 45, 932–934, 1994.
3. Goodchild, J., Zamecnik, P.C., and Kim, B., The clearance and degradation of oligodeoxynucleotide following intravenous injection into rabbits, *Ant. Res. Dev.*, 1, 153–160, 1991.
4. Agrawal, S., Temsamani, J., Galbraith, W., and Tang, J.-Y., Pharmacokinetics of antisense oligonucleotides, *Clin. Pharmacol.*, 28, 7–16, 1995.
5. Agrawal, S. and Iyer, R.P., Modified oligonucleotides as therapeutic and diagnostic agents, *Curr. Opin. Biotechnol.*, 6, 12–19, 1995.
6. Agrawal, S, Antisense oligonucleotides: Towards clinical trials, *Trends Biotechnol.*, 14, 376–387, 1996.
7. Akhtar, S. and Agrawal, S., *In vivo* studies with antisense oligonucleotides, *Trends Pharmacol. Sci.*, 18, 12–18, 1997.
8. Agrawal, S., Antisense oligonucleotides: A possible approach for chemotherapy of AIDS, *Prospects for Antisense Nucleic Acid Therapy of Cancer and AIDS*, Wickstrom, E., Ed., Wiley-Liss, New York, 1991, 143–158.
9. Agrawal, S. and Lisziewicz, J., Potential for HIV-1 treatment with antisense oligonucleotides, *J. Biotechnol. Health Care*, 1, 167–182, 1994.
10. Zhang, R., Yan, J., Shahinian, H., Amin, G., Lu, Z., Liu, T., Saag, M.S., Jiang, Z., Temsamani, J., Martin, R.R., Schechter, P.J., Agrawal, S., and Diasio, R.B., Pharmacokinetics of an anti-human immunodeficiency virus antisense oligonucleotide phosphorothioate (GEM 19) in HIV-infected subjects, *Clin. Pharmacol. Exp. Ther.*, 39, 929–939, 1995.
11. Tang, J.-Y., Temsamani, J. and Agrawal, S., Self-stabilized antisense oligonucleotide phosphorothioates: properties and anti-HIV activity, *Nucleic Acids Res.*, 21, 2729–2735, 1993.
12. Agrawal, S., Temsamani, J. and Tang, J.-Y., Self-stabilized oligonucleotides as a novel antisense agents, *Delivery Strategies for Antisense Oligonucleotide Therapeutics*, Akhtar, S., Ed., CRC Press, Boca Raton, FL, 1995, 105–122.

13. Metelev, V., Lisziewica, J., and Agrawal, S., Study of antisense oligonucleotide phosphorothioates containing segments of oligodeoxynucleotides and 2′-O-methyloligoribonucleotides, *Bioorg. Med. Chem. Lett.*, 4, 2929–2934, 1994.
14. Zhang, R., Lu, Z., Zhang, H., Diasio, R.B., Habus, I., Jiang, Z., Iyer, R.P., Yu, D., and Agrawal, S., *In vivo* stability and metabolism of a "hybrid" oligonucleotide phosphorothioate in rats, *Biochem. Pharmacol.*, 50, 545–556, 1995.
15. Agrawal, S., Zhang, X., Lu, Z., Hui, Z., Tamburin, M.J., Yan, J., Cai, H., Diasio, R.B., Habus, I., Iyer, R.P., Wu, D., and Zhang, R., Absorption, tissue distribution and *in vivo* stability in rats of a hybrid antisense oligonucleotide following oral administration, *Biochem. Pharmacol.*, 50, 571–576, 1995.
16. Agrawal S., Mayrand, S.M., Zamecnik, P.C., and Pederson, T., Site-specific excision from RNA by RNAse H and mixed phosphate backbone oligodeoxynucleotides, *Proc. Natl. Acad. Sci. U.S.A.*, 87, 1401–1405, 1990.
17. Zhang, R., Iyer, R.P., Yu, D., Tan, W., Zhang, X., Lu, Z., Zhao, H., and Agrawal, S., Pharmacokinetics and tissues disposition of a chimeric oligodeoxynucleotide phosphorothioate in rats after intravenous administration, *J. Pharmacol. Exp. Ther.*, 278, 971–979, 1996.
18. Agrawal, S., Temsamani, J., and Tang, J.-Y., Pharmacokinetics, biodistribution, and stability of oligodeoxynucleotide phosphorothioates in mice, *Proc. Natl. Acad. Sci. U.S.A.*, 88, 7595–7599, 1991.
19. Temsamani, J., Tang, J.-Y., Padmapriya, A.A., Kubert, M., and Agrawal, S., Pharmacokinetics, biodistribution and stability of capped oligodeoxynucleotide phosphorothioates in mice, *Antisense Res. Dev.*, 3, 277–284, 1993.
20. Sands, H., Gorey-Feret, L.J., Ho, S.W., Bao, Y., Cocuzza, A.J., Chidister, D., and Hobbs, F.W., Biodistribution and metabolism of internally ^{3}H-labeled oligonucleotides. II. 3′-, 5′-blocked oligonucleotides, *Mol. Pharmacol.*, 47, 636–646, 1995.
21. Saijo, Y., Perlaky, L., Wang, H., and Busch, H., Pharmacokinetics, tissue distribution and stability of antisense oligodeoxynucleotide phosphorothioate ISIS 33466 in mice, *Oncol. Res.*, 6, 243–249, 1994.
22. Chem, T.L., Miller, P., Ts'o, P.O.P., and Colvin, O.M., Disposition and metabolism of oligodeoxynucleoside methylphosphonate following a single i.v. injection in mice, *Drug Metab. Dispos.*, 18, 815–818, 1990.
23. Cossum, P.A., Sassmor, H., Delinger, D., Truong, L., Cumins, L., Owens, S.R., Markham, P.M., Shea, J.P., and Crooke, S., Disposition of the ^{14}C-labeled phosphorothioate oligonucleotide ISIS 2105 after intravenous administration to rats, *J. Pharmacol. Exp. Ther.*, 267, 1181–1190, 1993.
24. Cossum, P.A., Truong, L., Owens, S., Markaham, P.M., Shea, J., and Crooke, S.T., Pharmacokinetics of a ^{14}C-labeled phosphorothioate oligonucleotide ISIS 2105 after intradermal administration to rats, *J. Pharmacol. Exp. Ther.*, 267, 89–94, 1994.
25. Zhang, R., Diasio, R.B., Lu, Z., Liu, T., Jiang, Z., Galbraith, W.M., and Agrawal, S., Pharmacokinetics and tissue distribution in rats of an oligodeoxynucleotide phosphorothioate (GEM 91) developed as a therapeutic agent for human immunodeficiency virus type-1, *Biochem. Pharmacol.*, 49, 929–939, 1995.
26. Zhang, R., Lu, Z., Zhang, X., Diasio, R., Liu, T., Jiang, Z., and Agrawal, S., *In vivo* stability and disposition of a self-stabilized oligodeoxynucleotide phosphorothioate in rats, *Clin. Chem.*, 41, 836–843, 1995.
27. Iverson, P.L., Matta, J., Tracewell, W.G., and Zon, G., Pharmacokinetics of an antisense phosphorothioate oligodeoxynucleotide against rev from human immunodeficiency virus type 1 in adult male rat following single injections and continuous infusion, *Antisense Res. Dev.*, 4, 43–52, 1994.
28. Wu, D., Boado, R., and Partridge, W.M., Pharmacokinetics and blood-brain barrier transport of [^{3}H]-biotinylated phosphorothioate oligodeoxynucleotide conjugated to a vector-mediated drug delivery system, *J. Pharmacol. Exp. Ther.*, 276, 206–211, 1996.
29. Lee, W.A., Fishback, J.A., Shaw, J.-P., Bock, L.C., Griffin, L.C., and Cundy, K.C., A novel oligodeoxynucleotide inhibitor of thrombin. II. Pharmacokinetics in the cynomolgus monkey, *Pharm. Res.* 12, 1943–1947, 1995.
30. Bayever, E., Iverson, P.L., Bishop, M.R., Sharp, J.G., Tewary, H.K., Arneson, M.A., Pirruccello, S.J., Ruddon, R.W., Kessinger, A., Zon, G., and Armitage, J.O., Systemic Administration of a phosphorothioate oligonucleotide with a sequence complementary to p53 for acute myelodysplastic syndrome: Initial results of Phase I trials, *Antisense Res. Dev.*, 3, 383–390, 1993.
31. Crooke, S.T., Grillone, L.R., Tendolakr, A., Garrett, A., Franklin, M., Leeds, J., and Barr, W. H., A pharmacokinetic evaluation of ^{14}C-labeled afovirsen sodium in patients with genital warts, *Clin. Pharmacol. Ther.*, 56, 641–646, 1994.

32. Zhang, X., Lu, Z., Diasio, R.B., Jiang, Z., Tan, W., Agrawal, S., and Zhang, R., Plasma- and serum-protein binding of antisense oligodeoxynucleotide phosphorothioates in experimental animals and humans, *Proc. Am. Assoc. Cancer Res.*, 36, 411, 1995.
33. Zhao, H., Lu, Z., Diasio, R.B., Agrawal, S., and Zhang R., Biliary excretion of oligonucleotides: Previously unrecognized pathway in metabolism of antisense oligonucleotides, *FASEB J.*, 9 (3), A410, 1995.
34. Liu, T.-P., Lu, Z., Diasio, R.B., Agrawal, S., and Zhang, R., Mathematical modeling of biodistribution of an antisense oligodeoxynucleotide phosphorothioate, *Proc. Am. Assoc. Cancer Res.*, 36, 364, 1995.

FIGURE 4
Distribution in plasma (A) and tissues (B) and elimination in urine (C) of Oligo **1**, Oligo **2**, Oligo **3**, and Oligo **4**. Following i.v. administration, all oligos had similar plasma clearance and by 6-h post-dosing, the majority of the oligos were eliminated from the plasma. The oligos significantly accumulated in the vaious tissues tested. Elimination of oligos from the tissues was different for Oligos **1** and **2**, as compared to Oligos **3** and **4**, which are significantly more stable and have a slower elimination, suggesting that elimination from the tissues is mainly related to metabolism. Elimination in urine was time-dependent. Up to 65% of the administered dose was eliminated in urine for Oligos **1** and **2**, whereas only about 40% of the administered dose was eliminated for Oligos **3** and **4**.

Chapter **4**

Non-Antisense Effects of Antisense Oligonucleotides

Leonard M. Neckers and Kanak Iyer

CONTENTS

I. INTRODUCTION

Antisense RNA and DNA techniques have been developed as a relatively recent approach to the specific modulation of gene expression. The development of antisense RNA techniques began with observations from the labs of J. Tomizawa and N. Kleckner that bacteria can regulate gene replication and transcription by the elaboration of small complementary or "antisense" RNA molecules (for a review see Weintraub[1] or Inouye[2]). Evidence also now exists that eukaryotic cells elaborate antisense RNA transcripts,[3,4] but the physiologic role of these molecules remains controversial. Nevertheless, in 1984, Weintraub and Izant reported that a transfected expression vector could generate RNA capable of modulating eukaryotic gene expression in a target-specific manner.[5] Actually, prior to the discovery of regulatory RNAs, several laboratories had demonstrated that synthetic oligodeoxynucleotides complementary to mRNA sequences could downregulate mRNA translation *in vitro* and in cells.[6] A profusion of reports have followed describing the modulation of various oncogenes by both DNA and RNA antisense techniques. Such manipulations offer the possibility of combining the specificity of genetic approaches with the reversibility and temporal control of more pharmacologic approaches. The continued development of antisense technology and related delivery systems has led to initial explorations of the *in vivo* utility of antisense, particularly as it relates to oligonucleotides.

However, the excitement generated by initial *in vitro* successes has been tempered by the dawning realization that antisense technology is not as "clean" as previously thought. It is both more difficult and less appealing to publish one's experimental failures; reports of problems and difficulties with antisense techniques have been slow to appear in the scientific literature. However, understanding the problems associated with this technology is essential for the true promise of antisense to be ultimately achieved. The purpose of this brief review is to describe some of the more commonly observed problems associated with the use of antisense oligonucleotides *in vitro* and *in vivo*.

II. GENERAL CONSIDERATIONS

In the application of antisense techniques to the study of cellular systems we cannot stress enough the need for adequate controls and appropriate endpoints. Early studies targeted reporter gene constructs such as chloramphenicol acetyl transferase and thymidine kinase to explore the specificity and utility of antisense strategies.[5,7] These genes code for readily quantified protein products and, because they were extraneous to the cells into which they were introduced, their expression was not tied to normal cellular physiology. Interference with their expression had little impact on cell function and as a result interpretation of results was relatively clean and straightforward. In the case of cellular genes, the situation becomes more complex. Interference with expression can have far reaching and unexpected results which may be difficult to distinguish from nonspecific or toxic antisense effects. Many gene products are difficult to quantitate either because reagents do not exist or because expression is at such low levels that sensitivity becomes a problem. Investigators have occasionally been unable to document decreases in steady-state target mRNA levels even though target protein levels showed dramatic declines. The reasons for this are not clear. Likewise, it has often not been possible to document antisense RNA transcripts in transfected cells even though a pronounced biologic effect is observed. Biologic endpoints as an indication of true antisense effect can be very misleading. In particular, interference with genes critical to proliferation or survival may facilitate the overgrowth of resistant, mutant, or otherwise compensated populations which are not representative of the original system or its biology.

A recent editorial in the journal *Antisense Research and Development*[8] has called for the use of three types of control oligonucleotides: (1) a sense control, which maintains structural features of the oligonucleotide but not base composition; (2) a scrambled control, which maintains base composition but not structural features; and (3) a mismatch control to demonstrate target hybridization specificity. As will be seen below, even these controls may not be adequate to rule out non-antisense effects of oligonucleotides.

III. DOES OLIGONUCLEOTIDE LENGTH AFFECT SPECIFICITY?

Among the important variables in the use of antisense oligonucleotides is certainly the length of sequence required for adequate specificity and optimal efficacy. Based on an estimate of approximately 3 to 4 billion base pairs in the human genome and assuming a random distribution of bases, a number of investigators have calculated the minimum size needed to recognize a single specific sequence in the genome as between 12 and 15 bases.[9] Interestingly, longer may not be better. Antisense effects in *Xenopus* oocytes have been reported with an oligonucleotide as short as 10 bases.[10] Woolf et al.[9] have pointed out that increasing an oligonucleotide beyond that minimum length would be expected to decrease, rather than increase specificity, since a longer oligonucleotide would contain more internal sequences long enough to hybridize to other mRNAs. Thus, a 20-mer contains 9 different consecutive 12-mers, giving rise to approximately 11 different matches of 12 consecutive bases. Since antisense oligonucleotides as long as 21 bases are now commonly used as specific inhibitors of gene expression, the effect of mismatches on antisense efficacy becomes a very important and practical question.

In a recent study using microinjection into *Xenopus* oocytes, Woolf et al.[9] examined the degree to which mismatched antisense phosphodiester oligonucleotides could still cause degradation of their target mRNAs via RNase H. The results are disturbing. Using fibronectin as the target mRNA in *Xenopus*, the authors demonstrated that a perfectly complementary 25-mer antisense oligonucleotide produced 79% degradation of the target mRNA after 6 h. However, 25-mers with 17 and 14 centrally located complementary bases caused 32 and 37% degradation, respectively. The authors demonstrated that even internal mismatches did not prevent target sequence degradation. Using another target, Vg1 mRNA, they found that a single mismatch about one third of the way along a 13-mer antisense oligonucleotide reduced, but did not eliminate target degradation. Thus, the fully complementary 13-mer produced 90% degradation over 6 h, while the mismatch sequence caused 42% degradation over this time.

Because antisense-mediated degradation of a target sequence can be accomplished using a minimum of 10 consecutive complementary bases, and noncomplementary flanking sequences do not prevent antisense effects, Woolf et al.[9] reached the conclusion that any oligonucleotide long enough to be useful as an antisense reagent would be likely to cause at least partial degradation of a large number of mRNA species. Because *Xenopus* oocytes grow at a temperature of approximately 22°C, one could hope that the more stringent hybridization conditions under which mammalian cells grow (i.e., 37°C) might eliminate this problem. However, because antisense effects have been reported in mammalian cells with sequences as small as 11 bases,[11] one must at least consider the possibility of nonspecific mRNA cleavage.

IV. MOTIFS WITHIN OLIGONUCLEOTIDES CAN STIMULATE THE IMMUNE SYSTEM

In two reports, Yamamoto et al.[13] and Kuramoto et al.[12] found that certain 6-mer palindromic sequences potently induced interferon production in murine spleen cells. The most active palindromes were 5′-GACGTC-3′, 5′-AGCGCT-3′, and 5′-AACGTT-3′. Interferon production was accompanied by stimulation of natural killer cell activity, which could be blocked by antibodies to interferon. The authors noted that extra-palindromic sequences contributed to these effects. Thus, reducing a 45-mer oligonucleotide to a 15-mer while maintaining the 6-mer palindrome markedly reduced stimulatory activity.[14] An oligonucleotide with a repeated palindrome flanked by guanylate residues demonstrated the strongest activity.[12] The authors also concluded that a 5′-CpG-3′ motif was essential to the activity.

Interestingly, these authors initiated these studies because of earlier work demonstrating that a preparation of bacterial DNA displayed strong anti-tumor activity in mouse and guinea pig.[15,16] The original synthetic oligonucleotides tested were derived from sequences contained within the bacterial DNA preparation. In a more recent study, Krieg et al.[17] reported that unmethylated CpG motifs in bacterial DNA were responsible for B-cell activation, identifying this as a novel T-cell-independent B-cell activation pathway. Oligonucleotides with CpG-containing hexamers were also quite effective, resulting in the recruitment of more than 95% of all splenic B cells into the cell cycle. Not surprisingly, three of the four most active hexamers reported by Krieg et al.[17] were also found to be active in the earlier studies of Yamamoto et al. and Kuramoto et al.[12,13]

The importance of extra-palindromic sequence in this phenomenon is demonstrated in a study by McIntyre et al.[18] In this study, the authors showed that a sense control oligonucleotide to NF-kB caused massive splenomegaly and B-cell activation in mice. The sequence indeed contained a CpG hexamer. Although the antisense sequence also contained a CpG hexamer, it was without effect as were several other CpG-containing sequences. However, several additional unrelated CpG-containing oligonucleotides did produce B-cell activation.

Krieg et al.[17] conclude that "it may be desirable to avoid unmethylated CpGs in antisense oligonucleotides, or at least to include controls for these effects," particularly *in vivo*. However, given the difficulty of designing a proper mismatched control (see above), and given the dependence of immune stimulatory effects on extra-palindromic sequences, this may prove to be a difficult task.

V. OLIGONUCLEOTIDES NONSPECIFICALLY SUPPRESS [^{3}H]THYMIDINE INCORPORATION

Breakdown of thymidine-containing oligonucleotides and resultant alteration of nucleotide pools can have dramatic effects on assays of cellular proliferation and DNA synthesis, such as [^{3}H]thymidine incorporation.[19] This potential artifact is particularly relevant when using oligomers to study the regulation of proliferation. Because oligonucleotide degradation in serum is primarily due to 3′ exonuclease activity,[20] thymidines at or near the 3′ end of an oligonucleotide are more "inhibitory" than thymidines near the 5′ end of a sequence. While apparent inhibition can be as great as 90%, this is due solely to dilution of cellular thymidine pools (with a resultant decrease in specific activity of the radioactive tracer) and not to any true growth effects.

VI. OLIGONUCLEOTIDE-DRUG INTERACTIONS

Development of oligonucleotide-based therapeutics has raised the possibility of potential combination therapy with conventional chemotherapeutic agents. However, we and others have found that the class of anti-cancer drugs known collectively as DNA intercalators can bind directly to certain oligonucleotides.[21,22] This effect was initially observed while searching for an antisense oligonucleotide to the tumor necrosis factor (TNF) receptor. As a screening assay, we were assessing the ability of various sequences to block TNF-mediated *in vitro* cytotoxicity. This assay relies on small concentrations of actinomycin D to potentiate effects of TNF. To our surprise, many different oligonucleotides, related and unrelated to the TNF receptor mRNA sequence, reversed TNF toxicity. Upon closer examination, the effect could not be attributed to TNF receptor downregulation, but to interference with the activity of actinomycin D. Indeed, using a fluorescent derivative of actinomycin D, we were able to demonstrate direct binding of oligonucleotide to drug. Binding affinity was dependent on oligonucleotide length and guanosine content, but it was not sequence-dependent.[21]

The cytoprotective effect of all oligonucleotides was completely dependent on their ability to bind actinomycin. More importantly, these oligonucleotides also were able to abrogate the cytotoxicity of other DNA intercalators, including adriamycin and daunomycin. The toxicity of other DNA damaging agents, including mitomycin C, cisplatin, VP-16, and camptothecin, was not affected.[21] The mechanism by which single-stranded oligonucleotides bind to DNA intercalators appears to involve stacked complexes of drug and DNA.[23]

VII. PHOSPHOROTHIOATE OLIGONUCLEOTIDES DIRECTLY INTERACT WITH PROTEINS

A major hurdle in the development of antisense oligonucleotides has been the stability of the molecules themselves in serum-containing media and in cells. Unmodified phosphodiester (Po) oligonucleotides are very susceptible to degradation by cellular nucleases. Po oligonucleotides microinjected into a *Xenopus* embryo have half-lives of less than 30 min (see Neckers et al.[20] for review). Similar *in vivo* results were obtained when Po oligonucleotides were injected directly into the brains of rodents.[24,25] Studies of fluorescent oligonucleotides administered *in vitro* to mammalian cells have demonstrated degradation of Po compounds within 3 h.[26,27] In contrast, phosphorothioate (Ps) oligonucleotides are highly resistant to nuclease degradation[28] (for review see Neckers et al.[20]). Because this modification is relatively easy to make and is chemically stable, it has become the modification of choice for production of antisense oligonucleotides stable enough for *in vitro* and *in vivo* use.

Evidence has been accumulating, however, that incorporation of phosphorothioate moieties into oligonucleotides makes these molecules much "stickier" than unmodified oligonucleotides, particularly with respect to direct protein binding. An early study by Cazenave et al.[29] tested antisense phosphorothioates in both a frog oocyte system and a wheat germ extract *in vitro* translation system, and demonstrated that, while phosphorothioates were effective antisense molecules *in vitro* and *in vivo* at submicromolar concentrations, at 1 to 10 μM concentrations these oligonucleotides could nonspecifically inhibit protein synthesis. The authors concluded that nonspecific inhibition of protein synthesis was occurring because the Ps oligonucleotides were binding to enzymes involved in protein synthesis.

Ps oligonucleotides are strong sulfated polyanions. Naturally occurring polyanions bind to and sequester various growth factors to basement membranes. Synthetic sulfated polynanions, such as suramin, heparin, dextran, and pentosan polysulfate can mimic naturally occurring polyanions by themselves binding to a variety of growth factors including members of the fibroblast growth factor family (FGFs), platelet-derived growth factor (PDGF), and vesicular endothelial growth factor (VEGF).[30,31] These polyanions block the binding of growth factors to their cell surface receptors. Like these polyanions, Ps oligonucleotides also antagonize the binding of both FGF and PDGF to receptors on the surface of 3T3 fibroblasts and other cells.[8] Ps oligonucleotides, like heparin, also release growth factors already bound to extracellular matrix.[8]

Other proteins which interact with and are inhibited by both Ps oligonucleotides and other sulfated polyanions include recombinant soluble CD4, HIV-1 reverse transcriptase, HIV gp120, RNase H, DNA polymerase alpha and beta, and protein kinase C.[32-36] The interaction of Ps oligonucleotides with these proteins is somewhat length-dependent but seems not to depend on sequence. In all cases, when a similar effect is observed with unmodified phosphodiester oligonucleotides, it is much weaker and/or requires 10 to 100 times more oligonucleotide.

Ps oligonucleotide inhibition of protein kinase C or RNase H can be problematic for antisense experiments. Stein et al.[36] have found that SdC28, a Ps homopolymer of cytidine (28-mer), is able to directly inhibit the beta 1 isoform of protein kinase C with an IC_{50} of 1 μM. Other protein kinase C inhibitors appear to antagonize the cellular uptake of oligonucleotides, raising the possibility that, at low micromolar concentrations, Ps oligonucleotides will block their own cellular uptake.

At the same time, Gao et al.[35] have reported that SdC28 can inhibit RNase H, the enzyme thought to be primarily involved in mediating antisense activity. Using sequence-specific antisense Ps oligonucleotides, these authors found that, in the presence of the complementary mRNA, they could observe a biphasic effect dependent on the oligonucleotide concentration. At oligonucleotide concentrations less than or equal to the concentration of the target mRNA, RNA cleavage could be demonstrated, suggesting RNase H activity. However, when Ps oligonucleotide concentrations rose above the concentration of the target, RNA cleavage became progressively less, suggesting inhibition of RNase H activity by excess Ps oligonucleotide. Because it is impossible to precisely titrate antisense oligonucleotide concentrations in cells or *in vivo*, the possibility distinctly exists that a Ps antisense oligonucleotide would be likely to inhibit activity of the very enzyme responsible for mediating antisense effects.

Ps oligonucleotides also activate the nuclear transcription factor Sp1 in a sequence- and length-independent manner.[37] This effect is similar to that observed following treatment with the sulfated polyanion suramin. Induction occurs in both transformed and untransformed cells of both murine and human origin. Because Sp1 participates in transcriptional regulation of many diverse cellular promoters, nonspecific induction of this transcription factor by Ps oligonucleotides could lead to unexpected biological responses, whether or not specific antisense effects could be observed.

VIII. SEQUENCE-SPECIFIC PROTEIN RECOGNITION BY PHOSPHOROTHIOATE AND UNMODIFIED OLIGONUCLEOTIDES

Ps oligonucleotides cannot be as efficiently end-labeled with T4 polynucleotide kinase as can unmodified oligonucleotides. Teasdale et al.[38] have recently reported that this is partly due to direct inhibition of the kinase by phosphorothioates. Inhibition was dependent on both the length of the oligonucleotide (the longer the more inhibitory) and the number of Ps linkages in the molecule. Intriguingly, some sequence specificity to the inhibition was also noted. For example, a 12-base homopolymer of cytidine was 100 times more inhibitory than a 12-base heteropolymer. The inhibitory activity of several heteropolymers of identical length also was found to vary over 1000-fold. Potential sequence motifs responsible for inhibition remain to be identified.

Direct oligonucleotide inhibition of the oncogenic tyrosine kinase $p210^{bcr\text{-}abl}$ has recently been reported by Bergan et al.[39,40] While screening for an antisense oligonucleotide, the authors found instead a sequence which directly inhibited the enzymatic activity of the kinase *in vitro* and *in vivo* without affecting its protein level. Inhibition was length- and sequence-dependent, requiring at least one GGC motif in a 21-base molecule. Interestingly, while a Ps oligonucleotide of appropriate sequence was inhibitory, an ummodified version of the same sequence was even more inhibitory, with an IC_{50} of less than 1 μM. However, the same sequence (non-Ps) containing a 2′-methoxy modification of the sugar moiety was completely ineffective as a kinase inhibitor. Thus, negative charge alone, in the context of sequence, is not sufficient to achieve inhibition.

The kinase specificity of this oligonucleotide was demonstrated by the fact that several other tyrosine and serine/threonine kinases required at least one log more oligonucleotide before inhibition could be observed. Inhibition was noncompetitive with respect to ATP but could be antagonized by addition of a substrate protein, suggesting that the oligonucleotide bound to a substrate recognition site on the p210 protein.

Perhaps the finding of this study most relevant to antisense technology is that this direct protein-binding effect is dependent on both sequence and secondary structure of the oligonucleotide. Changing the character of the phosphate linkage or the sugar moiety without changing the sequence would not be expected to affect hybridization to target mRNA, but these alterations had profound effects on oligonucleotide inhibition of kinase activity.

Perhaps the most carefully controlled example of a physiologically significant direct oligonucleotide/protein interaction is a report by Bock et al.[41] describing identification of a consensus 15-base sequence capable of inhibiting thrombin activity. This sequence was identified by screening a random library containing approximately 10^{13} oligonucleotides. The consensus sequence, at 100 nM concentration, was able to increase clotting time nearly seven-fold, while a scrambled sequence was without effect. Thus, as in the example of $p210^{bcr\text{-}abl}$, although thrombin has at least two anion binding sites, electrostatic interactions cannot be solely responsible for the inhibitory effects observed.

IX. PHOSPHOROTHIOATE OLIGONUCLEOTIDES CAN INHIBIT ADHESION

Several groups have demonstrated an inhibitory effect of Ps oligonucleotides on cellular adhesion.[42-45] Watson, Pon, and Shiu[42] first reported that a Ps oligonucleotide targeting the c-myc oncogene inhibited the adhesion of MCF7 breast cancer cells.[42] This effect appeared to be sequence-specific, since the sense oligonucleotide and another irrelevant antisense oligonucleotide were without effect. However, the effect was not mediated via an antisense mechanism, since the authors could not demonstrate any alteration in either c-myc mRNA or protein.

More recently, Yaswen et al.[43] reported similar findings with a Ps c-myc antisense oligonucleotide and other Ps sequences. These authors extended the work of Watson, Pon, and Shiu[42] by making the observation that all oligonucleotides which inhibited adhesion had in common a so-called dG quartet, that is a motif of four contiguous guanosine residues, embedded in the overall sequence. They suggested that Ps oligonucleotides containing a dG quartet could somehow be inhibitory to cellular adhesion through undefined non-antisense mechanisms.

However, Maltese et al.[45] have found that sequences surrounding the dG quartet motif also contribute to an oligonucleotide's anti-adhesive properties, making the dG quartet essential, but not sufficient, for adhesion inhibition. Recent results of Chavany et al.[44] complicate the situation even further. These investigators found that both sequence and phosphorothioate content contribute to anti-adhesion phenomena. Working with the same c-myc antisense oligonucleotide as Watson, Pon, and Shiu,[42] and Yaswen et al.,[43] they observed no sequence specificity to the anti-adhesion effect if Ps oligonucleotides were used. As one might expect, oligonucleotides containing a dG quartet were more inhibitory to adhesion than were oligonucleotides lacking this motif. However, several oligonucleotides which did or did not contain a dG motif were equally inhibitory on cell growth in a sequence-nonspecific fashion.

In contrast, when the phosphorothioate content of these oligonucleotides was reduced to 53% (by capping the oligonucleotide on either end with phosphorothioate linkages but leaving the remainder of the molecule unmodified), a sequence-specific anti-adhesive effect became apparent. The c-myc antisense sequence was strongly anti-adhesive, but none of the control sequences were adhesive. Controls included dG quartet-containing oligonucleotides, including a 2-base mismatched antisense oligonucleotide. Thus, in these experiments, completely phosphorothioating the oligonucleotides masked a c-myc antisense sequence-specific anti-adhesive effect for which a dG quartet alone was not sufficient.

These results are in keeping with the findings of Brown et al.,[46] who recently reported strong and rather promiscuous intracellular protein binding by phosphorothioate oligonucleotides. These authors found that sequence-independent protein binding of Ps oligonucleotides was directly proportional to the degree of Ps content of the oligonucleotides. As in the study of Chavany et al.,[44] the authors found that reducing the Ps content of an oligonucleotide was sufficient to restore its sequence-specific protein interactions (i.e., sequence-specific double-stranded oligonucleotide interactions with transcription factors).

However, the anti-adhesive properties of the c-myc antisense oligonucleotide reported by Chavany et al.[44] are not mediated via antisense effects on c-myc because (1) washing pre-treated cells free of extracellular oligonucleotide completely abolished the effect without reversing the inhibition of c-myc protein and (2) addition of treated cells to fibronectin-coated culture dishes also abolished the effect without interfering in inhibition of c-myc protein. Also, neither unmodified phosphodiester oligonucleotides nor phosphoramidate-modified oligonucleotides were found to be anti-adhesive, although antisense effects toward c-myc could still be demonstrated.

X. DO SUITABLE CONTROLS EXIST FOR ANTISENSE EXPERIMENTS?

Given these examples of sequence-specific and nonspecific non-antisense effects of oligonucleotides, one must re-address the question of controls. At the beginning of this article we listed several proposals for appropriate controls made by the editors of the journal *Antisense Research and Development.* These included a sense control, a scrambled control, and a mismatch control.

The previous discussion has pointed out that sense and scrambled controls may not contain biologically active motifs found in the antisense sequence. At the same time, mismatch oligonucleotides, depending on their overall length, may not control for hybridization specificity. In addition, the relative position of mismatches within an oligonucleotide sequence is critical to loss of activity.[9,45] While a single mismatch nucleotide can in some cases abolish antisense activity, in many cases even several mismatches fail to abrogate activity.[45] The success or failure of mismatches in abrogating antisense activity is completely contextual, and no rules can be codified as to the proper method of choosing which bases to mismatch. Indeed, it is our opinion that each and every oligonucleotide be considered a unique drug, for which no ideal control exists. Thus, even those antisense experiments which apply the most stringent conditions to validate activity cannot unequivocally demonstrate that antisense is the sole mechanism mediating a given biological phenomenon.

XI. CONCLUSIONS

Although antisense inhibition in the absence of other activities may be difficult, if not impossible, to achieve, one should not ignore the ability of certain novel backbone-containing oligonucleotides to interact with proteins as well as RNA (and DNA). Chemically modified oligonucleotides represent a unique class of recombinatorial drugs whose true potential has yet to be fully realized.

REFERENCES

1. Weintraub, H. M., Antisense RNA and DNA, *Sci. Am.*, 262, 40, 1990.
2. Inouye, M., Antisense RNA: Its functions and applications in gene regulation — a review, *Gene*, 72, 25, 1988.
3. Kochbin, S. and Lawrence, J. J., An antisense RNA involved in p53 mRNA maturation in murine erythroleukemia cells induced to differentiate, *EMBO J.*, 8, 4107, 1989.
4. Krystal, G. W., Armstrong, B. C., and Battey, J. F., N-myc mRNA forms an RNA-RNA duplex with endogenous antisense transcripts, *Mol. Cell. Biol.*, 10, 4180, 1990.
5. Izant, J. G. and Weintraub, H., Constitutive and conditional suppression of exogenous and endogenous genes by anti-sense RNA, *Science*, 229, 345, 1985.
6. Zamecnik, P. C. and Stephenson, M. L., Inhibition of Rous sarcoma virus replication and cell transformation by a specific oligodeoxynucleotide, *Proc. Natl. Acad. Sci. U.S.A.*, 75, 280, 1978.
7. Izant, J. G. and Weintraub, H., Inhibition of thymidine kinase gene expression by antisense RNA: A molecular approach to genetic analyses, *Cell*, 36, 1007, 1984.
8. Stein, C. A. and Krieg, A. M., Problems in interpretation of data derived from *in vitro* and *in vivo* use of antisense oligodeoxynucleotides, *Antisense Res. Dev.*, 4, 67, 1994.
9. Woolf, T. M., Melton, D. A., and Jennings, C. G. B., Specificity of antisense oligonucleotides *in vivo*, *Proc. Natl. Acad. Sci. U.S.A.*, 89, 7305, 1992.
10. Shuttleworth, J., Matthews, G., Dale, L., Baker, C., and Colman, A., Antisense oligodeoxyribonucleotide-directed cleavage of maternal mRNA in *Xenopus* oocytes and embryos, *Gene*, 72, 267, 1988.
11. Chang, E. H., Miller, P. S., Cushman, C., Devadas, K., Pirollo, K. F., Ts'o, P. O. P., and Yu, Z. P., Antisense inhibition of ras p21 expression that is sensitive to a point mutation, *Biochemistry*, 30, 8283, 1991.
12. Kuramoto, E., Yano, O., Kimura, Y., Baba, M., Makino, T., Yamamoto, S., Yamamoto, T., Kataoka, T., and Tokunaga, T., Oligonucleotide sequences required for natural killer cell activation, *Jpn. J. Cancer Res.*, 83, 1128, 1992.
13. Yamamoto, S., Yamamoto, T., Kataoka, T., Kuramoto, E., Yano, O., and Tokunaga, T., Unique palindromic sequences in synthetic oligonucleotides are required to induce INF and augment INF-mediated natural killer activity, *J. Immunol.*, 148, 4072, 1992.

14. Tokunaga, T., Yano, O., Kuramoto, E., Kimura, Y., Yamamoto, T., Kataoka, T., and Yamamoto, S., Synthetic oligonucleotides with particular base sequences from the cDNA encoding proteins of *Mycobacterium bovis* BCG induce interferons and activate natural killer cells, *Microbiol. Immunol.*, 36, 55, 1992.
15. Tokunaga, T., Yamamoto, H., Shimada, S., Abe, H., Fukuda, T., Fujisawa, Y., Furutani, Y., Yano, O., Kataoka, T., Sudo, T., Makiguchi, N., and Suganuma, T., Antitumor activity of deoxyribonucleic acid fraction from *Mycobacterium bovis* GCG. I. Isolation, physicochemical characterization, and antitumor activity, *J. Natl. Cancer Inst.*, 72, 955, 1984.
16. Shimada, S., Yano, O., Inoue, H., Kuramoto, E., Fukuda, T., Yamamoto, H., Kataoka, T., and Tokunaga, T., Antitumor activity of the DNA fraction from *Mycobacterium bovis* BCG. II. Effects on various syngeneic mouse tumors, *J. Natl. Cancer Inst.*, 74, 681, 1985.
17. Krieg, A. M., Yi, A.-K., Matson, S., Waldschmidt, T. J., Bishop, G. A., Teasdale, R., Koretsky, G. A., and Klinman, D. M., CpG motifs in bacterial DNA trigger direct B-cell activation, *Nature*, 374, 546, 1995.
18. McIntyre, K. W., Lombard-Gillooly, K., Perez, J. R., Kunsch, C., Sarmiento, U. M., Larigan, J. D., Landreth, K. T., and Narayanan, R., A sense phosphorothioate oligonucleotide directed to the initiation codon of transcription factor NF-kB p65 causes sequence-specific immune stimulation, *Antisense Res. Dev.*, 3, 309, 1993.
19. Matson, S. and Krieg, A. M., Nonspecific suppression of [^{3}H]thymidine incorporation by "control" oligonucleotides, *Antisense Res. Dev.*, 2, 325, 1992.
20. Neckers, L., Whitesell, L., Rosolen, A., and Geselowitz, D., Antisense inhibition of gene expression, *Crit. Rev. Oncogen.*, 3, 175, 1992.
21. Blagosklonny, M. V. and Neckers, L. M., Oligonucleotides protect cells from the cytotoxicity of several anti-cancer chemotherapeutic drugs, *Anti-Cancer Drugs*, 5, 437, 1994.
22. Stull, R. A., Zon, G., and Szoka, F. C., Single-stranded phosphodiester and phosphorothioate oligonucleotides bind actinomycin D and interfere with tumor necrosis factor-induced lysis in the L929 cytotoxicity assay, *Antisense Res. Dev.*, 3, 295, 1993.
23. Wadkins, R. M. and Jovin, T. M., Actinomycin D and 7-aminoactinomycin D binding to single-stranded DNA, *Biochemistry*, 30, 9469, 1991.
24. Whitesell, L., Geselowitz, D., Chavany, C., Fahmy, B., Walbridge, S., Alger, J. R., and Neckers, L. M., Stability, clearance and disposition of intraventricularly administered oligodeoxynucleotides — implications for therapeutic application within the central nervous system, *Proc. Natl. Acad. Sci. U.S.A.*, 90, 4665, 1993.
25. Ogawa, S., Brown, H. E., Okano, H. J., and Pfaff, D. W., Cellular uptake of intracerebrally administered oligodeoxynucleotides in mouse brain, *Regul. Pept.*, 59, 143, 1995.
26. Akhtar, S., Kole, R., and Juliano, R. L., Stability of antisense DNA oligodeoxynucleotide analogs in cellular extracts and sera, *Life Sci.*, 49, 1793, 1991.
27. Iverson, P. L., Zhu, S., Meyer, A., and Zon, G., Cellular uptake and subcellular distribution of phosphorothioate oligonucleotides into cultured cells, *Antisense Res. Dev.*, 2, 211, 1992.
28. Campbell, J. M., Bacon, T. A., and Wickstrom, E., Oligodeoxynucleotide phosphorothioate stability in subcellular extracts, culture media, serum and cerebrospinal fluid, *J. Biochem. Biophys. Methods*, 20, 259, 1990.
29. Cazenave, C., Stein, C. A., Loreau, N., Thuong, N. T., Neckers, L. M., Subasinghe, C., Helene, C., Cohen, J. S., and Toulme, J.-J., Comparative inhibition of rabbit globin mRNA translation by modified antisense oligodeoxynucleotides, *Nucleic Acids Res.*, 17, 4255, 1989.
30. Wellstein, A., Zugmaier, G., Califano, J., Kern, F., Paik, S., and Lippman, M., Tumor growth dependent on Kaposi's sarcoma-derived fibroblast growth factor inhibited by pentosan polysulfate, *J. Natl. Cancer Inst.*, 83, 716, 1991.
31. Zugmaier, G., Lippman, M., and Wellstein, A., Inhibition by pentosan polysulfate (PPS) of heparin-binding growth factors released from tumor cells and blockage by PPS of tumor cell growth in animals, *J. Natl. Cancer Inst.*, 84, 1716, 1993.
32. Yakubov, L., Khaled, Z., Zhang, L.-M., Truneh, A., Vlassov, V., and Stein, C. A., Mode of interaction of oligodeoxynucleotides with recombinant sCD4, *J. Biol. Chem.*, 268, 18818, 1993.
33. Maury, G., Alaoui, A. E., Morvan, F., Muller, B., Imbach, J.-L., and Goody, R. S., Template-Phosphorothioate oligonucleotide duplexes as inhibitors of HIV-1 reverse transcriptase, *Biochem. Biophys. Res. Commun.*, 186, 1249, 1992.
34. Stein, C. A., Cleary, A., Yakubov, L., and Lederman, S., Phosphorothioate oligodeoxynucleotides bind to the third variable loop domain (V3) of HIV-1 gp120, *Antisense Res. Dev.*, 3, 19, 1993.
35. Gao, W.-Y., Han, F.-S., Storm, C., Egan, W., and Cheng, Y.-C., Phosphorothioate oligonucleotides are inhibitors of human DNA polymerases and RNase H: Implications for antisense technology, *Mol. Pharmacol.*, 41, 223, 1992.

36. Stein, C. A., Tonkinson, J. L., Zhang, L.-M., Yakubov, L., Gervasoni, J., Taub, R., and Rotenberg, S. A., Dynamics of the internalization of phosphodiester oligodeoxynucleotides in HL60 cells, *Biochemistry*, 32, 4855, 1993.
37. Perez, J. R., Li, Y., Stein, C. A., Majumder, S., Oorschot, A. V., and Narayanan, R., Sequence-independent induction of Sp1 transcription factor activity by phosphorothioate oligodeoxynucleotides, *Proc. Natl. Acad. Sci. U.S.A.*, 91, 5957, 1994.
38. Teasdale, R. M., Matson, S. J., Fisher, E., and Krieg, A. M., Inhibition of T4 polynucleotide kinase activity by phosphorothioate and chimeric oligodeoxynucleotides, *Antisense Res. Dev.*, 4, 295, 1994.
39. Bergan, R., Connell, Y., Fahmy, B., Kyle, E., and Neckers, L., Aptameric inhibition of $p210^{bcr\text{-}abl}$ tyrosine kinase autophosphorylation by oligodeoxynucleotides of defined sequence and backbone structure, *Nucleic Acids Res.*, 22, 2150, 1994.
40. Bergan, R. C., Kyle, E., Connell, Y., and Neckers, L., Inhibition of protein tyrosine kinase activity in intact cells by the aptameric action of oligodeoxynucleotides, *Antisense Res. Dev.*, 5, 33, 1995.
41. Bock, L. C., Griffin, L. C., Latham, J. A., Vermass, E. H., and Toole, J. J., Selection of single-stranded DNA molecules that bind and inhibit human thrombin, *Nature*, 355, 564, 1992.
42. Watson, P. H., Pon, R. T., and Shiu, R. P. C., Inhibition of cell adhesion to plastic substratum by phosphorothioate oligonucleotide, *Exp. Cell Res.*, 202, 391, 1992.
43. Yaswen, P., Stampfer, M. R., Ghosh, K., and Cohen, J. S. Effects of sequence of thioated oligonucleotides on cultured human mammary epithelial cells, *Antisense Res. Dev.*, 3, 67, 1993.
44. Chavany, C., Connell, Y., and Neckers, L., Contribution of sequence and phosphorothioate content to inhibition of cell growth and adhesion caused by c-myc antisense oligomers, *Mol. Pharmacol.*, 48, 738, 1995.
45. Maltese, J.-Y., Sharma, H. W., Vassilev, L., and Narayanan, R., Sequence context of antisense RelA/NF-kB phosphorothioates determines specificity, *Nucleic Acids Res.*, 23, 1146, 1995.
46. Brown, D. A., Kang, S.-H., Gryaznov, S. M., DeDionisio, L., Heidenreich, O., Sullivan, S., Xu, X., and Nerenberg, M. I., Effect of phosphorothioate modification of oligodeoxynucleotides on specific protein binding, *J. Biol. Chem.*, 269, 26801, 1994.

Chapter 5

Use of Antisense Oligodeoxynucleotides to Modulate Reproductive Behavior

Margaret M. McCarthy

CONTENTS

0-8493-8552-0/97/$0.00+$.50

I. INTRODUCTION

In theory, a small synthetic stretch of DNA (~13 to 22 nucleotides) designed to be complementary to a specific mRNA will selectively hybridize to this target and block its translation into protein. Two mechanisms of action predominate: hybridization arrest of translation by disruption of normal ribosomal functioning and activation of RNase H nuclease activity to degrade the hybridized mRNA. It is unlikely that antisense oligodeoxynucleotides (oligos) will act exclusively in this highly selective manner, and the potential for alternative mechanisms exists. Nonetheless, the *in vivo* use of antisense oligos to manipulate gene expression has proved a valuable and informative tool in behavioral neuroscience. Issues regarding experimental design, characteristics of the oligos, and appropriate use of controls have all been extensively reviewed and will not be considered further.[1-3] The purpose of this discussion will be to focus in detail on the collection of studies that have used antisense oligos to assess the neural control of reproductive behavior.

The use of antisense oligo technology in the analysis of female reproductive behavior has been particularly advantageous due to three inherent characteristics: (1) the behavior is induced by steroid hormones, (2) it is stimulus evoked, and (3) it is readily quantifiable. Female reproductive behavior has two phases, sexual behavior and maternal behavior. Each of these phases can be further subdivided into individual components. Sexual behavior consists of both proceptive and receptive responses. Proceptivity, broadly defined, is a collection of behaviors exhibited by the female to both elicit interest from the male and control aspects of the mating interaction.[4] For example, a female will use a combination of hopping and darting movements to advertise her state of sexual receptivity to specific males. Once a mating interaction begins, the female will regulate the timing of each mating bout by breaking away from the male and returning when she chooses. This behavioral phenomena, referred to as "pacing," is of physiological significance to the female on several levels.[5] In general, the proceptive behaviors are considered to reflect motivational components of sexual behavior. This is as opposed to the receptive component of sexual behavior, which in female rodents is called lordosis and is more in the nature of a reflex. The term lordosis refers to a stereotypical posture adopted by the female in response to somatosensory stimulation of the flanks and perineal region. This posture consists of arching of the back, elevation of the rump, and deflection of the tail and is required for the male to gain intromission into the vagina (Figure 1). The somatosensory stimulation that induces the reflex is provided by the male at the beginning of mounting. The neural circuitry as well as the neurochemistry regulating this complex behavioral reflex has been the topic of intensive investigation.[6]

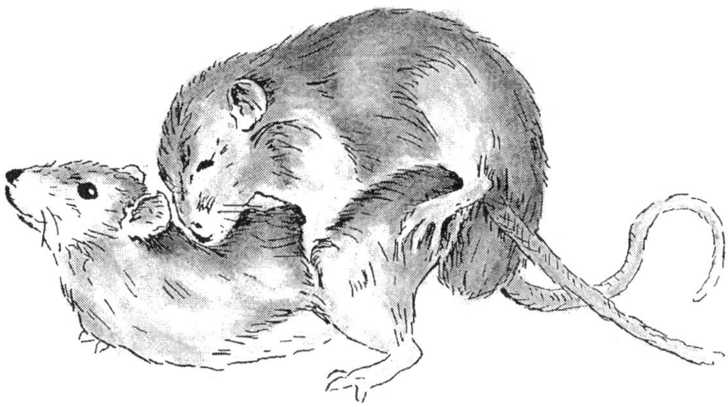

FIGURE 1
Illustration of the lordosis posture of the female rat. As a result of steroid hormone action in the brain, a receptive female rat exhibits lordosis in response to somatosensory stimulation from the male. The response is characterized by elevation of the head and rump and deflection of the tail. Many aspects of this behavior are reflexive in nature. (Redrawn from Barnett, S. S., *The Rat: A Study in Behavior,* Aldine Publishing, Chicago, IL, 1963.)

Maternal behavior also has several components. A simple division can be made in behaviors directed toward the pups vs. those directed toward other animals. Behaviors directed toward the pups include nest building, retrieving of the pups to the nest, crouching over the pups during feeding bouts, and grooming the pups to induce urination and defecation. Maternal aggression is considered a discrete form of aggression under unique neuroendocrine control and is only transiently expressed. When females stop lactating, maternal aggression dissipates. As with sexual behavior, a great deal is known about the neural circuitry and neurochemistry of maternal behavior. The induction of an intense aggression toward intruders into the nest area is a second specific aspect of maternal behavior.[7]

One of most important identifying features of reproductive behavior is steroid-hormone dependence. While female rats can be induced to show some components of maternal behavior with continuous exposure to pups during a process called sensitization, the normal induction of this behavior is the result of increasing estrogen levels followed by precipitous progesterone withdrawal. The induction of sexual behavior also requires sequential exposure to estrogen and progesterone, although the intensity and frequency of the behavior is highest when progesterone levels are also high. The dose and temporal aspects of steroid hormone induction of reproductive behavior are well characterized and this can be of considerable advantage when designing experiments involving antisense technology. As opposed to other hormonally modulated behaviors, such as aggression or anxiety, reproductive behavior is hormonally induced and this induction is temporary. For example, sexual behavior of naturally cycling animals is expressed during a 12- to 18-h period during each estrous cycle. The onset of maternal behavior is at the very end of gestation and will wane with the increasing development of the pups, only to be reinstated during the next pregnancy.

This behavioral plasticity induced by steroid hormones is dependent on the steroids binding to and activating their intracellular receptor. The activated receptor functions as a transcription factor to regulate gene expression.The induction of gene expression by steroid receptors is a key link in the chain of events leading to behavioral responses. The steroid receptors themselves are the transducers of peripheral endocrine profiles to changes in neuronal activity. Both the transducers (steroid receptors) and the effectors (neurotransmitters) have been the target of antisense oligo-mediated inhibition. This review will begin with a discussion of studies focused on steroid receptors, followed by those involving individual neurotransmitter systems.

II. ANTISENSE OLIGONUCLEOTIDES DIRECTED AGAINST STEROID RECEPTORS

A. Estrogen Receptor

1. *Effects of Antisense Oligos to Estrogen Receptor mRNA during Development*

The paramount importance of estrogen in reproductive behavior begins with its critical role in the differentiation of the developing brain. In rodents, gonadal steroids act on the brain during a critical or sensitive period to alter permanently the neuronal cytoarchitecture and patterns of synaptic connectivity in a process known as masculinization. This sensitive period begins with a surge of testosterone production by the embryonic testis of the male at gestational day 18. Circulating testosterone levels remain elevated until birth (day 22) and decline thereafter. It has been clearly established that testosterone gains access to the brain and serves as a substrate for the enzyme, P450 aromatase, which converts it to estrogen. It is estrogen that then induces masculine differentiation of the brain. The sensitivity of the brain to this masculinization process gradually decreases and ends by about postnatal day 10. If a female pup is given exogenous testosterone, her brain will also be masculinized and this is often referred to as androgenization. In adulthood, neonatally steroid-exposed animals will show male typical patterns of sexual behavior and gonadotropin secretion. If females are not treated with testosterone or if males are either neonatally castrated or treated with an aromatase inhibitor, they will exhibit female-typical behavior in adulthood. These early effects of steroids on the brain are essentially permanent and determine the steroid-responsiveness of the adult brain, a paradigm known as the organizational-activational hypothesis of steroid action. A consequence of this is that when adult males and females are given exogenous estrogen, only females will exhibit proceptive and receptive sexual behavior. By contrast, if adult males and females are treated with testosterone, only males will display stereotypical mounting and pelvic thrusting toward sexually receptive females.[8]

Steroid hormones exert their effect by binding to an intracellular receptor that translocates to the nucleus and interacts with the genome to alter gene activity. In other words, steroid receptors are transcription factors. However, steroids have been shown to exert effects independent of the genome, and growing evidence supports the concept of membrane-mediated steroid actions. One of the challenges in behavioral neuroendocrinology is differentiating between classic genomic steroid action and fast acting, membrane-mediated effects. Antisense technology has been useful in this endeavor. Substantial circumstantial evidence indicated that estrogen-mediated sexual differentiation of the brain was due to classical estrogen receptor action at the level of the genome. However, many of the strategies to distinguish genomic from membrane-mediated steroid effects that are used in the adult (see below) are not appropriate in the neonate. Therefore, antisense oligos directed against estrogen receptor mRNA was employed to address this issue.[9]

The experimental design was as follows. Male and female 3-day-old pups received a single intracerebral injection of either estrogen receptor antisense oligo, scrambled oligo, or vehicle. The oligos were unmodified, given at a dose of 2 μg, and were suspended in sesame oil. This dose and method of administration was well tolerated by the pups, with close to 100% survival. Half of the males were castrated at the same time as receiving the oligo injection. Half of the females were androgenized with a single injection of testosterone propionate (50 μg) given 6 h after the oligo infusion. The rationale for this time course was to allow the antisense oligos to gain access to the cell and hybridize with the estrogen receptor mRNA before testosterone was administered and aromatized to estrogen. The growth and development of the treated pups were closely monitored and no unusual patterns were observed. In adulthood, all the females were ovariectomized and treated with sequential estrogen plus progesterone before being tested for lordosis behavior. As predicted, the normal females showed very high levels of lordosis responding, and neonatal treatment with antisense to the estrogen receptor was without effect. Also as predicted, the androgenized females that had received control infusions (scrambled oligo or vehicle) showed low to nonexistent lordosis responding. However, the androgenized females that had received antisense oligo to the estrogen receptor showed significantly higher levels of lordosis responding, indicating that they had been partially protected from the masculinizing effect of neonatal testosterone administration (Figure 2). Wheel running is also a sexually differentiated behavior, and females will respond to estrogen treatment in adulthood with increased time spent running on a wheel. These animals were also tested for their sensitivity to estrogen-induced wheel running, and the data were again consistent with a protective effect of neonatal treatment with antisense oligos against the estrogen receptor. There was again no effect of antisense oligo treatment on normal females in this paradigm either. However, when we tested the same animals for the effects of estrogen on open field behavior, an indicator of endogenous anxiety levels, only the normal females showed an effect of antisense oligo treatment. A conclusion reached from these data is that masculinization of the brain in terms of sexual behavior and wheel running is mediated by the estrogen receptor. The data further suggest that the sexual differentiation of endogenous anxiety levels is also mediated by the estrogen receptor, but it involves an action in the female brain in the absence of testosterone.[9]

Sexual behavior was also tested in adult males that had been neonatally treated with antisense oligos. While sexual behavior was not completely disrupted, there were some significant differences. Gonadally intact adult males were tested on three separate occasions for ten minutes with a sexually receptive female. On the first trial, antisense-treated males had significantly longer latencies to the first mount, but by the third test it was significantly shorter compared to males in the other groups. However, a more indicative measure of the quality of male sexual behavior is the mount-to-intromission ratio. Higher performing males are more adept at gaining an intromission with each mount, and this is a parameter that improves with experience. In this experiment, the mount-to-intromission ratio significantly improved for the scrambled oligo and vehicle treated animals, as would be expected, but did not

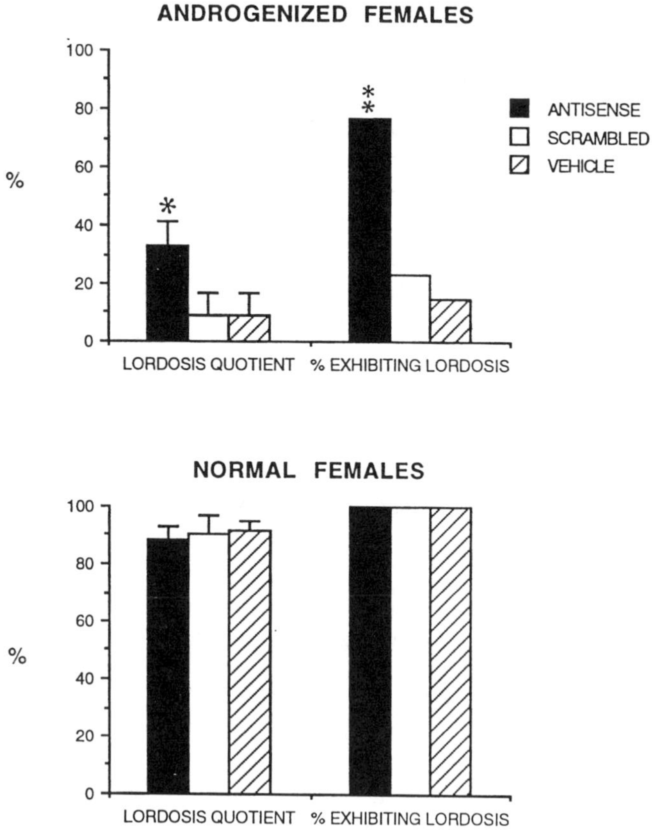

FIGURE 2
Three-day-old female rats received intracerebral infusions of either estrogen receptor antisense oligo, scrambled control oligo, or vehicle. Half the females were injected 6 h later with testosterone (ANDROGENIZED) or left untreated (NORMAL). In adulthood the females were ovariectomized and treated with estrogen and progesterone in a regimen known to induce a high level of lordosis responding. Normal females were unaffected by the neonatal oligo infusions. Androgenized females showed significantly reduced to absent female sexual behavior, unless they had been infused neonatally with antisense oligos to estrogen receptor mRNA (*p <0.05; ANOVA, **p <0.01; χ^2). These data demonstrate a protective effect of estrogen receptor antisense on masculinization of the brain, an effect known to be mediated by estrogen receptors. (From McCarthy, M. M., Schlenker, E. H., Pfaff, D. W., *Endocrinology*, 133, 433–439, 1993. ©The Endocrine Society, with permission.)

increase for the antisense oligo-treated males (Figure 3; McCarthy, Schlenker, and Pfaff, unpublished data). Thus, it appears that some aspects of the normal development of male sexual behavior had been disrupted by neonatal treatment with antisense oligos to the estrogen receptor.

At completion of the behavioral experiments, the animals were sacrificed and the brains collected for histological examination. The sexually dimorphic nucleus of the preoptic area (SDN-POA) is a sensitive marker for perinatal estrogen exposure. This collection of densely stained neurons within the medial preoptic nucleus is some five to seven times larger in males than females, and this volume difference appears to be entirely a function of the degree of estrogen exposure during the critical period.[10] Volumetric analysis indicated that the SDN was increased in androgenized females as compared to control females, except in androgenized females that were infused with antisense oligos to the estrogen receptor. In these animals the SDN volume was equal in size to that of normal females. Importantly, an additional

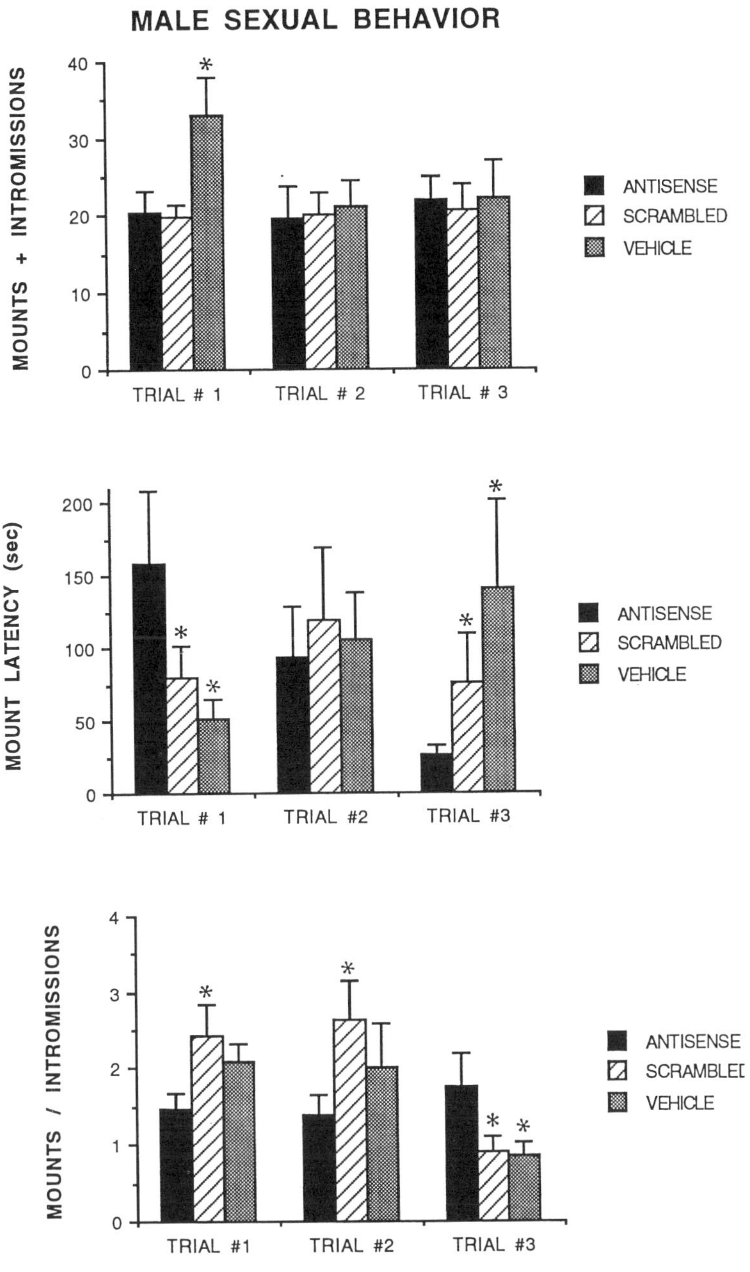

FIGURE 3
Three-day-old male rats received intracerebral infusions of either estrogen receptor antisense oligo, scrambled control oligo, or vehicle. In adulthood, they were tested for sexual behavior with hormonally primed stimulus females. Tests were conducted on three alternate days. On the first trial, antisense oligo-infused males had significantly longer mount latencies and lower mount-to-intromission ratios than control males. By the third trial, antisense oligo-infused males had shorter latencies to first mount but no improvement in the mount-to-intromission ratio. The latter measure is considered an indicator of the quality of male sexual behavior, and these data demonstrate that neonatal exposure to estrogen receptor antisense oligos interfered with the improvement in quality seen in control males, suggesting suboptimal masculinization (*p <0.05, ANOVA, McCarthy, M. M., Schlenker, E. H., and Pfaff, D. W., unpublished data).

nucleus in a region adjacent to the SDN, the parastrial nucleus, was found to be larger in the antisense-treated androgenized females. This would be predicted given that this nucleus is usually larger in females than males. The gonadally intact males did not show any effect of antisense treatment on SDN volume, but males that had been neonatally castrated did show a significant reduction if they had received an antisense infusion.

Taken together, these data offer definitive proof that estrogen acts on the brain during the critical period via its intracellular receptor. Furthermore, these findings contribute to evidence that different behavioral responses have distinct critical periods and hormone mediation. These data also demonstrate the feasibility of using antisense oligos during critical developmental windows and suggest that it might be particularly useful for questions regarding sexual differentiation of the brain.

2. *Effects of Antisense Oligos to Estrogen Receptor mRNA in the Adult*

At least three factors lead to the prediction that antisense oligos against estrogen receptor mRNA would be effective at reducing lordosis in adult females. These include the fact that (1) lordosis is absolutely dependent on estrogen exposure, (2) estrogen action restricted to the ventromedial nucleus (VMN) of the hypothalamus is sufficient to induce lordosis, and (3) antisense oligos against estrogen receptor mRNA work in neonates. Therefore, it was surprising that we found daily administration of phosphorothioated estrogen receptor oligos to be only weakly effective at reducing lordosis in females with subcutaneous estradiol capsules. Furthermore, the estrogen receptor antisense was completely ineffective in females that were primed with estrogen and progesterone (Figure 4; McCarthy and Mobbs, unpublished data), and there was no effect on estrogen-induced increases in oxytocin receptor binding.

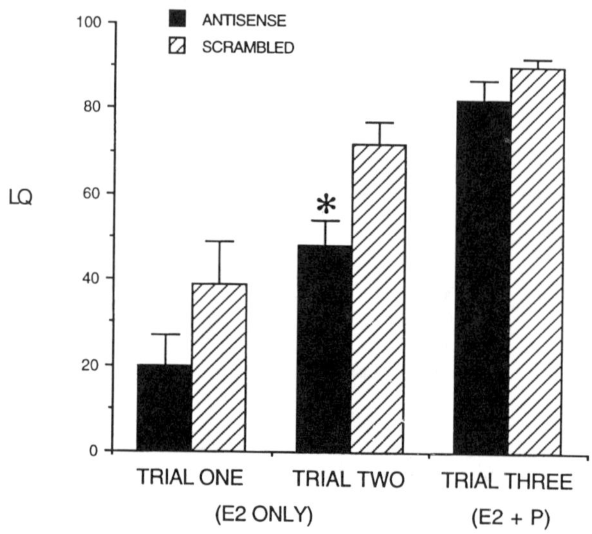

FIGURE 4
Estrogen-treated ovariectomized female rats bearing indwelling cannula aimed at the VMN were infused daily with antisense oligos to estrogen receptor mRNA. After two weeks of daily infusions, they were tested for sexual behavior with a stimulus male on three consecutive days. The data are expressed as a lordosis quotient (LQ), the percent of lordoses responses given to 10 mounts from the male. The behavioral tests on day one and two were done under conditions of E2 only. On the third day, they were injected with progesterone 4 h (E2 + P) prior to the behavioral test. Although there was significantly lower lordosis responding on the second trial (*$p < 0.05$, ANOVA), the effect was relatively weak given the importance of estrogen receptor to the induction of female sexual behavior. Furthermore, there was no difference between treatments when the females were injected with progesterone (McCarthy, M. M. and Mobbs, C. V., unpublished data).

The explanation for this lack of effect remains unclear. It is unlikely that the dose was insufficient as we gave daily infusions of phosphorothioated oligos for two consecutive weeks. Given the long half-life of these modified oligos,[2] the cumulative dose by the day of testing should have been quite large. There was no evidence of toxicity as all the animals showed very high to maximum levels of responding. Perhaps the explanation lies in the nature of the expression of the estrogen receptor gene. Estrogen is known to downregulate the expression of its own receptor.[11] As will be discussed further, there is increasing evidence that the most recently synthesized proteins are of the greatest significance to the cell. If the youngest estrogen receptors are the most potent at downregulation of estrogen receptor mRNA synthesis, antisense oligo disruption of translation might block the feedback pathway so that transcription of the estrogen receptor gene is maintained, or even increased. In this way, the cell might escape from antisense-mediated inhibition so that sufficient estrogen receptor protein is produced. Given that estrogen receptor activation mediates a cascade of responses that amplifies the initial event, estrogen binding, a little estrogen receptor may go a long way. This still begs the question of why the same antisense construct was effective in the neonatal brain, especially given that evidence suggests the same type of negative feedback exists in the newborn.[12] One possibility is that antisense oligos are more efficacious in the neonatal brain due to elevated RNase H activity,[13] resulting in degradation of the mRNA. Several studies have indicated a lack of RNase H activity as a major mechanism mediating antisense action in the adult brain, and this may be an important limiting factor in some systems.

B. Progesterone Receptor

As discussed previously, distinguishing between genomic and membrane-mediated steroid hormone effects is a constant challenge in behavioral neuroendocrinology. This has been especially true in the case of determining the influence of progesterone on female sexual behavior. Evidence has persisted that progesterone and/or its metabolites, acting at the neuronal membrane, may be an important mechanism in regulating behavior. Establishing a membrane-mediated progesterone action in the control of lordosis by female rats has proved elusive. However, the use of antisense oligos against the progesterone receptor has provided conclusive evidence for the importance of this intracellular receptor in the regulation of behavior. Three separate groups have reported significant inhibition of receptivity and proceptivity by antisense oligos to the progesterone receptor.[14-16] They have also reported reductions in progesterone receptor protein when assessed by immunocytochemistry,[15] *in vitro* exchange assay,[14] and enzymatic immunoassay in a T47D cell line.[16] It is notable that in no case was the magnitude of reduction of protein equal to the magnitude of the reduction in behavior. For example, a complete abolishment of lordosis responding was seen in females in which progesterone receptor binding was only reduced by 52%. This was in spite of the fact that estrogen treatment increased progesterone receptor binding by 161%, suggesting that the residual 80% increase in progesterone receptor binding was not sufficient to maintain any level of receptivity.[14]

Several factors were found to contribute to the efficacy of antisense oligos in these studies. Mani et al.[14] reported in a dose-response study with 0.8 and 1.6 nmol reducing behavior by 50% and 4 nmol reducing receptivity close to 100% (~260 ng; Figure 5). These investigators also used a 20-mer phosphorothioated antisense specific to the rat progesterone receptor A form. This may have contributed to the greater effect compared to the other studies which used either an 18-mer specific to the chicken progesterone receptor B-form[16] or a 15-mer specific to the rabbit B-form of

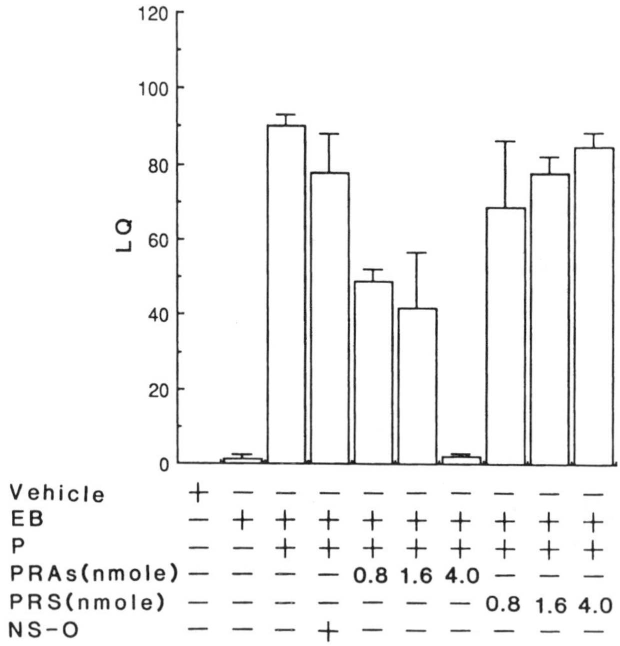

FIGURE 5
Adult ovariectomized rats were infused intraventricularly with varying doses of progesterone receptor antisense oligos (PRAs), progesterone receptor sense oligos (PRS), or nonspecific oligos (NS-O) at the same time they were primed with estrogen, and again 24 h later. They were tested for lordosis quotient (LQ) responding 3 h after progesterone. There was an almost 100% inhibition of lordosis in females receiving the highest dose of PRAs. (From Mani, S. K., Blaustein, J. D., Allen, J. M. C., Law, S. W., O'Malley, B. W., and Clark, J. H., *Endocrinology*, 135, 1409–1414, 1994. ©The Endocrine Society, with permission.)

the progesterone receptor.[15] All three studies used antisense constructs that spanned the translation initiation codon. In fact, a comparison of several constructs found this to be the only effective antisense oligo for reducing progesterone receptor protein.[16] The timing of antisense administration also proved a critical variable in all three studies. A single infusion given 12 h after estrogen treatment effectively reduced lordosis,[15,16] but single infusions at 0 h or 24 h after estrogen were not.[14,15] However, the combination of infusions at 0 and 24 h was extremely effective.[14] This timing schedule agrees well with the observation that estrogen induction of progesterone receptor mRNA is maximal at 24 h.[17]

Antisense to the progesterone receptor has also been used to help elucidate a novel mechanism by which progesterone receptor can facilitate lordosis. The neurotransmitter dopamine was found to activate the progesterone receptor in the absence of progesterone, presumably via phosphorylation of the receptor itself or a specific transcription cofactor.[18] In order to establish a physiological significance to this observation, progesterone receptor synthesis was blocked by infusion of antisense oligos to animals that were also infused intracerebroventricularly (i.c.v.) with specific dopamine receptor agonists and antagonists. Antisense to progesterone receptor reduced lordosis induced by either progesterone or the dopamine agonist, apomorphine, and to a selective D1 receptor agonist. These experiments confirmed that a reduction of progesterone receptor concentration by ~50% revealed a critical threshold that is essential for both progesterone and dopamine to induce lordosis.[19] More importantly, these data reveal a regulation of gene expression by means of cross-talk between membrane receptors for neurotransmitters and intracellular steroid receptors. The authors speculated that this could be a general aspect of integration of neural information in the neuroendocrine system.

III. ANTISENSE OLIGONUCLEOTIDES DIRECTED AGAINST NEUROTRANSMITTER SYSTEMS

A. Neurohypophyseal Neurotransmitters

1. *Oxytocin*

a. *Effects of Antisense Oligos against Oxytocin Receptor*

The neurohypophyseal hormone, oxytocin, is integrally involved in the regulation of lordosis in female rats. While there is evidence for behavioral significance of peripherally released oxytocin from the posterior pituitary, the majority of behavioral effects appear to be mediated by centrally released oxytocin binding to membrane receptors at distinct neuronal sites.[20] A critical brain area in the control of lordosis, the VMN, is also a site of high density of oxytocin receptor. More importantly, the density of binding in this brain region increases between 100 to 300% within hours of estrogen exposure. Binding is further influenced by the sequential administration of progesterone, resulting in a spreading of the receptor field into the lateral region of the VMN. Combinations of lesion studies and disruption of transport indicates that receptors are moving out into the dendrites of the VMN neurons and into the region of descending collaterals from oxytocin neurons in the periventricular nucleus.[21,22] Infusions of oxytocin into the vicinity of the ventrolateral VMN are particularly effective at inducing lordosis within 20 min of infusion in progesterone-primed females.[23] However, antagonists to oxytocin are only effective at reducing the behavioral response if given at the same time as progesterone, i.e., 4 h prior to behavioral testing.[24] The mechanism by which the antagonist blocks the behavior is unknown but does not seem to be due to a simple competition at the receptor.

The fact that oxytocin receptor synthesis is strongly induced within hours of estrogen treatment made this an ideal target for modulation by antisense oligonucleotides. An equimolar mix of two 15-mer fully phosphorothioated antisense oligonucleotides was infused into the vicinity of the VMN.[25] The experimental design was such that oligo administration would bracket the time period of steroid administration with the intention that sufficient quantities of oligo would be in the cells both prior to and during steroid exposure. Oligos were infused on three consecutive days, beginning with the first day of estradiol treatment, and preceded the estrogen injections by about 8 h and the progesterone injections by 2 to 3 h. The schedule of oligo infusion was based on previous observations that intact antisense oligo can be extracted from the brain 5 h post-infusion and the fluorescently labeled oligo is detectable in cells for up to 24 h post-infusion.[2]

There were two surprising findings from the behavioral tests. First was that antisense oligos were only effective at reducing lordosis in females primed with estradiol alone. Females treated with estrogen plus progesterone were not affected by antisense infusion. Behavioral specificity in the estrogen-only females was indicated by a concomitant increase in rejection behaviors, illustrating that the animals were not incapacitated or locomotorally impaired (Figure 6). A second surprising finding was a serendipitous observation that the antisense oligo-treated animals appeared to have lost weight after the first behavioral trial. On the second trial, the animals were reversed in their treatment, i.e., animals that previously received

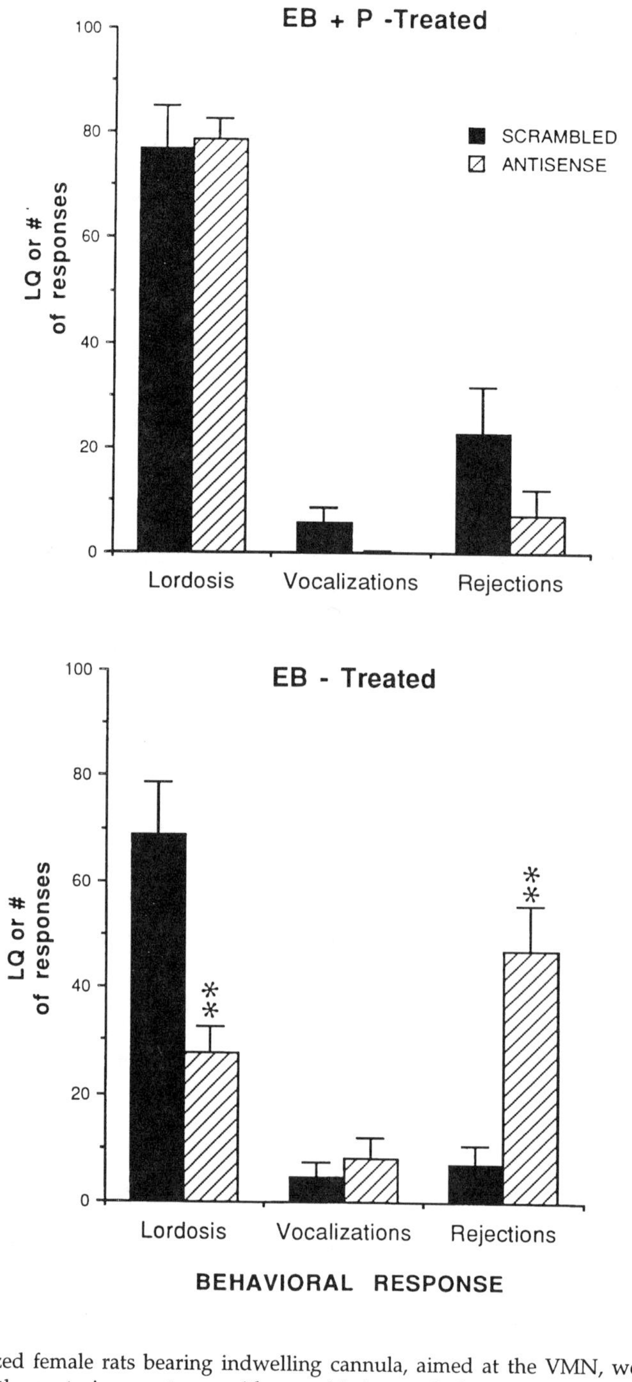

FIGURE 6
Adult ovariectomized female rats bearing indwelling cannula, aimed at the VMN, were infused with antisense oligos to the oxytocin receptor or with scrambled control oligos. Oligos were infused on three consecutive days beginning with the first day of estradiol benzoate (EB) treatment and preceded the estrogen injections by about 8 h and the progesterone (P) injections by 2 to 3 h. Antisense oligos to the oxytocin receptor significantly reduced lordosis responding expressed as lordosis quotient (LQ) and increased the frequency of rejection behaviors in EB treated females (**$p < 0.01$, ANOVA) but was without effect in females receiving EB + P. (From McCarthy, M. M., Kleopoulos, S. P., Mobbs, C. V., and Pfaff, D. W., *Neuroendocrinology*, 59, 432–440, 1994. With permission from Karger, Basel.)

scrambled oligo now received antisense, and they were tested for their appetite for sweet milk. Animals infused with antisense oligo showed a significantly reduced intake of sweet milk compared to controls. Although oxytocin is importantly involved in feeding, this effect is generally mediated peripherally at the level of the vagus nerve.[26] Furthermore, peripheral oxytocin inhibits feeding, and thus a reduction in the oxytocin receptor would be predicted to increase feeding. The hypothalamus is also of course importantly involved in feeding, and this observation may indicate a novel mechanism by which oxytocin acts in the brain to regulate food intake.

In vitro autoradiography indicated a significant reduction in oxytocin binding in the VMN, but there was no significant change in the amygdala of antisense oligo-treated animals compared to scrambled oligo-treated controls. However, the reduction in binding was on the order of 30% while the behavioral reduction was closer to 60%. Furthermore, in a situation analogous to that for estrogen induction of the progesterone receptor, there is a 100 to 300% increase in oxytocin binding in response to estrogen, so that at the very least there should be a residual 70% increase in oxytocin receptor binding. These data again support the notion that a threshold level of receptors is required for the maintenance of behavior, rather than a simple linear relationship between receptor concentration and behavioral response.

b. Effects of Antisense Oligos against Oxytocin

Given its abundance and stability, the neuropeptide oxytocin would not immediately present itself as an attractive target for antisense oligo-mediated knockdown. In fact, there are no reports of what would be considered a traditional antisense study involving repeated administration of large doses of oxytocin antisense oligo and eventually reducing peptide levels after several days of administration. However, there are fascinating reports of an unexpected rapid effect of antisense oligos against oxytocin, and the effect appears to be specific and physiologically relevant. Within 2 to 6 h of *in vivo* infusion of oxytocin antisense oligos, there is reduced electrophysiological responses of putative oxytocin, but not vasopressin, neurons in the supraoptic nucleus (SON). There is also a concomitant inhibition of the milk let-down response of the mammary gland, an effect known to be mediated by oxytocin.[27] Oxytocin antisense inhibited oxytocin release from the neurohypophysis in response to various stimulants and reversibly blocked CCK-induced expression of the neuronal activity marker, Fos, within the SON. Further specificity was demonstrated by the ability of vasopressin antisense to reduce the excitatory responses of vasopressin neurons, but not of oxytocin neurons.[28] However, as would be expected with this short period of antisense exposure, neuropeptide content within the SON and neurohypophysis remained unaltered, suggesting that a traditional antisense-mediated reduction in protein synthesis was not the causal mechanism. The authors propose that antisense may induce anticipatory, feed-forward alterations in electrical activity in order to conserve neuropeptide. The possibility was considered that a sequence-specific retention by oxytocin or vasopressin neurons of their respective antisense oligos might be responsible for the reduction in neuronal activity. However, the administration of antisense to β-actin had no affect on neuronal excitability, yet would surely be retained by the cell to an equivalent degree.[29]

Oxytocin is importantly involved in the onset of maternal behavior around parturition.[20] These investigators report no changes in maternal behavior despite a disruption of lactation. However, a change in maternal behavior, might not be predicted in this paradigm since oxytocin is only involved in the onset, not the maintenance of maternal behavior, as would be the case here. Secondly, the inhibition of peripherally released oxytocin may not be relevant to behavioral effects that are believed to be the result of centrally-acting oxytocin.

In a separate study designed to more carefully assess the behavioral effects of oxytocin antisense, an effect on maternal aggression was observed. As mentioned previously, female rats exhibit a specific and transient aggression during lactation. The mechanisms controlling this response are not well understood, and an observation that aggression levels were significantly reduced by oxytocin antisense infusion is intriguing.[30] Maternal aggression is not expressed until after maternal behavior has been established. The neurochemical control of the onset vs. the maintenance of maternal behavior appear to be distinct. These findings would suggest that oxytocin plays a dual role, first in helping to establish maternal behavior, and then in mediating the maintenance of maternal aggression. Many of the same brain areas are involved in both areas, for instance, the preoptic area and the amygdaloid complex, both of which show a high level of oxytocin receptor binding.

2. *Vasopressin*

a. *Effects of Antisense Oligos against Vasopressin*

Although they have not been related to reproduction per se, there have been several studies using vasopressin antisense. Rapid effects have also been seen for antisense directed against this neuropeptide. An increase in licking behavior and a decrease in urine osmolality were seen within hours of intraventricular infusion,[31] and changes in neuronal excitability analogous to that seen with oxytocin antisense have also been reported.[28] In these studies the effects were observed only acutely and could not be sustained with continued infusion. Again, these rapid effects are difficult to reconcile with what is assumed to be the mechanism of antisense action. As pointed out by others, vasopressin and oxytocin antisense oligos produced effects within 4 to 6 h, but transport of newly-synthesized prohormone from the hypothalamus to the posterior pituitary requires 12 to 24 h. It is possible that antisense oligos affect a separate, rapidly turning over pool of neuropeptide, but evidence for this is lacking.[3] It has been proposed that while basal levels of peptide in the plasma and pituitary remain unchanged, antisense oligo effects are revealed in response to challenges which activate the system, such as suckling or stress, suggesting that antisense treatment alters cellular responses.[3]

In a separate study, changes in urine osmolality and water intake were observed after daily infusions of phosphorothioated oligos to male rats, but there was also an unexplained mortality specific to antisense-treated animals.[32] This may have been related to toxicity of phosphorothioate oligos and the possibility that antisense oligos are retained in cells longer than scrambled control oligos. Other researchers report a significant increase in water intake 24 h after a single vasopressin antisense infusion.[33] As these investigators point out, given the large reserve of vasopressin in the neurohypophysis, it would be predicted that sufficient vasopressin is present to maintain water balance for an extended period, even in the absence of new synthesis. The fact that drinking behavior was altered within 24 h suggests that either ongoing synthesis is critical or that oligos exert other currently unidentified physiological effects. These researchers also observed a phenomenon seen by others, heterogeneity in cellular uptake of oligos. The potential mechanism for this remains completely unknown.

b. *Effects of Antisense Oligos against Vasopressin Receptor*

Noting that although there are potent and specific antagonists for the vasopressin receptor, Landgraf and colleagues[34] have exploited the specificity of antisense oligos against V1 vasopressin receptor because the potential for cross-reactivity with oxytocin receptors at high doses still exists. Olfactory cues often mediate social behavior in rodents, and both oxytocin and vasopressin had previously been implicated in this response. Using a social discrimination paradigm, adult male rats were tested for the duration of investigation of a novel or familiar juvenile male. Males that received four continuous days of V1 receptor antisense oligos infused into the lateral septum did not distinguish between novel or familiar stimulus animals. Blockade of V1 receptor synthesis by antisense oligos also caused a significant reduction in baseline anxiety levels, suggesting a role for endogenous vasopressin in anxiety. That receptor concentrations were in fact diminished was demonstrated by *in vitro* receptor autoradiography. Importantly, the receptor density was diminished only in the lateral septum, which was where the oligos were infused, and not in other vasopressin binding brain areas. Interestingly, these investigators reported a significant increase in the mRNA for the receptor, suggesting that transcription was maintained and that hybridization arrest, rather than RNase H-mediated degradation, was the only mechanism of antisense action. Of equal interest was the observation that the sense oligo at times had specific effects almost equivalent to that of the antisense oligo, whereas the effects of the scrambled control oligo were no different from that of the vehicle. This suggests that sense oligos may gain access to the nucleus and interact with the DNA to block transcription. Consistent with this interpretation, V1 receptor mRNA was slightly reduced in sense oligo infused animals.[34]

B. Amino Acid Neurotransmitters

1. *Gamma-Aminobutyric Acid (GABA)*

a. *Effects of Antisense Oligos against Glutamic Acid Decarboxylase (GAD)*

GABA is a predominant and ubiquitous inhibitory neurotransmitter that plays a key role in reproductive behavior. In females, GABA is known to exert distinct effects on lordosis depending on the brain area. In the preoptic area, GABA is inhibitory to lordosis responding and in the mediobasal hypothalamus and midbrain central gray (MCG), GABA facilitates lordosis.[35] GAD is the rate-limiting enzyme in GABA synthesis. The mRNA for GAD is modulated by estrogen, and tissue GABA levels change over the estrous cycle in a manner that is consistent with endogenous GABA modulation of behavior. Based on these observations, it was predicted that reduction of GAD protein by antisense oligonucleotides would reduce GABA and modulate lordosis in a brain region-specific manner.[36]

There are two forms of GAD protein which are coded by separate mRNAs. These are referred to as GAD_{65} and GAD_{67} due to the 2-kDa difference in molecular weight.[37] Both forms of the enzyme make GABA and, for the most part, both forms are found in the same neurons. The physiological significance of each remains unknown. Fortuitously, the highest degree of divergence between the mRNAs for the two forms is in the 5′ region near the translation start codon. Therefore, we were able to design antisense oligonucleotides that were specific to each form and would not be predicted to show any cross-hybridization. In view of the fact that there are no specific inhibitors distinct for each form of GAD, antisense technology in this instance appears particularly attractive.

Ovariectomized rats were implanted with indwelling cannula into either the POA, mHYP, or MCG and were also given subcutaneous silastic capsules containing estradiol. This regime of hormonal treatment is known to establish continuously high levels of lordosis responding for a period of weeks. After a postoperative recovery period, females were tested for sexual receptivity, and lordosis quotients of 90% or greater were verified for each animal. Immediately after behavioral testing, an injection cannula filled with crystalline GAD_{67} antisense or scrambled oligo was placed into the indwelling cannula. Two types of oligos were implanted: DNA with a normal phosphodiester backbone or DNA with a methylphosphonate modification to protect against degradation. The latter was mixed 1:10 with cholesterol and 24 h later animals were again behaviorally tested. As would be predicted, lordosis responding was significantly reduced in animals that received antisense oligo into the hypothalamus or MCG, but there was no decrease in animals infused into the POA (nor was there an increase since lordosis responding was already maximized). In some animals lordosis responding remained depressed when tested again 48 h post-infusion. Behavioral responding began to recover by 72 h, and all animals were back to preimplantation levels of receptivity by 4 days. Both the unmodified and methylphosphonate modified oligos were behaviorally effective, the latter being more so. This observation is of particular interest since the methylphosphonate modification not only protects the oligo against nuclease digestion, it also renders it insensitive to the actions of RNase H, suggesting the predominant mechanism of action in this case was hybridization arrest.[36]

An unsatisfactory aspect of the study using crystalline oligo tamped into the end of the injection cannula was the high degree of intra-animal variability. In a subsequent experiment, animals surgically and hormonally prepared in the same way were then infused with unmodified oligo that had been suspended in sesame oil. There was again a significant reduction in lordosis responding 24 h after antisense administration, with full recovery at 4 to 6 days. The variability in responsiveness was greatly reduced, and the previous observation that antisense administration into the hypothalamus resulted in greater inhibition of behavior than administration into the MCG was verified. This finding agrees quite well with pharmacological studies in which infusion of the $GABA_A$ antagonist, bicuculline, was substantially more effective in the hypothalamus than the midbrain.[38]

A third experiment compared the effects of antisense oligos specific for GAD_{65} vs. GAD_{67}, as well as the combination of the two. This experiment also used phosphorothioated oligos as an additional comparison. Antisense to GAD_{67} continued to be behaviorally effective within 24 h, whereas GAD_{65} antisense had no effect until 48 h post-infusion. The recovery from GAD_{65} infusion also lagged 24 h behind that for GAD_{67}. These data fit well with the protein half-lives of the two enzymes, on the order of 3 to 5 h for GAD_{67} and over 24 h for GAD_{65}. The combination of the two antisense oligos was not additive but was slightly more effective than either one alone. Lastly, the phosphorothioate oligos exerted the same or greater behavioral effects at half the doses used for unmodified oligos.

While these behavioral effects were specific and predicted, the measurement of biochemical indicators of antisense action proved more problematic. Attempts to show clear reductions in GABA levels by antisense oligos were unsuccessful, although the positive correlation between GABA levels and lordosis responding seen in control animals was lost in antisense-treated females. More importantly, however, was the quantification of GAD protein. Animals were infused with phosphorothioated antisense to GAD_{67} into the MCG, and 24 h later the brains were removed and tissue punches were taken near the infusion site. Tissue was assayed by Western blot with antiserum W887 which detects both GAD_{65} and GAD_{67}. As would be predicted, the GAD_{67} protein was significantly reduced in the antisense-infused animals compared to those receiving scrambled control. However, GAD_{65} protein was also reduced in the same tissue samples. This would not be predicted and to verify the effect, the blots were also probed with neuron-specific enolase which showed a nonsignificant reduction. Interpretating these data are difficult, but one possibility is to again relate these effects to possible toxicity of phosphorothioated oligos. Clearly the toxicity is not simply a matter of the oligo being phosphorothioated because the scrambled control was of the same length, given in the same dose, and in the same manner, yet was without effect. Therefore, there is something specific to the antisense oligo and it seems likely that these oligos are retained in the cell longer and are thus more likely to exert toxic effects. However, the precise nature of the toxicity remains unclear as there is no overt evidence for cell death or substantial lesions near the infusion sites (Figure 7). In addition, behavioral recovery after antisense infusion is relatively rapid, within days. It is possible that toxicity consists of a generalized disruption of transcription, translation, or both. This is not to say that the behavioral results have lost their significance; rather that the observed behavioral effects may be the result of a combination of specific and nonspecific mechanisms.[36]

Antisense oligos to GAD mRNA have been effective in other systems as well. The percentage of mice exhibiting cocaine-induced seizures was significantly increased 15 h after intraventricular infusion of GAD antisense oligos.[39] In a study involving female monkeys, GAD antisense oligos induced LH release from the pituitary within hours of administration to the arcuate-median eminence.[40] In this instance GAD antisense may be acting in a manner similar to that of oxytocin and vasopressin antisense when they exert rapid effects.

b. *Effects of Antisense Oligos against the $GABA_A$ Receptor*

The variety of subunits that constitute the heteroligomeric $GABA_A$ receptor have been cloned, making them suitable targets for antisense intervention. There have been reports of successful use of antisense oligos to block individual receptor subunits,[41,42] but not in the context of reproductive behavior. Benzodiazepine sensitivity of the $GABA_A$ receptor requires the presence of a $\gamma 2$ subunit.[43] We recently reported that benzodiazepine infused in the MCG facilitates lordosis behavior of estrogen-primed females,[44] and we subsequently found that estrogen increased the mRNA for the $\gamma 2$ subunit in this same brain region.[45] Ongoing experiments examining the effects of MCG infusion of antisense oligos to the $\gamma 2$ subunit on benzodiazepine enhancement of lordosis responding will provide evidence for a causal relationship between benzodiazepine-induced anxiolysis, $\gamma 2$ mRNA levels, and lordosis. Effectiveness of $\gamma 2$ subunit antisense oligos to reduce lordosis responding (in the absence of exogenous benzodiazepine) compared to GABA-facilitated behavior will suggest that endogenous benzodiazepine-like ligands are released in the MCG and that they support lordosis responding. This approach could also prove useful for determining the subunit specificity regulating the action of other compounds active at the $GABA_A$ receptor, such as neurosteroids.

2. *Glutamate*

Some of the first reports on the *in vivo* use of antisense oligonucleotides targeted a receptor subtype for the excitatory amino acid transmitter, glutamate.[46] Cortical neurons were protected from excitotoxicity after exposure to NMDA-R1 receptor channel mRNA. In a separate study, antisense against this same subunit enhanced neuronal survival and behavioral recovery following traumatic brain injury in rats.[47] This approach has not yet been used in studies regarding reproductive or related behaviors, but would likely prove informative.

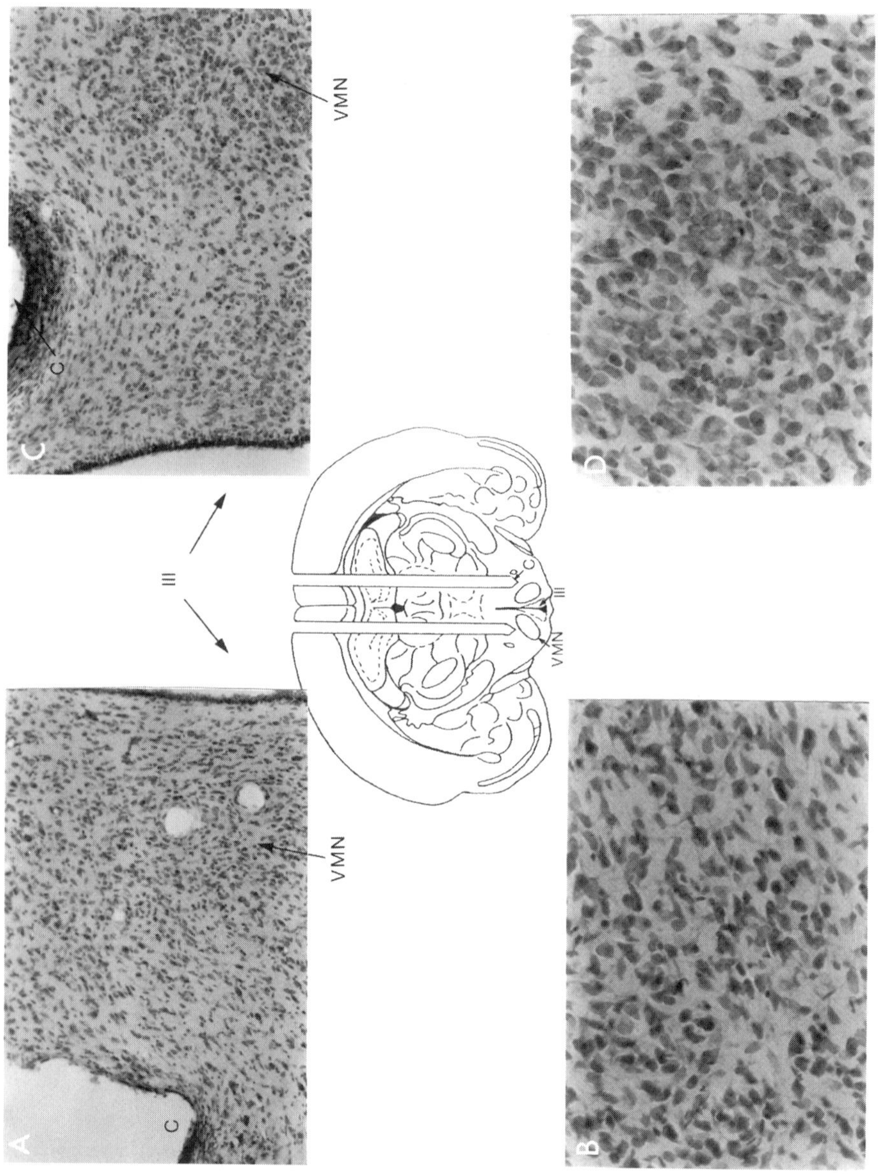

FIGURE 7

The possibility of toxic effects of infused oligos remains of serious concern in the *in vivo* use of antisense technology. Standard histological examination using a Nissl stain of brain tissue (ventromedial nucleus, VMN and third ventricle, III) near the tip of the injection cannula (C) show no overt signs of lesions or cellular damage after infusions of either antisense oligos to GAD (left panel) or scrambled control oligos (right panel). Nonetheless, the possibilty that a general disruption of translation or transcription has resulted from oligo infusion cannot be ruled out.

C. Serotonin

1. *Effects of Antisense Oligos against Tryptophan Hydroxylase*

The rate-limiting enzyme in serotonin synthesis is tryptophan hydroxylase. Serotonergic neurons are predominantly found in the raphe nuclei of the brain stem, and projections from there coalesce into three major ascending projections to the forebrain. Serotonin is intimately involved in several reproduction related behaviors, such as aggression and anxiety. The neuroanatomical localization of the tryptophan hydroxylase-containing cell bodies in the vicinity of the fourth ventricle, combined with the very low abundance of the mRNA for this enzyme, make this an ideal system to target with antisense oligonucleotides.

Male mice were infused with unmodified antisense or scrambled oligos, saline, or the irreversible tryptophan hydroxylase inhibitor, para-chlorophenylalanine (PCPA) into the fourth ventricle for four consecutive days.[48] Assay of brain tryptophan hydroxylase activity on the afternoon of the fourth day indicated a significant reduction (>50%) in enzyme activity in both the antisense oligo- and the PCPA-infused animals. A separate group of animals was behaviorally tested on the afternoon of the fourth day, and there was an increase in anxiety-related behavior as assessed by the elevated plus-maze in the antisense- and PCPA-infused males. The effects of the antisense oligo were of a similar magnitude to that of PCPA. In both cases confounding factors due to locomotor disturbances could not be ruled out. However, when tested on a rotorod apparatus, the antisense oligo-treated animals showed marked improvement on a second test, as did scrambled oligo-infused animals. This suggested they had retained good balance and coordination. Animals treated with the enzyme inhibitor failed to improve on the second test, suggesting that they had been seriously impaired by the treatment.[48] The observation that antisense oligo treatment appeared to produce less undesirable side effects than the PCPA supports the idea that therapeutic use of antisense oligos may offer additional advantages over pharmacological agents already available. A similar study in rats also reported an anxiogenic effect of tryptophan hydroxylase antisense, as well as a reduction in food intake.[49] However, there was no significant reduction in tissue serotonin content in these animals.

2. *Effects of Antisense Oligos against Serotonin Receptor*

The effects of the neurotransmitter serotonin are mediated via numerous receptor subtypes, and the physiological significance of each type is often difficult to discern. Some of these receptor subtypes have only been identified by molecular cloning techniques, making the establishment of a physiological role more difficult still. Recognizing this limitation, Bourson and colleagues[50] utilized antisense oligonucleotides against the 5-ht6 receptor in an attempt to assess the significance of this receptor subtype. Repeated intraventricular injections resulted in a behavioral syndrome of yawning, stretching, and chewing and was correlated with a 30% reduction in [^{3}H]-lysergic acid diethylamide binding, a nonselective serotonin agonist. This study illustrates a unique approach in the use of antisense oligos, an approach that may prove among the most useful in the future as issues of specificity and toxicity are clarified. The ability to discover new mechanisms for cellular proteins will be of particular advantage in behavioral neuroendocrinology.

D. Neuropeptides

1. *Effects of Antisense Oligos against Corticotrophin-Releasing Hormone*

Given that they tend to be relatively abundant and stable, neuropeptides do not seem to readily lend themselves to antisense approaches. However, given that specific receptor agonists and antagonists are notably scarce and that there are no rate-limiting synthetic enzymes, there is also a particular need for selective targeting of these behaviorally relevant neurotransmitters. For example, there has been no mechanism by which to block the synthesis of corticotrophin-releasing hormone (CRH), a neuropeptide critically involved in activation of the hypothalamic-pituitary-adrenal axis. Intraventricular infusions of CRH antisense oligos at three 12-h intervals resulted in significant increases in discriminative avoidance responses compared to controls. There was also a reduction in CRH immunoreactivity in the brain and decreases in plasma levels of ACTH and corticosterone, indicative of an overall anxiolytic effect. These data suggest that in addition to a selective arrest in translation of CRH, there may also have been an interruption of CRH secretion. The authors speculate that this approach may provide a new strategy for the treatment of affective disorders in which aberrant CRH responding has been implicated.[51]

2. *Effects of Antisense Oligos against Neuropeptide Y*

An additional study using anxiety as the behavioral endpoint involved antisense targeted at neuropeptide Y-Y1 receptors.[52] No specific neuropeptide Y receptor antagonists were available, making the functional significance of two receptor types difficult to distinguish. Repeated infusions of unmodified oligos into the lateral ventricles resulted in a significant elevation in an anxiety-like state compared to controls. Receptor binding assays showed a significant reduction in neuropeptide Y-Y1 receptor, but not the closely related Y2 receptor after antisense oligo infusions.

Endogenous neuropeptide Y itself has also been targeted by antisense oligos. Infusions into the arcuate nucleus significantly reduced carbohydrate and fat intake by 60 to 75%.[53] The levels of neuropeptide Y were reduced by ~35%, a relationship between behavioral effect and protein levels seen many times before.

IV. CONCLUSIONS

Although still a relatively new technique, there is now a substantial body of work on the *in vivo* use of antisense oligonucleotides. As with most new techniques, there was an initial honeymoon period followed by reassessment and refinement. When reviewing this literature it becomes apparent that the approach is a viable and constructive one; however, it is not without caveats and the variability in success rates remains high. The all too familiar scenario in science of negative findings and failures not being reported is particularly true in the case of antisense technology. Fortunately, it appears that investigators are becoming increasingly willing to report findings with the use of antisense techniques that may not be readily explainable; for instance, the rapid effects of oxytocin and vasopressin antisense oligos[27,28,31] and the discrepancies between protein levels and behavioral responses.[14,25]

However, there is still room for improvement in our application of the technique. A critical concern in behavioral studies utilizing antisense oligos is nonspecific disruption of protein synthesis. This caveat is perhaps of greatest concern in studies of hormonally induced reproductive behavior since it has been well established that disruption of RNA or protein synthesis in the hypothalamus will block the induction of lordosis.[54,55] A commonly used control in other *in vivo* antisense studies is the simultaneous quantification of both the targeted protein and another closely related protein that is not predicted to be affected by the antisense oligonucleotides.[52,56] This approach has not been routinely applied in studies of reproductive behavior, and the potential for nonspecific contributions to specific behavioral effects exists.[36] Nevertheless, there is reason for optimism regarding the continuing advances in the refinement of this technique. Furthermore, in addition to contributing to our understanding of the neural control of behavior, antisense experiments are beginning to reveal basic principles of cellular physiology. Such information will, in turn, be essential to our understanding of antisense action. As aptly put by others, "a complete understanding of the effects of oligonucleotides on mRNA translation will not be forthcoming until more is known about the natural control of cellular mRNA levels."[33]

ACKNOWLEDGMENTS

The author would like to thank Drs. S. Schwartz-Giblin and C. V. Mobbs for helpful comments on this manuscript and Ms. Rachael Kurzweil for her artistic assistance.

REFERENCES

1. McCarthy, M. M., Use of antisense oligonucleotides to block gene expression in the central nervous system, *Methods in Neurosciences: Neurobiology of Steroids*, Vol. 22, de Kloet, E. R. and Sutano, W., Eds., Academic Press, New York, 1994, 342–356.
2. McCarthy, M. M., Brooks, P. J., Pfaus, J., Brown, H. E., Flanagan, L. M., Schwartz-Giblin, S., and Pfaff, D. W., Antisense technology in behavioral neuroscience, *Neuroprotocols*, 2, 67–74, 1993.
3. Morris, M. and Lucion, A. B., Antisense oligonucleotides in the study of neuroendocrine systems, *J. Neuroendocrinol.*, 7, 493–500, 1995.
4. Erskine, M. S., Solicitation behavior in the estrous female rat: A review, *Horm. Behav.*, 23, 473–502, 1989.
5. Coopersmith, C. and Erskine, M. S., Influence of paced mating and number of intromissions on fertility in the laboratory rat, *J. Reprod. Fertil.*, 102, 451–458, 1994.
6. Pfaff, D. W., Schwartz-Giblin, S., McCarthy, M. M., and Kow, L.-M., Cellular mechanisms of female reproductive behaviors, *The Physiology of Reproduction*, 2nd edition, Knobil, E., Neil, E. et al., Eds., Raven Press, New York, Vol. 2, 1994, 107–220.
7. Numan, M., Maternal behavior, *The Physiology of Reproduction*, 2nd edition, Knobil, E., Neil, E. et al., Eds., Raven Press, New York, Vol. 2, 1994, 221–302.
8. Gerall, A. A. and Givon, L., Early androgen and age-related modifications in female rat reproduction, *Handbook of Behavioral Neurobiology: Sexual Differentiation*, Vol. 11, Gerall, A. A., Moltz, H., and Ward, I. L., Eds., Plenum Press, New York, 1992, chap. 10.
9. McCarthy, M. M., Schlenker, E. H., and Pfaff, D. W., Enduring consequences of neonatal treatment with antisense oligodeoxynucleotides to estrogen receptor messenger ribonucleic acid on sexual differentiation of rat brain, *Endocrinology*, 133, 433–439, 1993.
10. Gorski, R. A., Harlan, R. E., Jacobson, C. D., Shryne, J. E., and Sotham, A. M., Evidence for the existence of a sexually dimorphic nucleus in the preoptic area of the rat, *J. Comp. Neurol.*, 193, 529–439, 1980.
11. Lauber, A. H., Romano, G. J., Mobbs, C. V., and Pfaff, D. W., Estradiol regulation of estrogen receptor messenger ribonucleic acid in rat mediobasal hypothalamus: An *in situ* hybridization study, *J. Neuroendocrinol.*, 2, 605–611, 1990.
12. DonCarlos, L. L., McAbee, M., Ramer-Quinn, D. S., and Stancik, D. M., Estrogen receptor mRNA levels in the preoptic area of neonatal rats are responsive to hormone manipulation, *Dev. Brain Res.*, 84, 253–260, 1995.

13. Sawai, Y., Saito, J., and Tsukada, K., Developmental changes of two distinct ribonuclease H activities from rat brain and characterization of these enzymes, *Biochim. Biophys. Acta*, 630, 386–391, 1980.
14. Mani, S. K., Blaustein, J. D., Allen, J. M. C., Law, S. W., O'Malley, B. W., and Clark, J. H., Inhibition of rat sexual behavior by antisense oligonucleotides to the progesterone receptor, *Endocrinology*, 135, 1409–1414, 1994.
15. Ogawa, S., Olazabal, U. E., Parhar, I. S., and Pfaff, D. W., Effects of intrahypothalamic administration of antisense DNA for progesterone receptor mRNA on reproductive behavior and progesterone receptor immunoreactivity in female rat, *J. Neurosci.*, 14, 1766–1774, 1994.
16. Pollio, G, Xue, P., Zanisi, M., Nicolin, A., and Maggi, A., Antisense oligonucleotide blocks progesterone-induced lordosis behavior in ovariectomized rats, *Mol. Brain Res.*, 19, 135–139, 1993.
17. Romano, G. J., Krust, A., and Pfaff, D. W., Expression and estrogen regulation of progesterone receptor mRNA in neurons of the mediobasal hypothalamus: an *in situ* hybridization study, *Mol. Endocrinol.*, 3, 1295–1300, 1989.
18. Powers, R. F., Mani, S. K., Codina, J., Conneely, O. M., and O'Malley, B. W., Dopaminergic and ligand-independent activation of steroid hormone receptors, *Science*, 254, 1636–1639, 1991.
19. Mani, S. K., Allen, J. M. C., Clark, J. H., Blaustein, J. D., and O'Malley, B. W., Convergent pathways for steroid hormone-and neurotransmitter-induced rat sexual behavior, *Science*, 265, 1246–1249, 1994.
20. McCarthy, M. M., Estrogen modulation of oxytocin and its relation to behavior, *Oxytocin — Cellular and Molecular Approaches in Medicine and Research*, Ivell, R. and Russell, J., Eds., Plenum Press, New York, 1995, 235–246.
21. Coirini, H., Schumacher, M., Flanagan, L. M., and McEwen, B. S., Transport of estrogen-induced oxytocin receptors in the ventromedial hypothalamus, *J. Neurosci.*, 11, 3317–3324, 1991.
22. Johnson, A. E., Harbaugh, R., and Gelhard, R. E., Projections from the ventromedial nucleus of the hypothalamus contain oxytocin binding sites, *Brain Res.*, 567, 332–336, 1991.
23. Schumacher, M., Coirini, H., Pfaff, D. W., and McEwen, B. S., Behavioral effects of progesterone associated with rapid modulation of oxytocin receptors, *Science*, 250, 691–694, 1990.
24. Witt, D. M. and Insel, T. R., A selective oxytocin antagonist attenuates progesterone facilitation of female sexual behavior, *Endocrinology*, 128, 3269–3276, 1991.
25. McCarthy, M. M., Kleopoulos, S. P., Mobbs, C. V., and Pfaff, D. W., Infusions of antisense oligodeoxynucleotides to the oxytocin receptor in the ventromedial hypothalamus reduces estrogen-induced sexual receptivity and oxytocin receptor binding in the female rat, *Neuroendocrinology*, 59, 432–440, 1994.
26. Flanagan, L. M., Olson, B. R., Sved, A. F., Verbalis, J. G., and Stricker, E. M., Gastric motility in conscious rats given oxytocin and an oxytocin antagonist centrally, *Brain Res.*, 578, 256–260, 1992.
27. Neumann, I., Porter, D. W. F., Landgraf, R., and Pittman, Q. J., Rapid effect on suckling of an oxytocin antisense oligonucleotide administered into rat supraoptic nucleus, *Am. J. Physiol.*, 267, R852–R858, 1994.
28. Neumann, I., Kremarik, P., and Pittman, Q. J., Acute, sequence-specific effects of oxytocin and vasopressin antisense oligonucleotides on neuronal responses, *Neuroscience*, 69, 997–1003, 1997.
29. Pittman, Q. J., Takahasi, Y., and Wilson, B. C., Effect of bilateral administration of β-actin antisense into the supraoptic nuclei on the milk-ejection reflex in the conscious rat, *Soc. Neurosci. Abstr.*, 21, 450.3, 1995.
30. Lucion, A. B., Effects of antisense oligonucleotides against oxytocin mRNA on maternal aggression in the rat, *Ann. N.Y. Acad. Sci.*, 807, 1997.
31. Skutella, T., Probst, J. C., Engelmann, M., Wotjak, C. T., Landgraf, R., and Jirikowsi, G. F., Vasopressin antisense oligonucleotide induces temporary diabetes insipidus in rats, *J. Neuroendocrinol.*, 6, 121–125, 1994.
32. Flanagan, L. M., McCarthy, M. M., Brooks, P. J., Pfaff, D. W., and McEwen, B. S., Arginine vasopressin levels after daily infusions of antisense oligonucleotides into the supraoptic nucleus, *Ann. NY Acad. Sci.*, 689, 520–521, 1993.
33. Meeker, R., LeGrand, G., Ramierz, J., Smith, T., and Shih, Y.-H., Antisense vasopressin oligonucleotides: Uptake, turnover, distribution, toxicity and behavioral effects, *J. Neuroendocrinol.*, 7, 419–428, 1995.
34. Landgraf, R., Gertsberger, R., Montkowski, A., Probst, J. C., Wotjak, C. T., Holsboer, F., and Engelmann, M., V1 vasopressin receptor antisense oligodeoxynucleotide into septum reduces vasopressin binding, social discrimination abilities and anxiety-related behavior in rats, *J. Neurosci.*, 15, 4250–4258, 1995.
35. McCarthy, M. M., Functional significance of steroid modulation of GABAergic neurotransmission: Analysis at the behavioral, cellular and molecular level, *Horm. Behav.*, 29, 131–140, 1995.

36. McCarthy, M. M., Masters, D. B., Rimvall, K., Schwartz-Giblin, S., and Pfaff, D. W., Intracerebral administration of antisense oligodeoxynucleotides to GAD_{65} and GAD_{67} mRNAs modulate reproductive behavior in the female rat, *Brain Res.*, 636, 209–220, 1994.
37. Erlander, M. G., Tillakaratne, N. J. K., Feldblum, S., Patel, N., and Tobin, A. J., Two genes encode distinct glutamate decarboxylase, *Neuron*, 7, 91–100, 1991.
38. McCarthy, M. M., Pfaff, D. W., and Schwartz-Giblin, S., The role of steroid modulation of amino acid transmitters in the regulation of female reproduction, *Am. Zool.*, 33, 275–284, 1993.
39. Abel, M. S. and Kirages, T. J., Antisense oligonucleotide modulation of GAD alters cocaine-induced seizures in mice, *Soc. Neurosci. Abstr.*, 21, 624.20, 1995.
40. Mitsushima, D., Marzban, F., Hei, D. L., Golos, T. G., and Terasawa, E., Direct infusion of a glutamic acid decarboxylase (GAD1) antisense oligodeoxynucleotide into the stalk-median eminence increases the *in vivo* LHRH release in prepubertal female monkeys, *Soc. Neurosci. Abstr.*, 19, 258.1, 1993.
41. Karle, J., Hansen, S. E. W., Witt, M. R., and Nielsen, M., Small reduction of benzodiazepine receptor radioligand binding in rat brain following intracerebroventricular administration of antisense oligodeoxynucleotide to $GABA_A$ receptor γ2 subunit subtype, *Soc. Neurosci. Abstr.*, 21, 624, 24, 1995.
42. Peris, J. and Wielbo, D., Intraventricular injection of antisense oligonucleotides for $GABA_A$ receptor mRNA increases cocaine sensitivity in rats, *Soc. Neurosci. Abstr.*, 21, 286.15, 1995.
43. Prichett, D. B., Sontheimer, H., Shivers, B. D., Ymer, S., Kettenmann, H., Schofield, P. R., and Seeburg, P. H., Importance of a novel $GABA_A$ receptor subunit for benzodiazepine pharmacology, *Nature*, 338, 582–585, 1989.
44. McCarthy, M. M., Felzenberg, E., Robbins, A., Pfaff, D. W., and Schwartz-Giblin, S., Infusions of diazepam and allopregnanolone into the midbrain central gray facilitate open-field behavior and sexual receptivity in female rats, *Horm. Behav.*, 29, 279–295, 1995.
45. Schwartz-Giblin, S., Kaufman, L., Chan, K. Y. S., and McCarthy, M. M., Estrogen modulation of $GABA_A$ receptor and γ2 and β3 subunit mRNA in hypothalamus and midbrain central gray of the rat, submitted.
46. Wahlestedt, C., Golanov, E., Yamamoto, F., Yee, F., Ericson, H., Yoo, H. et al., Antisense oligodeoxynucleotides to NMDA-R1 receptor channel protect cortical neurons from excitotoxicity and reduce focal ischemic infarction, *Nature*, 363, 260–263, 1993.
47. Sun, F.-Y. and Faden, A. I., Pretreatment with antisense oligodeoxynucleotides directed against the NMDA-R1 receptor enhances survival and behavioral recovery following traumatic brain injury in rats, *Brain Res.*, 693, 163–168, 1995.
48. McCarthy, M. M., Nielsen, D. A., and Goldman, D., Antisense oligonucleotide inhibition of tryptophan hydroxylase activity in mouse brain, *Regul. Pept.*, 59, 163–170, 1995.
49. Hall, F. S., Pert, A., Nielsen, D. A., and Linnola, M., An antisense oligonucleotide to tryptophan hydroxylase has differing effects on indices of serotonin function, *Soc. Neurosci. Abstr.*, 21, 809.3, 1995.
50. Bourson, A., Borroni, E., Austin, R. A., Monsma, F. J., and Sleight, A. J., Determination of the role of the 5-ht6 receptor in the rat brain: A study using antisense oligonucleotides, *J. Pharmacol. Exp. Ther.*, 274, 173–180, 1995
51. Skutella, T., Criswell, H., Moy, S., Probst, J. C., Breese, G. R., Jirikowski, G. F., and Holsboer, F., Corticotropin-releasing hormone (CRH) antisense oligodeoxynucleotide induces anxiolytic effects in rat, *Neuroreport*, 5, 2181–2185, 1994.
52. Wahlestedt, C., Pich, E. M., Koob, G. F., Yee, F., and Heilig, M., Modulation of anxiety and neuropeptide Y-Y1 receptors by antisense oligonucleotides, *Science*, 259, 528–531, 1993.
53. Akabayashi, A., Wahlestedt, C., Alexander, J. T., and Leibowitz, S. F., Specific inhibition of endogenous neuropeptide Y synthesis in arcuate nucleus by antisense oligonucleotides suppresses feeding behavior and insulin secretion, *Mol. Brain Res.*, 21, 55–61, 1994.
54. Meisel, R. L. and Pfaff, D. W., RNA and protein synthesis inhibitors: Effects on sexual behavior in female rats, *Brain Res. Bull.*, 12, 187–193, 1989.
55. Rainbow, T. C., McGinnins, M. Y., Davis, P. G., and McEwen, B. S., Application of anisomysin to the lateral ventromedial nucleus of the hypothalamus inhibits the activation of sexual behavior by estradiol and progesterone, *Brain Res.*, 233, 417–423, 1982.
56. Zhou, L.-W., Zhang, S.-P., Qin, Z.-H., and Weiss, B., *In vivo* administration of an oligodeoxynucleotide antisense to the D_2 dopamine receptor mRNA inhibits D_2 dopamine receptor-mediated behavior and the expression of D_2 dopamine receptors in mouse striatum, *J. Pharmacol. Exp. Ther.*, 268, 1015–1023, 1994.
57. Barnett, S. S., *The Rat: A Study in Behavior*, Aldine Publishing, Chicago, IL, 1963.

Chapter 6

Establishing the Molecular Biology of Opioid Behavior through Antisense Approaches

Grace C. Rossi and Gavril W. Pasternak

CONTENTS

I. INTRODUCTION

Opiates are among the most widely used drugs in the world due to their ability to control pain. Opioids act upon the subjective perception of pain, leaving more objective sensations unaffected.[1,2] This ability to selectively target pain provides

0-8493-8552-0/97/$0.00+$.50

interesting insights into sensory processing as well as pain mechanisms themselves. A major goal in neuroscience is to uncover the molecular mechanisms of behavior. The recent explosion of cloned receptors and other proteins within the central nervous system (CNS) has opened the possibility of correlating functions with specific proteins. This correlation requires the selective elimination of the protein in question. Proteins can be "knocked out" in transgenic mice, providing animals completely lacking the gene of interest. However, the "knockout" of a protein can present a problem. If the gene of interest is important in development, significant structural/functional changes can result. Alternatively, other systems may "take over" the functions of the one which was deleted, making it difficult to assess the behavioral function(s) of the protein in question.

Antisense approaches[3-11] can avoid some of these problems. Developmental changes can be avoided by treating adult animals, and compensatory changes are usually not an issue over the short period of treatment. However, antisense approaches face other uncertainties.[3-6] Although the targeted protein in transgenic models is completely eliminated, antisense approaches typically give only a modest "knock down." There also are situations in which antisense methodologies simply do not work. The underlying reasons for success or failure are not completely understood. However, success seems to be more likely when targeting an mRNA of low abundance in cells readily accessible to the antisense. The CNS offers a number of advantages in antisense strategies, particularly the relative stability of the oligonucleotide within cerebrospinal fluid compared to blood. Diffusion into the brain and spinal cord may be the limiting factor, and care must be taken to ensure that the oligonucleotide gets to the region of interest. In recent years the utility of antisense approaches within the CNS has been clearly established in a number of systems.[8-11] Studies on the opioid system have been particularly fruitful, perhaps due to close proximity to the ventricular system of supraspinal opioid systems and the superficial localization of spinal systems, along with the relatively simple behavioral paradigms needed to assess the behavioral response.[6] The recent cloning of a number of opioid receptors has opened new avenues of research, including the relationship of the cloned receptors to opioid actions *in vivo*. Antisense approaches using short antisense oligodeoxynucleotides of approximately 20 bases has provided important insights into the molecular basis of opioid behavior.

II. OPIOID PHARMACOLOGY

Extensive pharmacological studies have suggested the presence of three major classes of opioid receptors, each with a number of putative subtypes (Table 1).[1,2] They can be differentiated by their selectivity for a panel of agonists and antagonists. While they have distinct regional localizations and mediate a wide range of activities, all the receptors share the ability to modulate pain perception. However, each receptor acts through independent mechanisms and in different regions. Opioid analgesia is easily demonstrated both spinally and supraspinally. Mu receptors mediate the actions of morphine and most clinically relevant opioid analgesics. Although morphine can act spinally or supraspinally, these systems can interact with each other synergistically.[12] Peripheral opioid mechanisms also are important,[13-16] as recently confirmed with antisense approaches described below.[17] Detailed studies have implied the presence of multiple classes of mu receptors, with the mu_1 receptor subtype acting supraspinally and the mu_2 receptor spinally.[1,2,18-26] Recent work also suggests that a morphine metabolite, morphine-6β-glucuronide (M6G), may elicit its analgesic actions through yet another receptor subtype.[27,28] M6G is particularly

TABLE 1

Opioid Receptor Subtypes and Their Actions

Receptor	Ligand	Analgesia	Other
Mu	Morphine DAMGO		
Mu_1	Naloxonazine	Supraspinal	Prolactin release Acetylcholine release in the hippocampus Feeding
Mu_2		Spinal	Respiratory depression Gastrointestinal transit Dopamine release by nigrostriatal neurons Guinea pig ileum bioassay Feeding
Kappa	Ketocyclazocine		Psychotomimesis Sedation
$Kappa_1$	Dynorphin A U50,488H	Predominantly spinal	Diuresis Feeding
$Kappa_2$		Unknown	Unknown
$Kappa_3$	NalBzoH Nalorphine	Predominantly supraspinal	
Delta	Enkephalins		Mouse vas deferens bioassay Dopamine turnover in the striatum Feeding
$Delta_1$		Supraspinal	
$Delta_2$		Spinal and supraspinal	

Note: Some actions assigned to general families have not yet been correlated with a specific subtype. NalBzoH refers to naloxone benzoylhydrazone.

interesting since it is over 100-fold more potent than morphine when administered centrally, despite its lower affinity at traditional mu receptors.[29,30] Morphine has other actions, including respiratory depression and inhibition of gastrointestinal transit.[1,2] Both actions appear to be mediated through the mu_2 receptor.

The kappa receptor family[31] has two pharmacologically relevant subtypes, $kappa_1$[32-34] and $kappa_3$.[1,2,32,35-41] Although included within the kappa receptor family, these two receptors appear quite distinct pharmacologically and biochemically, as discussed below. A number of highly selective $kappa_1$ ligands have been developed, including U50,488H.[33] Dynorphin A, an endogenous opioid peptide, has very high affinity for this site and is thought to be the endogenous ligand. $Kappa_1$ analgesia is most easily demonstrated spinally. $Kappa_3$ analgesia, on the other hand, is mediated predominantly supraspinally. Unlike the $kappa_1$ receptor, no highly selective $kappa_3$ ligands have been developed yet, and the endogenous ligand is unknown.

The delta receptor system[1,2,42] was discovered soon after the identification of the enkephalins, the endogenous ligands for these receptors. Over the years a wide variety of stabilized enkephalin derivatives have been developed, some of which are extremely selective for these receptors. With the development of these agents, evidence also has accumulated for two subtypes of delta receptor based upon their pharmacology.[2,43-47] DPDPE acts predominantly through $delta_1$ receptors, but its selectivity is limited and it also can work through $delta_2$ receptors. [D-Ala^2,Glu^4]deltorphin, on the other hand, is more active on $delta_2$ receptors. Antagonists which selectively reverse the actions of one subtype also have been developed. Like the mu system, delta analgesic systems are readily demonstrated both spinally and supraspinally.

This wide variety of opioid receptors and potential subtypes illustrates the complexity of these systems and underscores the difficulty in deciphering the actions of each of the receptors *in vivo*. This is a particularly challenging problem since all these receptors are active in the same behavioral assay.

III. MOLECULAR BIOLOGY OF OPIOID RECEPTORS

In 1992 two groups cloned a delta opioid receptor (DOR-1),[48,49] followed soon afterward by clones encoding mu (MOR-1) and $kappa_1$ (KOR-1) receptors.[50-62] All of these receptors fall into the G-protein receptor family with seven transmembrane regions and show high homology to each other. The MOR-1 gene contains four coding exons while the DOR-1 and KOR-1 genes have three. However, the fourth coding exon of MOR-1 encodes only a very short sequence, and the positions of the other splice sites are similar among all three genes. Two splice variants of the fourth coding exon of MOR-1 (MOR-1A and MOR-1B) have been described,[61,62] but they do not demonstrate any significant pharmacological differences thus suggesting they do not represent the putative mu receptor subtypes described above. All of these clones have been expressed and characterized pharmacologically. They all show the anticipated binding profiles and activities in cyclase assays.

A fourth member of the opioid receptor family has been reported by several laboratories.[63-73] It shows the same homology toward the other opioid receptors as they demonstrate to each other. Like DOR-1 and KOR-1, this receptor has three coding exons with splice sites in the same general location as DOR-1 and KOR-1. However, this clone does not encode a traditional opioid receptor. When expressed, opiates bind with very poor affinity. The endogenous ligand for this clone has now been isolated and identified and found to have many structural similarities to dynorphin A. Termed orphanin FQ[74] or nociceptin[75] (OFQ/N), this heptadecapeptide labels this clone with very high affinity (K_D 50 pM), but does not bind to any of the traditional opioid receptors. However, other evidence suggests that this clone is closely related to the $kappa_3$ receptor, leading us to term it KOR-3. A monoclonal antibody which blocks $kappa_3$ binding *in vitro* and analgesia *in vivo* also recognizes the expressed KOR-3 clone. Further evidence supporting the association of these two receptors comes from the antisense studies described below. However, the receptor encoded by KOR-3 is not identical to the $kappa_3$ receptor.

IV. INITIAL OPIOID RECEPTOR ANTISENSE STUDIES

We first examined the actions of antisense in a model system, the NG108 neuroblastoma cell line, from which the original DOR-1 cDNA was cloned.[76,77] Treatment paradigms must take into consideration the turnover time of the protein when looking for its downregulation. Blocking new synthesis will not reduce protein levels until pre-existing proteins are cycled out. Since prior work had suggested a turnover time *in vivo* of approximately 3 to 4 days for opioid receptors, cells were grown with an oligodeoxynucleotide (0.25 μM) in the absence of serum for five days and then examined. In control studies we observed a rapid uptake of a ^{32}P-labeled oligodeoxynucleotide.[77] Once taken into the cell, a significant proportion of the oligodeoxynucleotide remained intact for several days, as determined by a size. However, the amount of intact oligodeoxynucleotide was still only a fraction of the amount added despite the absence of serum. Having established the uptake and stability of the oligodeoxynucleotide in the cell, we then proceeded to assess the effects of antisense treatment using several different parameters. Antisense treatment lowered the levels of both mRNA and protein, as determined by a Western blot using a monoclonal antibody directed against the delta receptor. Binding studies confirmed a decrease in delta opioid receptor binding (Figure 1).[76] To ensure the selectivity of the action, we also examined α_2-adrenergic receptor binding in the same membranes and found no decrease. Additional controls included using a mismatch sequence in which the sequence of four bases was altered while maintaining the same base composition and a sense oligodeoxynucleotide. Neither the mismatch nor the sense probe lowered binding.

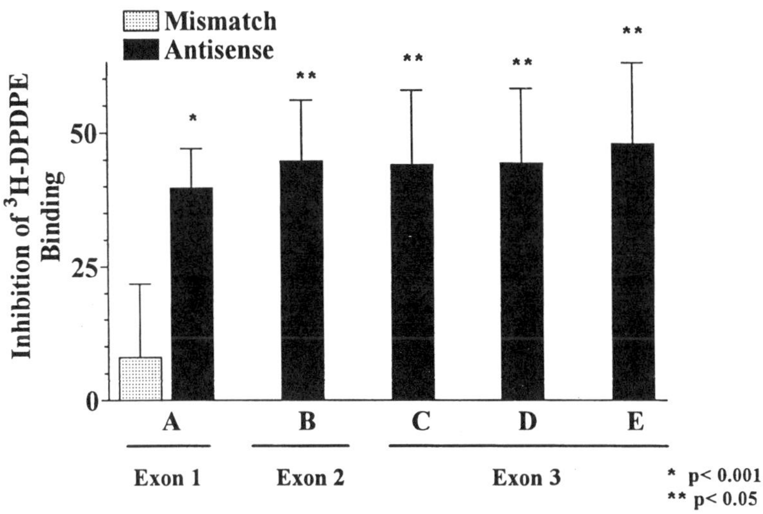

FIGURE 1
Inhibition of ^{3}H-DPDPE binding in NG108 cells by DOR-1 antisense treatment. Results are summarized from published reports.[76] Cells were treated with antisense oligodeoxynucleotides targeting the indicated exons and binding assessed with the delta-selective radioligand ^{3}H-DPDPE.

To determine whether the cloned DOR-1 receptor mediated enkephalin analgesia *in vivo*, we treated mice intrathecally with antisense (5 μg) on days 1, 3, and 5.[76] We chose this paradigm based upon the estimated turnover time of the receptors. Given intrathecally, ^{32}P-labeled oligodeoxynucleotide was taken up into cells of the spinal cord and remained relatively stable for over two days, permitting the alternate day dosing. We tested the mice for enkephalin analgesia on day 6 and observed a highly significant decrease in mice treated with antisense (Figure 2A). Mice given the mismatch oligodeoxynucleotide were unaffected. The decreased analgesic sensitivity of the antisense-treated mice gradually resolved over the next four days, indicating that the antisense effects were reversible and could not be explained by simple toxicity. The effects of the antisense also were highly selective. Although it potently decreased enkephalin analgesia, it had no affect upon the analgesic actions of the mu opioid DAMGO or the kappa$_1$ drug U50,488H. Similar results were subsequently reported by other groups as well.[78-82]

The first mu receptor was cloned from the rat.[50,52,53,67,83] Using this sequence, we designed an antisense probe targeting the 5′ untranslated region, which was administered into the periaqueductal gray (PAG), a region important in mediating morphine analgesia. Administering a MOR-1 antisense probe directly into the PAG on the same alternative day schedule effectively lowered the tailflick latency to baseline levels, completely blocking morphine's analgesic response (Figure 2B).[84] A mismatch

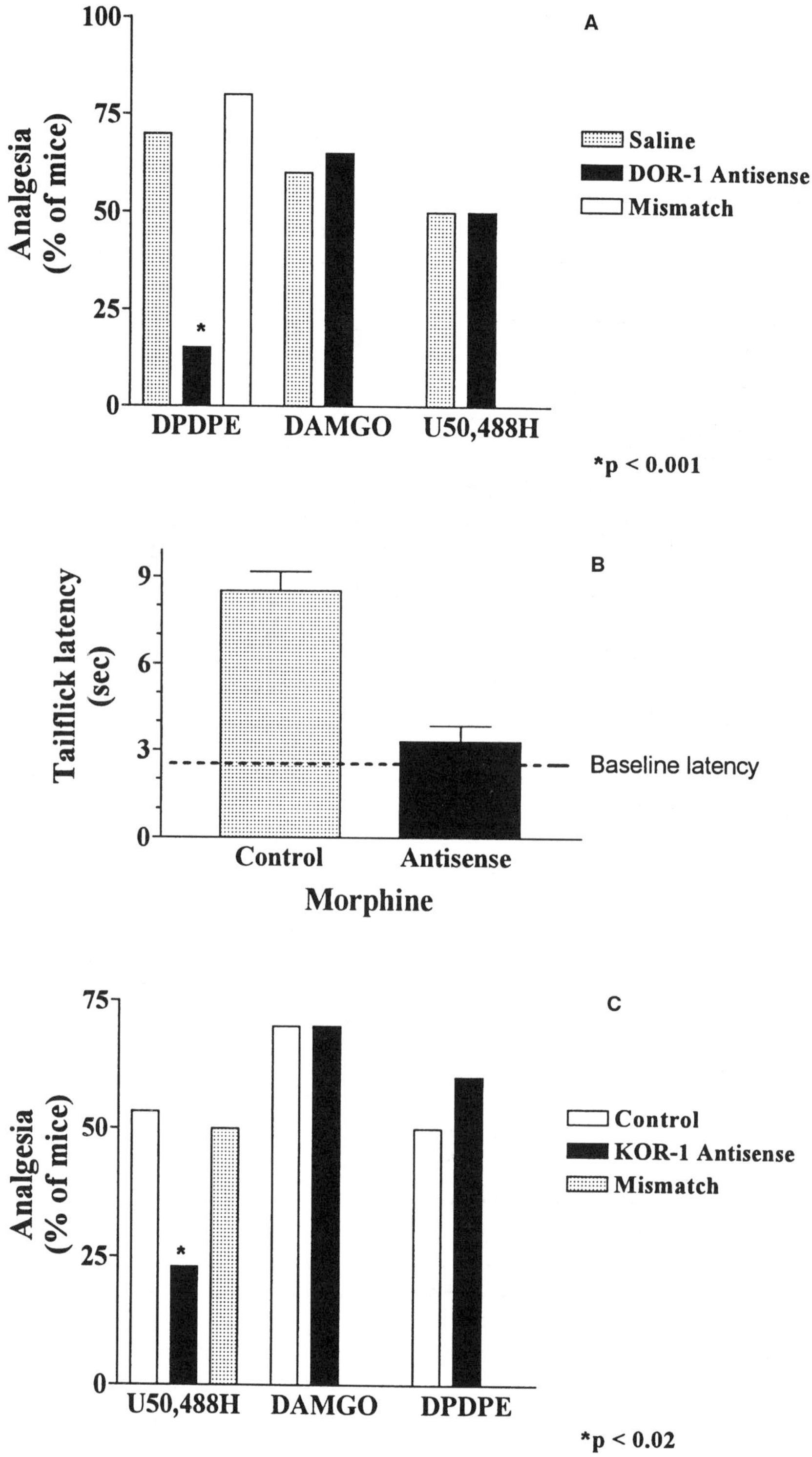

FIGURE 2
Summary of antisense treatment on opioid analgesia. Mice were treated with antisense oligodeoxynucleotide based upon (A) DOR-1,[76] (B) MOR-1,[84] or (C) KOR-1[85] on days 1, 3, and 5. Analgesia was assessed on day 6 with the delta drug DPDPE, the mu drug DAMGO, or the $kappa_1$ drug U50,488H.

control was inactive. Thus, this study implicated a major role for MOR-1 in morphine analgesia. A similar approach confirmed the importance of the KOR-1 clone in $kappa_1$ analgesia (Figure 2C),[85,86] and results were confirmed by others.[87,88] Administered spinally, an antisense oligodeoxynucleotide against this clone selectively blocked the analgesic actions of the highly selective $kappa_1$ agent U50,488H without interfering with the mu drug DAMGO or the delta drug DPDPE. Thus, these early studies quickly confirmed the relevance of the cloned traditional opioid receptors.

V. ANTISENSE MAPPING DOR-1

Next, we tried to assess whether any specific region along the mRNA was particularly sensitive to targeting with antisense. We designed five different oligodeoxynucleotides targeting various regions along the DOR-1 mRNA corresponding to all three exons and treated NG108 cells in tissue culture.[76] All the antisense oligodeoxynucleotides lowered ^{3}H-DPDPE binding equally well after five days of treatment (Figure 1), implying that any exon could be targeted using antisense approaches. It is important to note that the antisense-induced reductions were quite modest, ranging from only 40 to 50%. The effects were specific since the sense probe and the mismatch antisense probes were both inactive, and the treatment did not influence α_2-adrenergic receptor levels.[76] Furthermore, incubating the antisense probe with its corresponding sense probe prior to treating the cells also rendered the treatment ineffective.

The tissue culture studies indicated that antisense approaches could target any of the exons comprising the mRNA. Thus, antisense approaches can be used to explore the presence of individual exons in a functional receptor, permitting the assessment of potential alternative splicing. Although studies from several groups implied the existence of delta receptor subtypes,[2,43-47] only a single clone has been identified. These studies examining delta receptor subtypes utilized a series of agonists and antagonists to distinguish between the two putative receptors. However, the selectivity of the various agents for one site compared to the other was only modest. For example, DPDPE is more active at $delta_1$ receptors while [D-Ala^2,Glu^4]deltorphin is more active at $delta_2$. Because several groups had suggested that the NG108 cells contain $delta_2$ receptors, it was likely that DOR-1 encoded this receptor. Could these two subtypes represent isoforms of DOR-1?

Antisense oligodeoxynucleotides targeting exons 1, 2, or 3 of DOR-1 all blocked [D-Ala^2,Glu^4]deltorphin analgesia both spinally and supraspinally, implying that these actions were mediated through the DOR-1 receptor (Figure 3).[89] Spinally, all the antisense probes also blocked DPDPE analgesia, consistent with prior suggestions that this compound acts spinally through $delta_2$ receptors. Supraspinally, DPDPE appears to act through a different receptor mechanism. Despite the ability of all the antisense probes to block supraspinal [D-Ala^2,Glu^4]deltorphin analgesia, the oligodeoxynucleotide targeting exon 1 did not interfere with supraspinal DPDPE analgesia. Thus, the supraspinal analgesic receptor mechanisms subserving these two delta ligands appear to be quite distinct at the molecular level, consistent with true subtypes. The mapping studies are consistent with the possibility of alternatively spliced isoforms, but they have not yet been identified.

VI. ANTISENSE MAPPING MOR-1

Pharmacological studies have suggested subtypes of mu receptors.[1,2,18-26] Antagonists, such as naloxonazine, selectively block specific opioid actions without altering

DOR-1	exon 1	exon 2	exon 3
Binding (NG108)	1 / 1	1 / 1	3 / 3
Analgesia			
Deltorphin (i.t.)	2 / 2	1 / 1	2 / 2
DPDPE (i.t.)	2 / 2	1 / 1	2 / 2
Deltorphin (i.c.v.)	2 / 2	1 / 1	2 / 2
DPDPE (i.c.v.)	0 / 2	0 / 1	2 / 2

FIGURE 3
Antisense mapping DOR-1. Summary of antisense mapping studies of DOR-1 against ^{3}H-DPDPE binding in NG108 cells[76] or the analgesic actions of the delta$_1$ drug DPDPE or the delta$_2$ agent [D-Ala^2,Glu^4]deltorphin.[89] Shaded exons indicate that the antisense probes blocked the indicated response while clear ones indicate that the antisense probes were inactive. Inside each exon is given (the number of active antisense probes)/(number of antisense probes tested against that exon).

others. For example, naloxonazine blocks supraspinal morphine analgesia without interfering with either morphine-induced respiratory depression, inhibition of gastrointestinal transit, or even most signs of morphine dependence. Even morphine analgesia itself appears to be mediated through distinct subtypes. Although supraspinal morphine analgesia is sensitive to naloxonazine, spinal morphine analgesia is not. These traditional pharmacological approaches suggested two subtypes of mu receptors, subsequently termed mu$_1$ (naloxonazine sensitive) and mu$_2$. Binding correlates of these sites have been proposed. A very high affinity site of low abundance identified in brain tissue correlates with mu$_1$ receptors while the mu$_2$ receptor corresponds to the traditional mu opioid binding site. The concept of mu receptor subtypes was extended further by detailed studies with M6G.[27-30] M6G labels the traditional mu receptors in binding assays with an affinity slightly less than morphine; yet, when given centrally in mice, its analgesic potency is 100-fold greater. Efficacy differences between the two drugs cannot explain these observations since they both behave as partial agonists with similar intrinsic activities in cyclase studies. These observations raised the possibility that M6G might act through yet another subtype of the mu receptor. Although the pharmacology suggesting these designated subtypes was quite convincing, only a single mu receptor has been cloned, raising questions about its relationship to these pharmacologically defined subtypes. Detailed antisense mapping of MOR-1 now raises the possibility that these subtypes might represent isoforms of MOR-1 generated by alternative splicing.

After sequencing the mouse MOR-1 cDNA, we designed a series of eleven antisense oligodeoxynucleotides targeting each of the four exons (Figure 4) with exon 4 being quite short.[28] Three different probes were used against each of the first three exons. One probe was designed targeting the coding region while a second probe was made based upon the 3′ untranslated region. Using a paradigm similar to that previously established with DOR-1, we then treated groups of mice with these individual antisense probes. Animals received antisense treatment on days 1, 3, and 5 with pharmacological testing performed on day 6. The results were quite intriguing. The supraspinal analgesic actions of morphine were effectively blocked by all three antisense probes targeting exon 1, including the original probe used in the rat study.

However, these same probes were inactive against spinal morphine analgesia. The possibility of technical problems in these studies is very unlikely since the probe targeting the coding region of exon 4 blocked both spinal and supraspinal morphine analgesia. These results distinguishing between a mu_1 and mu_2 action were interesting since they provided the first molecular evidence supporting discrete mu receptor subtypes. To explore this possibility further, we examined another mu_2 action, the inhibition of gastrointestinal transit by morphine. Like the first two actions, the antisense based upon the coding region of exon 4 effectively blocked this response, but the probes targeting exon 1 were ineffective. Thus, the antisense mapping profile of gastrointestinal transit activity corresponded closely to that of spinal analgesia with both pharmacologically defined as mu_2 actions (Figure 4).

MOR-1	exon 1	exon 2	exon 3	exon 4
Analgesia				
Morphine (i.c.v.)	3 / 3	0 / 3	1 / 3	1 / 1*
Morphine (peripheral)	1 /1	0 / 1	0 / 1	1 / 1*
Morphine (i.t.)	0 / 3	0 / 3	1 / 3	1 / 1*
M 6 G (i.c.v)	0 / 3	3 / 3	3 / 3	0 / 1*
GI Transit	0/ 3	0 / 3	0 / 3	1 / 1*
Feeding	1 / 1	1 / 1	1 / 1	1 / 1*

* Coding region

FIGURE 4
Antisense mapping MOR-1. Summary of antisense mapping studies of MOR-1 against morphine and M6G analgesia in mice.[27,28] Gastrointestinal transit was assessed in mice with morphine given i.c.v.[28] Free feeding was tested in rats.[90] Shaded exons indicate that the antisense probes blocked the indicated response while clear ones indicate that the antisense probes were inactive. Inside each exon is given (the number of active antisense probes)/(number of antisense probes tested against that exon).

The probes targeting exons 2 and 3 provided very interesting insights into the pharmacology of these mu receptors. None of the probes based upon exon 2 influenced morphine actions. Of the three based upon exon 3, only one was effective against supraspinal morphine analgesia. These findings varied enormously from those observed against M6G analgesia which was effectively blocked by all six probes targeting exons 2 and 3. At the same time, the antisense oligodeoxynucleotides from exons 1 and 4 active against supraspinal morphine analgesia were without effect against M6G analgesia. The activity of multiple probes within an exon greatly enhances the likelihood of a selective effect. Furthermore, the fact that all the antisense probe's targets exons 1, 2, 3, and the coding region of exon 4 were active in at least one functional assay strongly argues that these differences among behaviors cannot result from technical problems with the approach. Yet, the sensitivity of morphine and M6G analgesia to the various antisense probes was quite different. The only antisense inactive in all assays targeted the 3′ untranslated region of exon 4. This complete inactivity of the probe precludes any judgments regarding its actions. These results strongly suggest that different receptors mediate the analgesic effects of morphine and M6G and that they probably respresent isoforms of MOR-1. Ironically, MOR-1 itself does not appear to be responsible for any of these analgesic actions.

These results have been observed in rats as well.[27] Morphine analgesia is blocked by exon 1 and 4 probes, but not those from exons 2 and 3. M6G analgesia shows the exact opposite sensitivities, as previously observed in mice. Most recently, we have examined free feeding behavior in rats.[90] These results differed from the others in that probes targeting all four exons effectively blocked the behavior. Thus, free feeding behavior appears to involve MOR-1.

VII. KAPPA$_3$ RECEPTORS AND THE ORPHAN CLONE

Using a variety of opioid drugs, evidence strongly suggests the presence of a subtype of kappa receptor, termed kappa$_3$, which mediates analgesia through entirely distinct mechanisms.[1,2,32,35-41] Using a series of novel opiates, including naloxone benzoylhydrazone (NalBzoH), we demonstrated that kappa$_3$ analgesia has a different sensitivity to a variety of selective opioid antagonists and shows no cross-tolerance to traditional opioid drugs. Subsequent studies suggest that this receptor probably corresponds to the nalorphine site first suggested by Martin[91] in his proposal of receptor dualism. The relationship of this pharmacologically defined receptor to the cloned receptors has proven elusive. Like many other groups, we designed a series of degenerate primers based upon DOR-1 for use in RT-PCR to look for additional opioid receptor subtypes. We quickly identified a cDNA fragment of approximately 500 bp. To assess whether it might be related to an opioid receptor before cloning out the full length cDNA, we designed an antisense oligdeoxynucleotide and examined its effects upon a series of opioid analgesics. It was inactive against all the traditional opioid analgesics, including morphine (mu), DPDPE (delta), and U50,488H (kappa$_1$); (Figure 5).[63,66] However, it potently blocked the analgesic actions of the kappa$_3$-analgesic NalBzoH. A mismatch control was inactive, further supporting the specificity of the response. Based upon these results, we then cloned the full length cDNA from mouse, termed KOR-3. The association of this cDNA with the kappa$_3$ receptor is further supported by the ability of a monoclonal antibody recognizing the kappa$_3$ receptor to recognize the protein encoded by KOR-3 in both traditional expression systems utilizing CHO cells, as well as *in vitro* translation. Together, these studies suggested a close association between this receptor and kappa$_3$ receptor.

Despite this strong evidence correlating KOR-3 with the kappa$_3$ receptor, further study has confirmed that KOR-3 does not encode the kappa$_3$ receptor. When expressed, the KOR-3 receptor has poor affinity for traditional opiates, including those active against kappa$_3$ receptors. More recently several groups isolated the novel peptide OFQ/N, which has very high affinity for the KOR-3 receptor in binding and functional assays and presumably is the endogenous ligand for this receptor. In contrast to the subnanomolar affinity of OFQ/N for this receptor, OFQ/N has no appreciable affinity at any of the traditional opioid receptors in binding assays. Thus the relationship between the kappa$_3$ receptor and this fourth member of the cloned opiate receptor family identified by our group and numerous others is somewhat ambiguous.

Antisense mapping has opened several possibilities to explain these results (Figure 6).[63] Our initial probe targeted the third coding exon. An additional five probes targeting exons 2 and 3 also effectively blocked the analgesic actions of NalBzoH. In contrast, five probes based upon the first exon were inactive. The strong demarcation between exons 1 and the other two strongly raise the possibility that kappa$_3$ receptors may be isoforms of KOR-3 generated by alternative splicing.

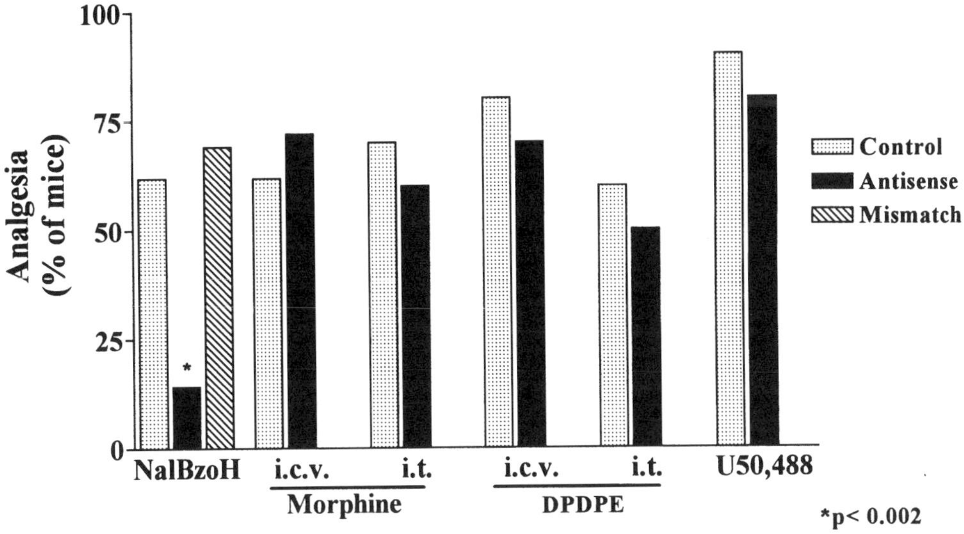

FIGURE 5
Selectivity of a KOR-3 antisense probe on opioid analgesia. Effects of an antisense oligodeoxynucleotide based upon KOR-3 on opioid analgesia.[6,63,66] Mice received the antisense probes on days 1, 3, and 5. Analgesia was tested with the indicated analgesic. The kappa$_3$ drug NalBzoH was given intracerebroventricularly (i.c.v.), the mu drug morphine and the delta drug DPDPE were both given i.c.v. and intrathecally (i.t.), and the kappa$_1$ drug only i.t.

Antisense approaches also have proven valuable in looking at OFQ/N. OFQ/N has a biphasic action when given supraspinally in mice. There is an initial hyperalgesia[92,93] followed by analgesia. These two actions can be easily distinguished pharmacologically. For example, the hyperalgesia is resistant to opioid antagonists while the analgesic actions are readily reversed by naloxone, naltrexone, or diprenorphine. An antisense probe targeting exon 1 which is ineffective against kappa$_3$ analgesia blocks the hyperalgesia without interfering with the analgesic response (Figure 6). This is important for two reasons. First, it confirms that the antisense itself is active in at least one assay. Second, it supports the possibility that OFQ/N is producing analgesia and hyperalgesia through distinct receptor systems.

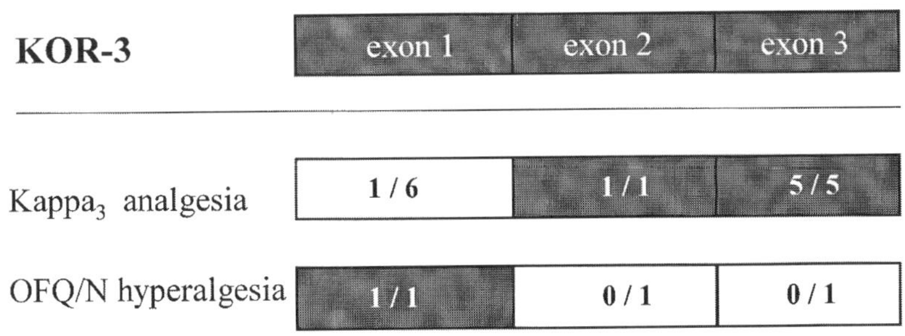

FIGURE 6
Antisense mapping KOR-3. Summary of antisense mapping studies of KOR-3 in mice against kappa$_3$ analgesia using NalBzoH[63] and OFQ/N hyperalgesia.[92] Shaded exons indicate that the antisense probes blocked the indicated response while clear ones indicate that the antisense probes were inactive. Inside each exon is given (the number of active antisense probes)/(number of antisense probes tested against that exon).

VIII. SECOND MESSENGER SYSTEMS IN OPIOID ANALGESIA

Antisense probes also have proven effective in investigating the role of specific G protein α subunits in opioid actions.[94-97] Antisense probes based upon the various different Gα proteins can selectively downregulate individual Gα proteins without affecting the expression of others, as determined by immunoblots.[95,96] Time action studies reveal significant reductions after a single injection of these antisense probes, with a maximal effect between 24 to 48 h after injection. A wide variety of Gα proteins have been examined in this model against a large number of opioid receptor systems. Overall, the G proteins involved with the various opioid receptor systems vary in their needs for individual G proteins. Downregulation of $G_i\alpha2$ inhibits morphine analgesia, while oligodeoxynucleotides directed against $G_i\alpha1$ or $G_i\alpha3$ are ineffective (Table 2). In contrast, the probes against $G_i\alpha1$ or $G_i\alpha3$ block M6G and κ_3-opioid receptor analgesia. The overall profile of each opioid receptor system to the battery of G-protein antisense probes is consistent with independent and distinct systems. In these studies, however, it is important to keep in mind that interruption anywhere along the circuit may block the response. Thus, activity of a specific antisense does not necessarily imply that the opioid receptor actually couples to the specific G protein being targeted. Alternatively, it may play a role downstream in the circuit.

TABLE 2

Summary of the Sensitivity of Opioid Analgesia to G-protein α Subunits

	Blockade of Analgesia by Antisense ODN						
	$G_i\alpha1$	$G_i\alpha2$	$G_i\alpha3$	$G_o\alpha$	$G_q\alpha$	$G_{x/z}\alpha$	$G_s\alpha$
Supraspinal							
Morphine	–	++	–	+	–	–	+
M6G	++	–	–	–	–	+	+
NalBzoH	++	–	+	–	+	+++	+++
Spinal	–	–	–	–	–	–	–
Morphine	–	+	–	–	–	+	–
M6G	++	–	+	+	–	+	–
U50,488	–	–	–	–	++	–	–
DPDPE	+++	++	++	++	++	+	+++

Note: Results summarize the ability of treatment with an antisense oligodeoxynucleotide targeting the indicated G-protein α subunit.[95] Increasing degrees of blockade of the analgesic response is indicated by increasing numbers of "+". Treatments which did not significantly lower the response are denoted by "–". All drugs were tested with all antisense treatments.

IX. CONCLUSION

Antisense approaches have proven very valuable in understanding the relationship of various opioid receptors with their functional correlates and have provided valuable information regarding various analgesic systems, although the suggestion of alternative splicing still requires the isolation of the various cDNAs. The possibility of looking for specific exons and alternative splicing with this approach may prove to be very valuable as a basic approach toward understanding CNS function.

REFERENCES

1. Pasternak, G.W., Pharmacological mechanisms of opioid analgesics, *Clin. Neuropharmacol.*, 16, 1, 1993.
2. Reisine, T. and Pasternak, G.W., Opioid analgesics and antagonists, *Goodman & Gilman's: The Pharmacological Basis of Therapeutics*, 9th ed., Hardman, J.G. and Limbird, L.E., Eds., McGraw-Hill, 1996, 521.
3. Wagner, R.W., Gene inhibition using antisense oligodeoxynucleotides, *Nature*, 372, 333, 1994.
4. Crooke, S.T., Progress toward oligonucleotide therapeutics: pharmacodynamic properties, *FASEB J.*, 7, 533, 1993.
5. Crooke, S.T. and Bennett, C.F., Progress in antisense oligonucleotide therapeutic, *Annu. Rev. Pharmacol. Toxicol.*, 36, 107, 1996.
6. Pasternak, G.W. and Standifer, K.M., Mapping of opioid receptors using antisense oligodeoxynucleotides: Correlating their molecular biology and pharmacology, *Trends Pharmacol. Sci.*, 16, 344, 1995.
7. Wahlestedt, C., Antisense oligonucleotide strategies in neuropharmacology, *Trends Pharmacol. Sci.*, 15, 42, 1994.
8. Holopainen, I. and Wojcik, W.J., A specific antisense oligodeoxynucleotide to mRNAs encoding receptors with seven transmembrane spanning regions decreases muscarinic m_2 and gamma-aminobutyric $acid_B$ receptors in rat cerebellar granule cells, *J. Pharmacol. Exp. Ther.*, 264, 423, 1993.
9. Wahlestedt, C., Pich, E.M., Koob, G.F., Yee, F., and Heilig, M., Modulation of anxiety and neuropeptide Y-Y1 receptors by antisense oligodeoxynucleotides, *Science*, 528, 1993.
10. Wahlestedt, C., Golanov, E., Yamamoto, S., Yee, F., Ericson, H., Yoo, H., Inturrisi, C.E., and Reis, D.J., Antisense oligodeoxynucleotides to NMDA-R1 receptor channels protect cortical neurons from excitotoxicity and reduce focal ischaemic infactions, *Science*, 363, 260, 1993.
11. Zhang, M. and Creese, I., Antisense oligodeoxynucleotide reduces brain dopamine D2 receptors: behavioral correlates, *Neurosci. Lett.*, 161, 223, 1993.
12. Yeung, J.C. and Rudy, T.A., Multiplicative interaction between narcotic agonisms expressed at spinal and supraspinal sites of antinociceptive action as revealed by concurrent intrathecal and intracerebroventricular injections of morphine, *J. Pharmacol. Exp. Ther.*, 215, 633, 1980.
13. Stein, C., Schäfer, M., and Hassan, A.H.S., Peripheral opioid receptors, *Ann. Med.*, 27, 219, 1995.
14. Barber, A. and Gottschlich, R., Opioid agonists and antagonists: an evaluation of their peripheral actions in inflammation, *Med. Res. Rev.*, 12, 525, 1992.
15. Joris, J.L., Dubner, R., and Hargreaves, K.M., Opioid analgesia at peripheral sites: a target for opioids released during stress and inflammation?, *Anesth. Analg.*, 66, 1277, 1987.
16. Junien, J.L. and Wettstein, J.G., Role of opioids in peripheral analgesia, *Life Sci.*, 51, 2009, 1992.
17. Kolesnikov, Y.A., Jain, S., Wilson, R., and Pasternak, G.W., Peripheral morphine analgesia: Synergy with central sites and a target of morphine tolerance, *J. Pharmacol. Exp. Ther.*, 279, 502, 1996.
18. Pasternak, G.W. and Snyder, S.H., Identification of a novel high affinity opiate receptor binding in rat brain, *Nature*, 253, 563, 1975.
19. Wolozin, B.L. and Pasternak, G.W., Classification of multiple morphine and enkephalin binding sites in the central nervous system, *Proc. Natl. Acad. Sci. U.S.A.*, 78, 6181, 1981.
20. Pasternak, G.W., Childers, S.R., and Snyder, S.H., Opiate analgesia: Evidence for mediation by a subpopulation of opiate receptors, *Science*, 208, 514, 1980.
21. Nishimura, S., Recht, L.D., and Pasternak, G.W., Biochemical characterization of high affinity ^{3}H-opioid binding: Further evidence for mu_1 sites, *Mol. Pharmacol.*, 25, 29, 1984.
22. Bodnar, R.J., Williams, C.W., and Pasternak, G.W., Role of mu_1 opiate receptors in supraspinal opiate analgesia: A microinjection study, *Brain Res.*, 447, 45, 1988.
23. Heyman, J.S., Williams, C.L., Burks, T.F., Mosberg, H.I., and Porreca, F., Dissociation of opioid antinociception and central gastrointestinal propulsion in the mouse: Studies with naloxonazine, *J. Pharmacol. Exp. Ther.*, 245, 238, 1988.
24. Pasternak, G.W., Childers, S.R., and Snyder, S.H., Naloxazone, long-acting opiate antagonist: Effects in intact animals and on opiate receptor binding *in vitro*, *J. Pharmacol. Exp. Ther.*, 214, 455, 1980.
25. Ling, G.S.F., Spiegel, K., Lockhart, S.H., and Pasternak, G.W., Separation of opioid analgesia from respiratory depression: evidence for different receptor mechanisms, *J. Pharmacol. Exp. Ther.*, 232, 149, 1985.
26. Goodman, R.R. and Pasternak, G.W., Visualization of mu_1 opiate receptors in rat brain using a computerized autoradiographic subtraction technique, Proc. Natl. Acad. Sci. U.S.A., 82, 6667, 1985.

27. Rossi, G.C., Standifer, K.M., and Pasternak, G.W., Differential blockade of morphine and morphine-6β-glucuronide analgesia by antisense oligodeoxynucleotides directed against MOR-1 and G-protein α subunits in rats, Neurosci. Lett., 198, 99, 1995.
28. Rossi, G.C., Pan, Y.-X., Brown, G.P., and Pasternak, G.W., Antisense mapping the MOR-1 opioid receptor: Evidence for alternative splicing and a novel morphine-6ß-glucuronide receptor, *FEBS Lett.*, 369, 192, 1995.
29. Pasternak, G.W., Bodnar, R.J., Clark, J.A., and Inturrisi, C.E., Morphine-6-glucuronide, a potent mu agonist, *Life Sci.*, 41, 2845, 1987.
30. Paul, D., Standifer, K.M., Inturrisi, C.E., and Pasternak, G.W., Pharmacological characterization of morphine-6β-glucuronide, a very potent morphine metabolite, *J. Pharmacol. Exp. Ther.*, 251, 477, 1989.
31. Martin, W.R., Eades, C.G., Thompson, J.A., Huppler, R.E., and Gilbert, P.E., The effects of morphine and nalorphine-like drugs in the nondependent and morphine-dependent chronic spinal dog, *J. Pharmacol. Exp. Ther.*, 197, 517, 1976.
32. Clark, J.A., Liu, L., Price, M., Hersh, B., Edelson, M., and Pasternak, G.W., Kappa opiate receptor multiplicity: Evidence for two U50,488-sensitive $kappa_1$ subtypes and a novel $kappa_3$ subtype, *J. Pharmacol. Exp. Ther.*, 251, 461, 1989.
33. VonVoightlander, P.F., Lahti, R.A., and Ludens, J.H., U50,488: a selective and structurally novel non-mu (kappa) opioid agonist, *J. Pharmacol. Exp. Ther.*, 224, 7, 1983.
34. Kosterlitz, H.W., Paterson, S.J., and Robson, L.E., Characterization of the kappa subtype of opiate receptor in the guinea pig brain, *Br. J. Pharmacol.*, 68, 333, 1986.
35. Standifer, K.M., Cheng, J., Brooks, A.I., Honrado, C.P., Su, W., Visconti, L.M., Biedler, J.L., and Pasternak, G.W., Biochemical and pharmacological characterization of mu, delta and $kappa_3$ opioid receptors expressed in BE(2)-C neuroblastoma cells, *J. Pharmacol. Exp. Ther.*, 270, 1246, 1994.
36. Paul, D., Levison, J.A., Howard, D.H., Pick, C.G., Hahn, E.F., and Pasternak, G.W., Naloxone benzoylhydrazone (NalBzoH) analgesia, *J. Pharmacol. Exp. Ther.*, 255, 769, 1990.
37. Price, M., Gistrak, M.A., Itzhak, Y., Hahn, E.F., and Pasternak, G.W., Receptor binding of ^{3}H-naloxone benzoylhydrazone: A reversible kappa and slowly dissociable μ opiate, *Mol. Pharmacol.*, 35, 67, 1989.
38. Gistrak, M.A., Paul, D., Hahn, E.F., and Pasternak, G.W., Pharmacological actions of a novel mixed opiate agonist/antagonist, naloxone benzoylhydrazone, *J. Pharmacol. Exp. Ther.*, 251, 469, 1990.
39. Cheng, J., Standifer, K.M., Tublin, P.R., Su, W., and Pasternak, G.W., Demonstration of $kappa_3$-opioid receptors in the SH-SY5Y human neuroblastoma cell line, *J. Neurochem.*, 65, 170, 1995.
40. Cheng, J., Roques, B.P., Gacel, G.A., Huang, E., and Pasternak, G.W., $Kappa_3$ opiate receptor binding in the mouse and rat, *Eur. J. Pharmacol.*, 226, 15, 1992.
41. Paul, D., Pick, C.G., Tive, L.A., and Pasternak, G.W., Pharmacological characterization of nalorphine, a $kappa_3$ analgesic, *J. Pharmacol. Exp. Ther.*, 257, 1, 1991.
42. Lord, J.A.H., Waterfield, A.A., Hughes, J., and Kosterlitz, H.W., Endogenous opioid peptides: multiple agonists and receptors, *Nature*, 267, 495, 1977.
43. Vanderah, T., Takemori, A.E., Sultana, M., Portoghese, P.S., Mosberg, H.I., Hruby, V.J., Haaseth, R.C., Matsunaga, T.O., and Porreca, F., Interaction of [D-Pen^2,D-Pen^5]enkephalin and [D-Ala^2,Glu^4]deltorphin with δ-opioid receptor subtypes *in vivo*, *Eur. J. Pharmacol.*, 252, 133, 1994.
44. Fang, L., Knapp, R.J., Horvath, R., Matsunaga, T.O., Haaseth, R.C., Hruby, V.J., Porreca, F., and Yamamura, H.I., Characterization of [^{3}H]naltrindole binding to delta opioid receptors in mouse brain and mouse vas deferens: Evidence for delta opioid receptor heterogeneity, *J. Pharmacol. Exp. Ther.*, 268, 836, 1994.
45. Takemori, A.E. and Portoghese, P.S., Enkephalin antinociception in mice is mediated by δ_1- and δ_2-opioid receptors in the brain and spinal cord, respectively, *Eur. J. Pharmacol.*, 242, 145, 1993.
46. Jiang, Q., Takemori, A.E., Sultana, M., Portoghese, P.S., Bowen, W.D., Mosberg, H.I., and Porreca, F., Differential antagonism of opiate delta antinociception by [D-Ala^2,Cys^6]enkaphalin and naltrindole-5′-iosothiocyanate: evidence for subtypes, *J. Pharmacol. Exp. Ther.*, 257, 1069, 1991.
47. Mattia, A., Vanderah, T., Mosberg, H.I., and Porreca, F., Lack of antinociceptive cross tolerance between [D-Pen^2,D-Pen^5]enkephalin and [D-Ala^2]deltorphin II in mice: evidence for delta receptor subtypes, *J. Pharmacol. Exp. Ther.*, 258, 583, 1991.
48. Kieffer, B.L., Befort, K., Gaveriaux-Ruff, C., and Hirth, C.G., The δ-opioid receptor: Isolation of a cDNA by expression cloning and pharmacological characterization, *Proc. Natl. Acad. Sci. U.S.A.*, 89, 12048, 1992.
49. Evans, C.J., Keith, D.F., Morrison, H., Magendzo, K., and Edwards, R.H., Cloning of the delta opioid receptor by functional expression, *Science*, 258, 1952, 1992.
50. Chen, Y., Mestek, A., Liu, J., Hurley, J.A., and Yu, L., Molecular cloning and functional expression of a μ-opioid receptor from rat brain, *Mol. Pharmacol.*, 44, 8, 1993.

51. Minami, M., Toya, T., Katao, Y., Maekawa, K., Nakamura, S., Onogi, T., Kaneko, S., and Satoh, M., Cloning and expression of a cDNA for the rat kappa-opioid receptor, *FEBS Lett.*, 329, 291, 1993.
52. Thompson, R.C., Mansour, A., Akil, H., and Watson, S.J., Cloning and pharmacological characterization of a rat μ opioid receptor, *Neuron*, 11, 903, 1993.
53. Eppler, C.M., Hulmes, J.D., Wang, J.-B., Johnson, B., Corbett, M., Luthin, D.R., Uhl, G.R., and Linden, J., Purification and partial amino acid sequence of a μ opioid receptor from rat brain, *J. Biol. Chem.*, 268, 26447, 1993.
54. Reisine, T. and Bell, G.I., Molecular biology of opioid receptors, *Trends Neurosci.*, 16, 506, 1993.
55. Wang, J.B., Johnson, P.S., Persico, A.M., Hawkins, A.L., Griffin, C.A., and Uhl, G.R., Human μ opiate receptor: cDNA and genomic clones, pharmacologic characterization and chromosomal assignment, *FEBS Lett.*, 338, 217, 1994.
56. Raynor, K., Kong, H., Chen, Y., Yasuda, K., Yu, L., Bell, G.I., and Reisine, T., Pharmacological characterization of the cloned kappa-, δ-, and μ-opioid receptors, *Mol. Pharmacol.*, 45, 330, 1994.
57. Yasuda, K., Raynor, K., Kong, H., Breder, C., Takeda, J., Reisine, T., and Bell, G., Cloning and functional comparison of kappa and δ opioid receptors from mouse brain, *Proc. Natl. Acad. Sci. U.S.A.*, 90, 6736, 1993.
58. Kozak, C.A., Filie, J., Adamson, M.C., Chen, Y., and Yu, L., Murine chromosomal location of the μ and kappa opioid receptor genes, *Genomics*, 21, 659, 1994.
59. Min, B.H., Augustin, L.B., Felsheim, R.F., Fuchs, J.A., and Loh, H.H., Genomic structure and analysis of promoter sequence of a mouse μ opioid receptor gene, *Proc. Natl. Acad. Sci. U.S.A.*, 91, 9081, 1994.
60. Knapp, R.J., Malatynska, E., Fang, L., Li, X., Babin, E., Nguyen, M., Santoro, G., Varga, E.V., Hruby, V.J., Roeske, W.R., and Yamamura, H.I., Identification of a human delta opioid receptor: Cloning and expression, *Life Sci.*, 54, PL463, 1994.
61. Bare, L.A., Mansson, E., and Yang, D., Expression of two variants of the human μ opioid receptor mRNA in SK-N-SH cells and human brain, *FEBS Lett.*, 354, 213, 1994.
62. Zimprich, A., Bacher, B., and Höllt, V., Cloning and expression of an isoform of the rmu-opioid receptor (rmuOR1B), *Regul. Pept.*, 54, 347, 1994.
63. Pan, Y.-X., Cheng, J., Xu, J., Rossi, G.C., Jacobson, E., Ryan-Moro, J., Brooks, A.I., Dean, G.E., Standifer, K.M., and Pasternak, G.W., Cloning and functional characterization through antisense mapping of a kappa$_3$-related opioid receptor, *Mol. Pharmacol.*, 47, 1180, 1995.
64. Chen, Y., Fan, Y., Liu, J., Mestek, A., Tian, M., Kozak, C.A., and Yu, L., Molecular cloning, tissue distribution and chromosomal localization of a novel member of the opioid receptor gene family, *FEBS Lett.*, 347, 279, 1994.
65. Keith, D., Jr., Maung, T., Anton, B., and Evans, C., Isolation of cDNA clones homologous to opioid receptors, *Regul. Pept.*, 54, 143, 1994.
66. Pan, Y.X., Cheng, J., Xu, J., and Pasternak, G.W., Cloning, expression and classification of a kappa$_3$-related opioid receptor using antisense oligodeoxynucleotides, *Regul. Pept.*, 54, 217, 1994.
67. Uhl, G.R., Childers, S., and Pasternak, G.W., An opiate-receptor gene family reunion, *Trends Neurosci.*, 17, 89, 1994.
68. Wick, M.J., Minnerath, S.R., Lin, X., Elde, R., Law, P.-Y., and Loh, H.H., Isolation of a novel cDNA encoding a putative membrane receptor with high homology to the cloned μ, δ, and kappa opioid receptors, Mol. *Brain Res.*, 27, 37, 1994.
69. Wang, J.B., Johnson, P.S., Imai, Y., Persico, A.M., Ozenberger, B.A., Eppler, C.M., and Uhl, G.R., cDNA cloning of an orphan opiate receptor gene family member and its splice variant, *FEBS Lett.*, 348, 75, 1994.
70. Mollereau, C., Parmentier, M., Mailleux, P., Butour, J.L., Moisand, C., Chalon, P., Caput, D., Vassart, G., and Meunier, J.C., ORL-1, a novel member of the opioid family: cloning, functional expression and localization, *FEBS Lett.*, 341, 33, 1994.
71. Lachowicz, J.E., Shen, Y., Monsma, F.J., Jr., and Sibley, D.R., Molecular cloning of a novel G protein-coupled receptor related to the opiate receptor family, *J. Neurochem.*, 64, 34, 1995.
72. Bunzow, J.R., Saez, C., Mortrud, M., Bouvier, C., Williams, J.T., Low, M., and Grandy, D.K., Molecular cloning and tissue distribution of a putative member of the rat opioid receptor gene family that is not a μ, δ or kappa opioid receptor type, *FEBS Lett.*, 347, 284, 1994.
73. Fukuda, K., Kato, S., Mori, K., Nishi, M., Takeshima, H., Iwabe, N., Miyata, T., Houtani, T., and Siguimoti, T., cDNA cloning and regional distribution of a novel member of the opioid receptor family, *FEBS Lett.*, 343, 42, 1994.
74. Reinscheid, R.K., Nothacker, H.P., Bourson, A., Ardati, A., Henningsen, R.A., Bunzow, J.R., Grandy, D.K., Langen, H., Monsma, F.J., and Civelli, O., Orphanin FQ: a neuropeptide that activates an opioidlike G protein-coupled receptor, *Science*, 270, 792, 1995.

75. Meunier, J.C., Mollereau, C., Toll, L., Suaudeau, C., Moisand, C., Alvinerie, P., Butour, J.L., Guillemot, J.C., Ferrara, P., Monsarrat, B., Mazargull, H., Vassart, G., Parmentier, M., and Costentin, J., Isolation and structure of the endogenous agonist of the opioid receptor like ORL_1 receptor, *Nature*, 377, 532, 1995.
76. Standifer, K.M., Chien, C.-C., Wahlestedt, C., Brown, G.P., and Pasternak, G.W., Selective loss of δ opioid analgesia and binding by antisense oligodeoxynucleotides to a δ opioid receptor, *Neuron*, 12, 805, 1994.
77. Standifer, K.M., Jenab, S., Su, W., Chien, C.-C., Pan, Y.-X., Inturrisi, C.E., and Pasternak, G.W., Antisense oligodeoxynucleotides to the cloned δ receptor, DOR-1: Uptake, stability and regulation of gene expression, *J. Neurochem.*, 65, 1981, 1995.
78. Tseng, L.F., Collins, K.A., and Kampine, J.P., Antisense oligodeoxynucleotide to a δ-opioid receptor selectively blocks the spinal antinociception induced by δ-, but not μ- or kappa-opioid receptor agonists in the mouse, *Eur. J. Pharmacol.*, 258, R1, 1994.
79. Lai, J., Bilsky, E.J., Rothman, R.B., and Porreca, F., Treatment with antisense oligodeoxynucleotide to the opioid δ receptor selectively inhibits δ_2-agonist antinociception, *Neuroreport*, 5, 1049, 1994.
80. Lai, J., Bilsky, E.J., Bernstein, R.N., Rothman, R.B., Pasternak, G.W., and Porreca, F., Antisense oligodeoxynucleotide to the cloned delta opioid receptor selectively inhibits supraspinal, but not spinal, antinociceptive effects of [D-Ala^2,Glu^4]deltorphin, *Regul. Pept.*, 54, 159, 1994.
81. Bilsky, E.J., Bernstein, R.N., Pasternak, G.W., Hruby, V.J., Patel, D., Porreca, F., and Lai, J., Selective inhibition of [D-Ala^2,Glu^4]deltorphin antinociception by supraspinal, but not spinal, administration of an antisense oligodeoxynucleotide to an opioid delta receptor, *Life Sci.*, 55, 37, 1994.
82. Cha, X.Y., Xu, H., Ni, Q., Partilla, J.S., Rice, K.C., Matecka, D., Calderon, S.N., Porreca, F., Lai, J., and Rothman, R.B., Opioid peptide receptor studies: Antisense oligodeoxynucleotide to the delta opioid receptor delineates opioid receptor subtypes, *Regul. Pept.*, 59, 247, 1995.
83. Wang, J.B., Imai, Y., Eppler, C.M., Gregor, P., Spivak, C.E., and Uhl, G.R., μ opiate receptor: cDNA cloning and expression, *Proc. Natl. Acad. Sci. U.S.A.*, 90, 10230, 1993.
84. Rossi, G.C., Pan, Y.-X., Cheng, J., and Pasternak, G.W., Blockade of morphine analgesia by an antisense oligodeoxynucleotide against the mu receptor, *Life Sci.*, 54, PL375, 1994.
85. Chien, C.-C., Brown, G., Pan, Y.-X., and Pasternak, G.W., Blockade of U50,488H analgesia by antisense oligodeoxynucleotides to a kappa-opioid receptor, *Eur. J. Pharmacol.*, 253, R7, 1994.
86. Chien, C.C. and Pasternak, G.W., (-)-Pentazocine analgesia in mice: Interactions with a α receptor system, *Eur. J. Pharmacol.*, 294, 303, 1995.
87. Adams, J.U., Chen, X.H., Deriel, J.K., Adler, M.W., and Liu-Chen, L.-Y., *In vivo* treatment with antisense oligodeoxynucleotide to kappa-opioid receptors inhibited kappa-agonist-induced analgesia in rats, *Regul. Pept.*, 54, 1, 1994.
88. Adams, J.U., Chen, X., Deriel, J.K., Adler, M.W., and Liu-Chen, L.-Y., Intracerebroventricular treatment with an antisense oligodeoxynucleotide to kappa-opioid receptors inhibited kappa-agonist-induced analgesia in rats, *Brain Res.*, 667, 129, 1994.
89. Rossi, G.C., Leventhal, L., and Pasternak, G.W., Antisense mapping DOR-1: Evidence for delta receptor subtypes, *Brain Res.*, in press.
90. Leventhal, L., Bodnar, R.J., Cole, J.L., Rossi, G.C., Pan, Y.X., and Pasternak, G.W., Antisense oligodeoxynucleotides against the MOR-1 clone alter weight and ingestive responses in rats, *Brain Res.*, 719, 78, 1996.
91. Martin, W.R., Opioid antagonists, *Pharmacol. Rev.*, 19, 463, 1967.
92. Rossi, G., Leventhal, L., Boland, E., and Pasternak, G.W., Pharmacological characterization of orphanin FQ/nociceptin and its fragments, submitted.
93. Rossi, G.C., Leventhal, L., and Pasternak, G.W., Naloxone-sensitive orphanin FQ-induced analgesia in mice, *Eur. J. Pharmacol.*, 31, R7, 1996.
94. Raffa, R.B., Martinez, R.P., and Connelly, C.D., G-protein antisense oligodeoxyribonucleotides and μ-opioid supraspinal antinociception, *Eur. J. Pharmacol.*, 258, R5, 1994.
95. Standifer, K.M., Rossi, G.C., and Pasternak, G.W., Differential blockade of opioid analgesia by antisense oligodeoxynucleotides directed against various G-protein α subunits, *Mol. Pharmacol.*, 50, 293, 1996.
96. Raffa, R.B., Goode, T.L., Martinez, R.P., and Jacoby, H.I., $AG_i2\alpha$ antisense oligonucleotide differentiates morphine antinociception, constipation and acute dependence in mice, *Life Sci.*, 5, PL73, 1996.
97. Sanchez-Blazquez, P., Garcia-Espana, A., and Garzon, J., *In vivo* injection of antisense oligodeoxynucleotides to Gα subunits and supraspinal analgesia evoked by mu and delta opioid agonists, *J. Pharmacol. Exp. Ther.*, 275, 1590, 1995.

Chapter 7

Antisense Oligodeoxynucleotides Targeted to the Angiotensin System as a Novel Strategy to Treat Hypertension

M. Ian Phillips and Robert Gyurko

CONTENTS

0-8493-8552-0/97/$0.00+$.50

I. INTRODUCTION

Hypertension is one of the most important risk factors for myocardial infarction, stroke, congestive heart failure, end-stage renal disease, and peripheral vascular disease.[1,2] An estimated 43 million (24%) of the adult, civilian, noninstitutionalized population of the U.S. has hypertension.[3] The incidence of hypertension is slightly more prevalent among men than women. Both pharmacological and nonpharmacological interventions have been used to lower blood pressure in the treatment of hypertension. Many drugs have been successful in controlling hypertension. Among the most successful are the beta-blockers, the angiotensin converting enzyme inhibitors, and the diuretics. More recently, new drugs have been introduced which inhibit the angiotensin receptor or inhibit calcium channels. All present drug regimens suffer from one obvious disadvantage. Since the disease of hypertension is life-long, treatments have to be constantly repeated. In the case of drug treatment, compliance with a daily ration of medicine by patients is difficult to maintain. Our goal in developing antisense for the treatment of hypertension is to find effective sequences and a delivery system which allows a single dose to have prolonged effects over several days or weeks or months. To reach that point, we have to understand hypertension and briefly explain the theory behind the antisense approach.

Hypertension is not a single disease, but a manifestation of high blood pressure due to multiple causes. Unfortunately, less than 10% of all cases of hypertension are due to a known cause. A few of those known factors can be cured, but in the majority of cases, hypertension is an incipient progressive disease, often without obvious symptoms until one or more of the risk factors becomes evident. For example, hypertension can result from excess production of catecholamines as in pheochromocytoma, which if successfully removed by surgery, can cure the hypertension, but in most cases the causes are multiple and cannot be so easily removed. Lifton[4] has contributed greatly to identifying rare examples of single genes as causes of hypertension and isolated various defects in the fundamental cellular processes such as the Na^+-Cl^- transporter gene (Gitelman's syndrome) and epithelial Na^+ channel subunits (Liddle's syndrome and pseudohypoaldosteronism-1). In cases of polygenic hypertension, high steroid levels and high circulating peptides are associated with hypertension. One such peptide is angiotensin II (Ang II). Ang II is the product of the kidney producing renin, the liver producing the renin substrate, angiotensinogen, and the lungs, which have the largest amount of angiotensin converting enzyme, which converts the angiotensin I (Ang I) formed by renin from angiotensinogen to Ang II. Ang II acts on receptors, principally the angiotensin type 1 (AT_1) receptor subtype in blood vessels, to cause vasoconstriction and in other tissues to have local effects on growth leading to vascular and cardiac hypertrophy. Studies by Jeunemaitre et al.[5] have correlated hypertension in several families to a genetic defect in the angiotensinogen gene. Inserting genes, such as the renin gene, into rats in transgenic animals results in their developing hypertension. Furthermore, direct measurements of Ang II in the plasma and in tissues of hypertensive rat models, show increased levels of Ang II. In one model, the spontaneously hypertensive rat (SHR), Ang II is increased in the brain and slightly elevated in the periphery.[6] In addition, AT_1 receptors are overabundantly expressed in the brain of the SHR, compared to the brains of normotensive rats.

The apparent increased activity of angiotensin in brain tissue of SHRs, gave us a starting point for testing the effectiveness of antisense in lowering blood pressure in hypertensive animals. Earlier experiments[7] had shown that a single injection into the brain of the nonspecific angiotensin antagonist Sar^1ile^8Ang II brain produced a significant decrease in blood pressure at a dose which was ineffective when given peripherally. Normotensive rats did not respond to the central injections of Ang II antagonists. Therefore, it was hypothesized that in the SHR hypertension is associated with an overactive brain angiotensin system. Although the decreases in blood pressure noted lasted only a few minutes, they were sufficient to indicate a role for the angiotensin receptors in these rats. Sar[1]ile[8]Ang II is not a selective antagonist and we now know that there are two receptor subtypes, AT_1 and AT_2. We considered that an antisense approach could lead to the specific inhibition of brain Ang II receptors and would have the advantage of producing longer-lasting effects than a single injection of the pharmacological antagonist.

Antisense inhibition has been used in a number of studies and is particularly well developed in cell culture conditions, to the point where it is currently being tested in clinical trials for HIV and cancer.[8,9] Before 1992, however, antisense had not been applied *in vivo* with any success. As so often happens in science, several laboratories simultaneously and independently made and tested antisense by injecting it into the brain. Chiasson et al.[10] showed the effectiveness of antisense designed to inhibit c-*fos* expression in the brain nuclei. Wahlestedt et al.,[11] using antisense designed to inhibit neuropeptide Y-Y1 receptors, demonstrated the effectiveness of an antisense injection in the brain on neural behavior activity. Weiss and his coworkers[12-15] demonstrated that the intraventricular injection of antisense directed against the D_1 or D_2 dopamine receptor mRNAs selectively inhibited the behavioral effects modified by D_1 and D_2 dopamine agonists, respectively. Wahlestedt et al.[16] showed the effectiveness of an antisense to NMDA-R1 receptor channels in protecting cells during cerebral ischemia. McCarthy and Pfaff and colleagues[17] produced evidence for an antisense inhibition of estrogen receptors in neonates and employed antisense to GAD_{65} and GAD_{67} to modulate the reproductive behavior of female rats. The first demonstration of antisense in hypertension was the use of an antisense designed to inhibit angiotensinogen mRNA and angiotensin and the AT_1 receptor RNA by Gyurko et al.[18]

II. DESIGNING ANTISENSE MOLECULES

The original concept of antisense inhibition assumes that the antisense molecules bind to the mRNA of the target protein in the cytoplasm and prevent either ribosomal assembly or read-through.[19] Most oligonucleotides, therefore, are targeted to the initiation codon AUG or a part of the downstream coding region. When designing such an antisense oligodeoxynucleotide (AS-ODN), one has to consider two major factors: the affinity of the oligonucleotide for its target sequence, which is dependent on the number and composition of complementary bases, and the availability of the target sequence, which is dependent on the folding of the mRNA molecule.[20]

Several reports have suggested that AS-ODNs targeted to different regions of the RNA have unequal efficiencies.[21,22] These differences may be related to the predicted secondary structure of the target mRNA.[23-25] The folding of the mRNA influences target sequence availability. The RNA double helices which are responsible for the secondary structure of the mRNA incorporate a weaker G-U base pairing in addition to the A-U and G-C motifs, and are generally short and rarely stable. Therefore, an ODN that has the potential to form strong (Watson-Crick) base pairing with 100% complementarity will form the thermodynamically more favorable structure with its target RNA.[26]

Besides inhibition of translation, other possible antisense mechanisms of action have been proposed. Based on studies of cellular uptake of labeled oligonucleotides, a picture has emerged that most AS-ODNs quickly migrate to the cell nucleus, suggesting an intranuclear site of action.[27] This suggests a more direct action on gene expression: antisense molecules might inhibit pre-RNA splicing, transport of mRNA from the nucleus to the cytoplasm, or bind to the DNA, thus inhibiting transcription. Based on this, effective AS-ODNs have been designed which are targeted to exon-intron splicing sites[28] or to the major groove of the DNA.[29]

The three regions that are considered to be the best targets for designing effective AS-ODNs are the 5′ cap region, the AUG translation initiation codon, and the 3′ untranslated region of the mRNA.[20,30,31] Because most mRNAs have an AUG initiator codon site, targeting of the 12-15 of the bases neighboring the initiation codon should produce inhibitory ODNs. Routinely, all designed oligonucleotides must be checked for homology with the existing sequences in the GeneBank databank to avoid any complementarity with nontarget mRNAs. Essentially, antisense design comes down to trial and error testing in an appropriate model. A general rule, suggested by our own experience, is that for a 15-mer oligonucleotide, of three different sites tested, only one will work. Obviously, a rapid screening test for changes in the levels of the specific protein for which the AS-ODN has been designed to inhibit is desirable.

A. Stability of Oligonucleotides

Oligonucleotides, in their natural form as phosphodiesters, are subject to rapid degradation in the blood, intracellular fluid, or cerebrospinal fluid by exo- and endonucleases. The half-life of phosphodiester oligonucleotides is in the range of minutes in blood and tissue culture media. The half-life of oligonucleotides is somewhat longer in cerebrospinal fluid, and intact oligonucleotides can be detected 24 h after injection into the cerebral ventricles.[32] Several chemical modifications have been proposed that prolong the half-life of oligonucleotides in biological fluids while retaining their activity and specificity.

The most widely used modified oligonucleotides are phosphorothioates, in which one of the oxygen atoms in the phosphodiester bond between nucleosides is replaced by a sulfur atom. These phosphorothioate oligonucleotides have greater stability in biological fluids than normal oligonucleotides. The half-life of a 15-mer phosphorothioate oligonucleotide is 9 h in human serum, 4 days in tissue culture media,[33] and 19 h in cerebrospinal fluid.[34] Phosphorothioate oligonucleotides can be synthesized with automated DNA synthesizers, but the product may contain impurities unless purified on an affinity gel. Oligonucleotides should be checked by polyacrylamide gel to ensure that they are pure.

One or more of the oxygen atoms in the phosphodiester bond can be replaced with a variety of other groups, such as methyl (methylphosphoniate), alkyl phosphotriester, phosphoramidate, or boranophosphate, all of which expand the half-life of oligonucleotides in *in vivo* experiments. Some clever new designs are being tested in which the ODN has a dumbbell shape produced by a hairpin extension at the 3′ end.[35]

B. Cellular Uptake of Oligonucleotides

In order to hybridize with the target mRNA, AS-ODNs have to cross the cell membrane. Saturable uptake of oligonucleotides plateauing within 50 h occurs rapidly and, depending on the cell type, the uptake can be efficient.[36] Uptake is faster for shorter oligonucleotides than for longer ones. Decreasing the temperature prevents oligonucleotide uptake, indicating that there is an active uptake mechanism. An 80-kDa oligonucleotide-binding protein has been proposed to be the receptor molecule for oligonucleotide uptake.[36] An efflux mechanism has also been described, indicating temperature-dependent secretion of the oligonucleotides from the cells to the extracellular space.

C. Mechanism of Antisense Action

AS-ODNs have several potential sites of action. AS-ODNs inhibit translation by hybridizing to the specific mRNA that they are designed to inhibit, and the hybridization prevents either ribosomal assembly or ribosomal sliding along the mRNA. This kind of action assumes that AS-ODNs are acting in the cytosol and do not measurably affect the mRNA levels. Indeed, there are several articles reporting antisense effects without detectable changes in the target mRNA levels.[16]

Alternatively, the mechanism can be by reduction of mRNA. Decreased mRNA levels can occur of the RNA portion of the mRNA-antisense DNA hybrid by RNase H digestion. RNase H is found in the cytoplasm as well as in the nucleus, and it is normally involved in DNA duplication. The role of RNase H is to cleave RNA that has bound to DNA. Activation of RNase H is advantageous, because the enzyme leaves the AS-ODN intact, so it is free to hybridize with another mRNA, making the reaction catalytic rather than stoichiometric.

AS-ODNs can be taken up by the nucleus, suggesting they may have other possible mechanisms of action. Antisense DNA can hybridize to its target mRNA or pre-mRNA in the nucleus, thereby forming a partially double-stranded structure which would inhibit the transport of mRNA out of the nucleus into the cytoplasm, and, thus, prevent translation. AS-ODNs, targeted to intron-exon junction sites, prevent the splicing process and, consequently, the maturation of the transcript.

Theoretically, AS-ODNs can bind to the DNA and form a triple helix or bind to the opened loop created by RNA polymerase.[37] However, triple helix formation by oligonucleotides to provide long-term inhibition of transcription has not proven effective, because DNA cleavage is corrected in the cell by various repair mechanisms.

D. Pharmacology of AS-ODNs

Antisense inhibition can be considered pharmacologically as a drug-receptor interaction where the oligonucleotide is the drug and the target sequence is the receptor. For binding to occur between the two, a minimum level of affinity is required, which is provided by hydrogen bonding between the Watson-Crick base pairs and base stacking in the newly formed double helix. In order to achieve pharmacological activity, a minimum number of 12 to 15 bases can provide the minimum level of affinity.[38] Longer sequences are more specific, but above 20 bases the problems of cell uptake begin to reduce the effectiveness of ODNs.

The specificity of the AS-ODN target sequence interaction is provided by the Watson-Crick base pairing. Considering that roughly 1% of the human genome contains coding regions, an oligonucleotide 12 to 15 nucleotides long is specific enough statistically to be complementary to a single sequence.[9] Increasing the length of the antisense should result in a higher level of specificity, but it decreases their uptake into cells.

AS-ODNs can inhibit protein synthesis in cultured cells in millimolar doses. The therapeutic window for AS-ODNs is rather narrow; when testing for the optimal dose, small increments in the low millimolar range should be tested.[32] High concentrations may produce nonspecific binding to cytosolic proteins and give misleading results.

E. Toxicity

Phosphodiester oligonucleotides are degraded to their naturally occurring nucleotide building blocks relatively quickly; therefore, no toxic reactions are expected even from high doses of phosphodiester oligonucleotides. Studies on phosphorothioated oligonucleotides in rats have shown that following intravenous injection, they are taken up from the plasma mainly by the liver, fat, and muscle tissues. Phosphorothioated oligonucleotides are excreted through the urine in three days, mainly in their original form. An apparent mild increase in plasma LDH, and to a lesser extent, in the liver enzymes AST and ALT, indicated a possible transient liver toxicity with high doses.[39] The prolonged presence of the phosphorothioated oligonucleotides in the organism is promising from a pharmacological point of view, because sufficient tissue levels could be maintained with infrequent administration.

III. ANTISENSE AND HYPERTENSION

The role of candidate genes in the pathogenesis of hypertension can be approached by the inhibiting of an overexpressed target gene with AS-ODNs. This approach is being developed in rat models of hypertension. Table 1 lists all the current *in vivo* studies reported to date in which blood pressure has been measured.

TABLE 1

Use of Antisense Oligodeoxynucleotides to Reduce Hypertension *In Vivo*

Protein target	Antisense type	Delivery	Ref.
Angiotensinogen	phosphorodiester	i.c.v.	14
Angiotensin AT_1 receptor	phosphorothioate		67
Angiotensinogen	phosphorothioate	i.c.v.	41
Angiotensinogen	phosphorothioate		42
	Sendai virus and liposomes	hepatic v.	
Angiotensinogen	phosphorothioated in liposome	i.a.	44
c-fos	phosphorothioated	i.c.v. brainstem	47
Thyrotropin-releasing hormone	phosphodiester	i.c.v.	46

The first study on antisense and hypertension was by Gyurko et al.[18] who used synthetic antisense ODN, delivered intracerebroventricularly (i.c.v.), in SHR with established hypertension. They designed and constructed an antisense ODN to be complementary to bases –5 to +13 of the angiotensinogen mRNA (18-mer) and a 15-mer oligonucleotide, to be complimentary to bases +63 to +77 of AT_1 receptor mRNA. The AT_1 receptor antisense ODN was phosphothioated and the angiotensinogen mRNA antisense ODN was a phosphodiester. In both cases, hypertension was significantly reduced by the injection of 50 µg of antisense ODN. The blood pressure was reduced by up to 35 mmHg, in most cases lowering the high blood pressure to normotensive levels. These effects, which were measured 8 and 24 h after treatment, began at 8 h and were significant at 24 h. It was later found that the antisense ODN to the AT_1 receptor produced long-lasting 7-day decreases in blood pressure. AT_1 receptors were measured to determine whether this treatment decreased the targeted protein AT_1_R as reduced in the paraventricular nucleus (PVN) and in the anterior third ventricle area (AV3V). Following angiotensinogen antisense treatment, brain Ang II levels were significantly reduced, (p <0.05), confirming decreased Ang II

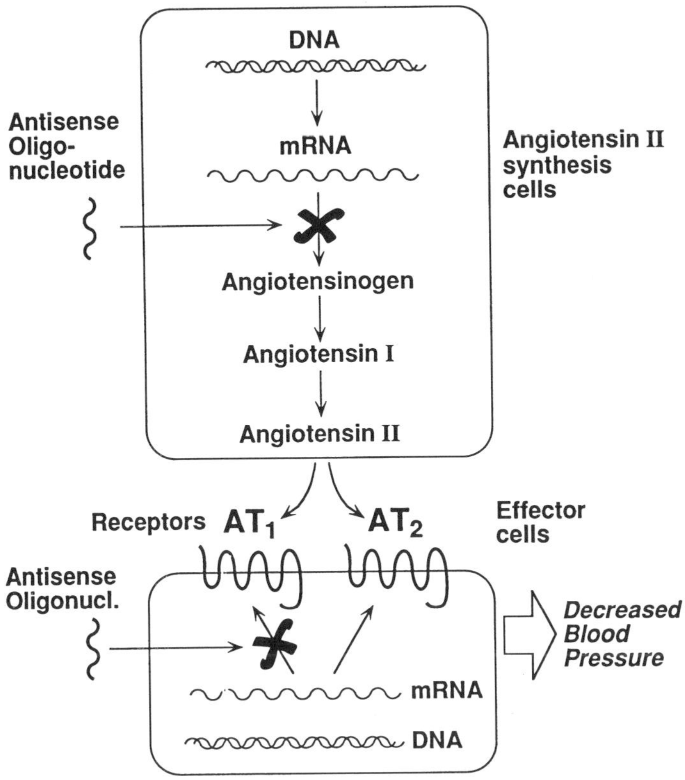

FIGURE 1
The principal of antisense inhibition applied to the renin-angiotensin system to decrease blood pressure in hypertension. Top: Angiotensin is synthesized in the cells of various tissues and secreted or released into the blood. An antisense oligonucleotide targeted to angiotensinogen mRNA will block the synthesis of angiotensinogen, which is ordinarily converted by renin to Ang I. The reduction of Ang II results in the lowering of blood pressure by reducing activation of the effector cells. Bottom: Activation of angiotensin receptors on the effector cells lead to the vasoconstrictor actions of Ang II. These cells include not only contractile cells, such as vascular smooth muscle cells, but also noncontractile cells such as brain and glial cells, which trigger physiological circuits leading to an increase in blood pressure. Application of antisense directed to the angiotensin type 1 (AT_1) mRNA specifically inhibits the synthesis of AT_1 receptors. (Phillips, M. I., *Hypertension*, 29, 177, 1997. With permission.)

synthesis. The results indicated that inhibiting the brain renin-angiotensin system (RAS) through the use of AS-ODNs targeted to either the major substrate, angiotensinogen, or to the major receptor involved in this process, the AT_1 receptor, effectively lowered the high blood pressure (Figure 1).

Follow-up studies investigated the extent of the decrease in the levels of the AT_1 receptor and angiotensinogen caused by these oligonucleotides, as well as other effects of Ang II. Ambühl et al.[40] quantified the reduction in angiotensin receptor following treatment with an antisense ODN against the mRNA for the AT_1 receptor by means of autoradiography, quantitative analysis, and membrane binding. The control injections contained sense or scrambled oligonucleotides or saline vehicle. Three daily injections of antisense ODN into the third ventricle of Sprague-Dawley (SD) rats significantly decreased the levels of AT_1 receptors by 25% as determined in hypothalamic tissue blocks. The AT_2 receptors were not affected by the AT_1 antisense. Autoradiography showed a decrease in the levels of AT_1 receptors in the hypothalamic nuclei and in the AV3V after the antisense treatment. Because the AT_2 receptors were not reduced, the effect of AT_1 AS-ODN was shown to be specific.

In a second series of experiments, single injections of antisense ODN into the lateral ventricles of SHR rats were tested. Antisense ODN produced a significant decrease in the target receptor numbers in the hypothalamic area. Sense and scrambled oligonucleotides did not decrease the receptor numbers significantly. The extent of the decrease following injections of antisense ODN was between 15 to 30%. These relatively modest changes apparently accounted for the physiological effects on hypertension seen by Gyurko et al.[18] Wielbo et al.[41] followed up the initial findings with a phosphodiester antisense ODN to angiotensinogen mRNA by developing a phosphorothioated ODN. This agent was administered i.c.v. in SHR rats while recording blood pressure. The antisense lowered hypertensive blood pressure significantly, while the sense ODN had no effect. The phosphothioated antisense produced a decrease in blood pressure that lasted several days, in contrast to the shorter one-day effect of phosphodiesters. This likely reflects the longer-lasting action of the phosphothioated ODN due to its resistance to nucleases. Direct measurements of angiotensinogen showed there was a significant decrease in the hypothalamus and also a decrease in the brain stem. Again, this supported the concept of centrally mediated regulation of hypertension by an overactive brain angiotensin system. The study also included an experiment using FITC-labeled oligonucleotides to locate the sites at which the cellular uptake of the oligonucleotide occurred. Much of the uptake was close to the site of injection and the surrounding brain nuclei. Because no decreases in mRNA were found, it was concluded that the angiotensinogen antisense inhibited mRNA translation, not transcription.

Injections into the brain, however, are hardly the most attractive route for administering agents for hypertension therapy. A more practical route is by oral intake or injections into the peripheral blood. Two studies have achieved this. Tomita et al.[42] demonstrated a decrease in high blood pressure by antisense ODN against rat angiotensinogen mRNA, delivered by injections of three antisense ODNs into the portal vein. The ODNs were encapsulated in liposomes that contained viral agglutins. The viral carrier, in this case, was a Sendai virus which had been shown to be efficient in promoting fusion with target cells by Kaneda et al.[43] The effect of the ODNs was to produce a transient decrease in plasma angiotensinogen levels in SHR. This decrease in protein correlated with a decrease in blood pressure and a reduction in hepatic angiotensinogen mRNA. The plasma Ang II concentration also decreased in these rats. The reduction in blood pressure, however, was shorter lasting (1 to 4 days) than the reductions in hormone (1 to 7 days). This discrepancy has not been explained. Recently Wielbo et al.,[44] in a follow-up study, have succeeded in showing a reduction in blood pressure after a single intra-arterial (i.v.) injection of an angiotensinogen ODN encapsulated in a liposome. Using an FITC label (cholesterol + phospholipids), they showed by using the i.v. route that the ODN was delivered mainly to the liver. The liver angiotensinogen was reduced after antisense treatment. This study shows the possibility of direct antisense delivery by means of an i.v. injection of an antisense prepared in a simple liposome. Preliminary work in a different model of hypertension indicates that naked DNA is also effective. Valera et al.[45] injected antisense ODN to angiotensinogen in two kidney-1 clip (2K-1C) rats. These rats have high circulating Ang II which causes hypertension. The AS-ODN administered in a single dose (100 μg) lowered blood pressure significantly.

Antisense thyrotropin-releasing hormone (TRH) receptor has also been shown by Suzuki et al.[42] to reduce arterial blood pressure in SHR They used an intrathecal administration approach to deliver an antisense ODN complimentary to TRH receptor mRNA in order to study the pressor response to intrathecal administration of TRH and on the effect of resting arterial blood pressure. The rats used were Wistar Kyoto (WKY) and SHR rats. The antisense was an 18-base phosphodiester, and the rats received a dose of 100 μg per day for 3 days. Twenty-four hours after the last injection, the magnitude of the response to the intrathecal injection of TRH (10 μg) was significantly reduced in the antisense-treated group. In separate experiments, it was shown that the mean resting arterial blood pressure was significantly reduced by the antisense treatment in SHR, but the arterial blood pressure not affected in WKY. The blood pressure in these SHR rats was relatively low (156 ± 4.8 mmHg) but was reduced to 119 ± 8.8 mmHg ($p < 0.01$). No efforts were made to measure any changes in the TRH receptors following this treatment. Without showing that the protein levels are reduced, one cannot definitely conclude that the mechanism by which the antisense has reduced blood pressure was inhibiting receptor protein synthesis.

In another study done by the same group, Suzuki et al,[47] injected an antisense into c-*fos* mRNA in the rostral ventral medulla of SHR rats and the mean arterial pressure in anesthetized rats was significantly reduced at 6 h, compared to the sense-treated controls. In this experiment, the protein (FOS) was shown to be reduced in the brains of the antisense-treated rats. In all of the studies using SHR in which WKY have been used as normotensive controls, no effects of the antisense have been found on the WKYs. This indicates that antisense is useful for reducing overactive hormonal systems, such as the RAS, but does not interfere with the normal physiological functions of the normal hormonal system.

Several studies have reported on the application of AS-ODNs in cellular culture models relevant to hypertensive mechanisms. Smooth muscle cell proliferation is a critical feature of many forms of hypertension. The oncogenes c-myb and the cyto-skeletal protein myosin are believed to be involved in this process. Simons et al.[48] used phosphorothioate ODN antisense to non-muscle myosin heavy chain (NMMHC) or to c-myb phosphorothioate in order to inhibit the proliferation of SMCs *in vitro*. The growth suppression correlated with reductions in the levels of the RNAs for NMMHC and c-myb and of their corresponding proteins. The sense controls were without effect. The effects were long-lasting up to 72 h. Transforming growth factor beta (TGF-β) has also been implicated in the faster growth observed in vascular smooth muscle cells (VSMC) from SHR rats compared to their normotensive controls. Antisense ODN complimentary to TGF-β-1 mRNA significantly suppressed the VSMC number in SHR but not in WKY rats. Plasmin, an activator of TGF-β, did not stimulate DNA synthesis in the presence of the antisense ODN. This cellular study suggests that endogenous TGF-β plays a role in hypertension in the SHR through the increased growth of VSMC.

Important pathophysiological events such as arterial restenosis after balloon catheterization have been effectively influenced by AS-ODNs. Inhibition of two cell cycle regulatory enzymes, cyclin-dependent kinase 2 kinase and cell division cycle 2 kinase, with AS-ODNs resulted in a nearly complete abolition of neointima formation, which is thought to be responsible for arterial restenosis.[49] Application of c-myc AS-ODNs in apluronic gel to the outside of a balloon-catheter injured blood vessel resulted in 75% decrease in c-myc expression and significantly reduced neointima formation.[50] This result also suggests the oligonucleotides' remarkable penetrating ability by which they reached the neointima of the rat carotid from the outside of the vessel.

The outcome of cerebral infarction can be influenced with AS-ODNs. The synthesis of NMDA receptors, which are thought to be responsible for the neuronal death following cerebral vascular occlusion, can be inhibited by antisense treatment. Such an inhibition reduces the volume of the infarction produced experimentally by occlusion of the middle cerebral artery.[16]

IV. DELIVERY OF ANTISENSE

A. Naked DNA

Table 2 shows the currently used methods of delivering antisense for the treatment of hypertension and some of their advantages and disadvantages.

TABLE 2

Vectors for Gene Transfer in Hypertension

Vector	Advantages	Disadvantages	Refs.
Naked DNA	Administered directly into tissue by injection Easy to produce	Difficult to control sites of uptake Preferential take-up by some tissues, e.g., liver, kidney, blood vessels, muscle DNA copy number unquantifiable	51
Liposome-encapsulated	Easy to produce	DNA copy number unquantifiable Preferential uptake in certain tissues, e.g., liver Toxic to some tissues, e.g., brain	44 42
Adenovirus	Produced without difficulty to high titers Infects broad range of cells	Invokes inflammatory response Copy number not controlled Does not integrate into the genome (episomal)	68
Adeno-associated virus	Integrates into the genome	Difficult to produce high titers	66
	Non-pathogenic Effective	Small loading capacity (4.5 Kb)	69
Retrovirus	Efficient transfer Single-copy gene delivery Efficient uptake	Only useful in dividing cells May damage non-target dividing cells	57

Direct injection of the antisense DNA has been used in the experiments described above. For injections into the brain, naked DNA appears to be very successful. A number of studies, using different AS-ODNs, have demonstrated efficient uptake and effective reduction in protein and inhibition of the physiological parameters studied. Although uptake is very efficient, there is one difficulty encountered with i.c.v. injections; there is a tendency for DNA to be taken up close to the injection site and not to spread to other parts of the brain. While this has little impact on the use of antisense ODNs for hypertension therapy, it is an important consideration in antisense strategies for the treatment of brain diseases, such as Parkinson's disease, thalamic pain, Alzheimer's disease, and gliomas.

Direct injection of DNA into the blood is still being studied, and only a few reports have been published. Chao and colleagues[51] have reported outstanding success in reducing blood pressure of SHRS with direct gene delivery of human tissue kallikrein. They used two naked DNA constructs, one with a metallothionine response element, the other with a Rous sarcoma virus 3′ long terminal repeat (LTR) promoter and they were injected i.v. As a result, expression of human kallikrein was identified in several tissues. Blood pressure was significantly reduced for 6 weeks reaching a maximum reduction of 46 mmHg.[51] Our preliminary work using a single i.v. injection of antisense ODN directed to angiotensinogen mRNA in the 2K-1C rat to reduce renovascular hypertension is encouraging.[45] We found that this treatment decreased blood pressure for six days. However, it is difficult to determine precisely where in the body tissues the antisense is having its major effect and whether this effect is direct or indirect.

B. Liposomes

Liposomes, which are self-assembling particles of lipid bilayers, have been used for encapsulating antisense ODN for delivery in blood. Antisense directed to angiotensinogen mRNA and administered using liposomes has yielded successful results. In this study, Tomita et al,[42] utilized liposome encapsulation and a Sendai virus containing the antisense and injected these complexes into the portal vein. As a result, blood pressure decreased over several days. However, these authors did not compare their results to those seen after injection of naked DNA. In contrast to this study, Wielbo et al.[44] compared the effects of intra-arterially (i.a.)-administered liposome encapsulated antisense and naked DNA, and they found that under the same conditions only the liposome-encapsulated DNA was effective, whereas the naked DNA was not. Twenty-four hours after the administration of 50 μg liposome-encapsulated (25 mg) antisense ODN, blood pressure decreased by 25 mmHg. The empty liposomes or the liposomes encapsulating a scrambled ODN had no significant action. Unencapsulated antisense ODN also did not have any significant effect on blood pressure. Confocal micrographs of rat liver tissue obtained 1 h after an i.a. injection of 50 μg unencapsulated FITC antisense or liposome-encapsulated FITC-conjugated antisense showed the presence of intense fluorescence in liver tissue sinusoids only when the liposome-encapsulated ODN was used. The levels of protein (angiotensinogen and Ang II in the plasma) were significantly reduced in the liposome-encapsulated ODN group. Antisense alone, lipids alone, or scrambled ODN in liposomes were without effect.

The development of liposomes with cationic lipids has allowed high transfection efficiencies of plasmid DNA. In contrast to double-stranded DNA vectors the short, single-stranded AS-ODNs are not actually encapsulated, but they are complexed with the lipid milamellar vesicles by electrostatic interactions. This simplifies the production of the lipid based-antisense delivery systems in comparison to the delivery systems for viral vectors and allows the use of a variety of delivery routes, such as aerosol nasal sprays, and parenteral injections.

C. Viral Vectors

There are several viruses which have been tested for gene delivery, and each of them has its advantages, but none fits perfectly into the requirements for an "ideal" viral vector. To be an ideal vector, a virus should fulfill all of the following criteria.

1. The vector should be safe. This means that it cannot be a virus known to cause disease, or it has to be re-engineered to be harmless. The viral vector should not elicit an immune response, and it should not integrate into the genome randomly, which would carry the risk of disrupting other cellular genes. It also has to be replication-deficient in order to avoid the risk of the spread of the virus to unwanted tissues or subjects. An ideal viral vector would deliver a defined gene copy number into each infected cell.

2. The vector must be efficient. The virus has to infect the target cells with high frequency in order to achieve a biological effect.
3. The vector should be easy to manipulate. The virus should be able to accommodate the gene of interest, along with its regulatory sequences (such as the promoter), and the recombinant DNA has to be packaged with high efficiency into the viral capsid proteins.

D. Retroviruses

Retroviruses have been used primarily because of their high efficiency in delivering genes to cells.[52] Retroviruses permit the insertion and stable integration of single-copy genes. Although effective in cell culture systems, they integrate randomly into the genome, which raises concerns about their safety for practical use *in vivo*. Retroviruses can only act in dividing cells, which makes them ideal vectors for tumor therapy but less desirable when other dividing cells have to be protected. Experiments done by Katovich et al.[53] have tested the effectiveness of retroviral delivery of antisense DNA to AT_1-R mRNA. Injections into the heart of 6-week-old SHRs resulted in effective long-term inhibition of AT_1 receptor mRNA and significant inhibition of the development of hypertension.

E. Adenoviruses

Adenovirus vectors have been tested successfully in their natural host cells, the respiratory endothelium, as well as in other tissues such as muscle and brain.[54-56] Most adenovirus vectors in their current form are episomal in the cell and do not integrate into the host DNA. They provide high levels of expression for a significant amount of time, but the episomal DNA will invariably turn inactive. Repeated infections, on the other hand, result in an inflammatory response with consequent tissue damage. This is because the adenoviruses express genes which can lead to immune cell attack. This limitation makes adenoviruses unsuitable for long-term treatment. Although preliminary studies with adenovirus vectors for the delivery of AT_1-R antisense mRNA have been successful in reducing AT_1-R in neurons of SHRs,[57] the toxicity limits adenovirus vectors for *in vivo* studies.

F. Adeno-Associated Viruses (AAV)

AAVs have been gaining attention because of their safety and efficiency.[58] An AAV vector has been successfully used for delivering antisense RNA against alpha-globin[59] and HIV LTR,[60] and AAV is our vector of choice for delivering antisense targeted to the AT-1 receptor.

AAV is a parvovirus, discovered as a contaminant of adenoviral stocks. It is a ubiquitous virus (antibodies against AAV are present in 85% of the U.S. human population), which has not been linked to any disease. It is also classified as a dependovirus, because its replication is absolutely dependent on the presence of a helper virus, such as adenovirus. Five AAV serotypes have been isolated, of which AAV-2 is the best characterized. AAV has a single-stranded linear DNA, which is encapsidated into the capsid proteins VP1, VP2, and VP3 to form an icosahedral virion of 20 to 24 nm in diameter.

The AAV DNA is approximately 4.7 kb long. It contains two open reading frames and it is flanked by two terminal repeats. Each terminal repeat can form a T-shaped hairpin structure. These terminal repeats are the only essential components of the

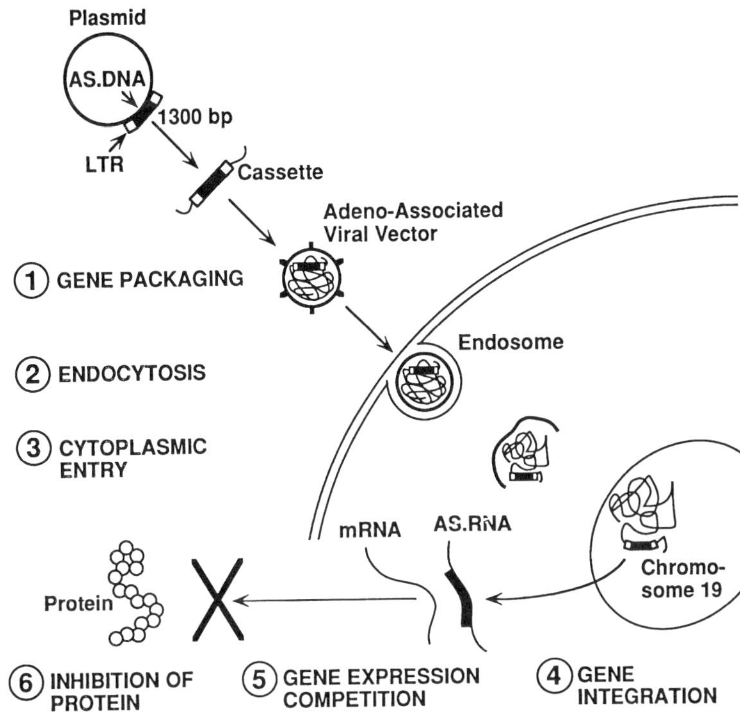

FIGURE 2
Gene delivery of antisense by means of an AAV vector. **1.** Gene packaging. The plasmid containing the ITR characteristic of an AAV is recombined with a 1300-bp DNA in the antisense direction. The final cassette also contains promoters such as a cytomegalovirus promoter. The AAV are grown in cells in the presence of adenovirus and a helper virus, and the cassette is packaged into the AAV. **2.** Endocytosis. The viral vector fuses with the cell membrane by binding to adhesion molecules and becomes an endosome within the bilipid layer. **3.** Cytoplasmic entry. The vesicle opens in the cytoplasm releasing the vector which is transported to, and enters, the nucleus. **4.** Gene integration. AAV integrates with chromosome 19 in culture. It is not known if the addition of foreign DNA interferes with this integration. **5.** Gene expression competition. The inserted genomic message in chromosome 19 produces an antisense RNA. This competes with the natural mRNA and prevents it from producing its product. **6.** Inhibition of protein. Binding of the antisense RNA to the target mRNA prevents translation through the ribosomal assembly to produce the protein. (From Phillips, M. I., *Hypertension,* 22, 177, 1997. With permission.)

AAV for chromosomal integration. They also serve as origins of replication. There are two major genes in the AAV genome: *rep* and *cap*. The *rep* codes for proteins are responsible for viral replication, whereas *cap* codes are responsible for the capsid proteins VP1-3. Three promoters have been identified and named p5, p19, and p40, according to their position in the map of the viral genome. Transcription from p5 and p19 results in production of *rep* proteins, and transcription from p40 produces the capsid proteins.[61] For more powerful expression we have inserted cytomegalo virus in place of the P40 virus. Other promoters are being tested which are specific to certain tissues.

Upon infection of a human cell, the wild-type AAV integrates to the q arm of chromosome 19.[62] For chromosomal integration the only essential components are the terminal repeats. The viral components responsible for site-specific integration have yet to be identified. Without a helper virus present, AAV infection remains latent indefinitely. Upon superinfection of the cell with helper virus, the AAV genome is excised, replicated, packaged into virions, and released to the extracellular fluid.

There are several factors that prompted researchers to study the possibility of using AAV as an expression vector. One is that the requirements for delivering a gene to integrate into the host chromosome are surprisingly few. All that is necessary is the presence of the terminal repeats, which are only 6% of the AAV genome. This leaves room in the vector to assemble into it an antisense insertion of reasonable length in the range of 1 to 2 kb, a length that is more likely to produce a specific response.

The second characteristic that makes AAV a good vector candidate is its relatively complicated rescue mechanism. The spread of recombinant AAV vectors to nontarget areas can therefore be limited to only certain tissues.

AAV is a good candidate for gene therapy because it has a very broad host range. AAV infects all mammalian tissues tested, with the only apparent exception being vascular endothelial cells.[63] Preparation of recombinant AAVs is relatively easy — 94% of the genome can be replaced with the gene(s) of interest.

Despite some problems which are currently being investigated, AAV appears to be one of the best candidates for gene delivery. Recently Flotte and colleagues[64] have established gene therapy for cystic fibrosis using AAV in patients. The AAV does not induce an inflammatory reaction (unlike the adenoviral vectors), and this makes the AAV suitable for human use and long-term gene therapy.

G. Expression of Antisense Sequences with Vectors

We have constructed expression vectors for both AT_1 receptor antisense and angiotensinogen antisense into the AAV-derived expression vector, pJDT95, downstream from the promoter in the antisense direction. The resulting antisense vectors were transfected into NG108-15 cells (for the vector $paAT_1$) or into hepatoma H4 cells (for the pa angiotensinogen [Ao] vector).[65,66] In both cases, there were significant reductions in the protein levels and by using markers for AAV, such as the *rep* gene. The results indicated that the effects of the constructs were specific. Currently we are testing the AAV antisense vectors by injecting them into rats. Preliminary tests *in vivo* have shown that the antisense vectors produced reductions in high blood pressure in some, but not all of the SHRs.[70] We believe that the major problem at present is the consistency of delivery, and we are currently addressing this issue.

Long-term suppression of the synthesis of individual proteins is desirable in conditions where overexpression of endogenous genes or the expression of foreign genes is thought to be the cause of the disease. Inhibition of the synthesis of certain proteins for extended periods of time is also useful when studying protein function, e.g., in development.

Antisense expression vectors produce antisense RNA, which can hybridize with the target mRNA and prevent its translation by either promoting its degradation, preventing its transport from the nucleus to the cytoplasm, or interfering with ribosomal function.

AAV-derived expression vectors have been successfully used to inhibit alpha-globin expression in an erythroleukemia cell line; where a 1-kb fragment of the alpha-globin gene was inserted in the antisense direction under the control of either thymidine kinase, SV40, or alpha-globin promoters. Ninety-one percent inhibition in the production of alpha-globin mRNA was achieved using the alpha-globin promoter, whereas two other unrelated promoters proved to be less efficient.[59]

A much shorter antisense sequence (64 bp long) targeted to the HIV LTR was expressed in 293 cells by means of an AAV vector containing the SV40 promoter.

Greater than 99% reduction in the production of the infectious HIV-1 and the absence of cellular toxicity were observed over a period of 20 days.[60]

V. SUMMARY

Many problems have to be overcome in the use of antisense technology as a treatment for hypertension, but thus far AS-ODNs to either the AT_1 receptor mRNA or to the angiotensinogen mRNA, have been effective at lowering hypertension in the SHR to normotensive levels. One injection of a naked antisense ODN into the brain or an antisense ODN in a lipid-encapsulated form i.a., is effective for several days. The antisense appears to be working through the expected antisense mechanisms as the appropriate proteins are reduced in correlation to the physiological effects. More studies need to be done in different models of hypertension and need the effectiveness of repeated doses. The answer to the long-term goal of prolonged blood pressure control by means of antisense may lie in the delivery of antisense DNA using viral vectors. Preliminary results with AAV vectors *in vitro* suggest that *in vivo* injections will also be effective and will permit the antisense DNA to be integrated into the genome in order to achive long-lasting reduction in blood pressure.

REFERENCES

1. Whelton, P.K., Epidemiology of hypertension, *Lancet*, 334, 101–106, 1994.
2. Stamler, J., Stamler, R., and Neaton, J.D., Blood pressure, systolic and diastolic and cardiovascular risks: U.S. population data, *Arch. Intern. Med.*, 153, 598–615, 1993.
3. Burt, V.L., Whelton, P.K., Roccella, E.J., Brown, C., Cutler, J.A., Higgins, M., Horan, M.J., and Labarth, D., Prevalence of hypertension in the U.S. adult population: results from the 3rd National Health and Nutrition Examination Survey, 1988-1991, *Hypertension*, 25, 305–313, 1995.
4. Lifton, R.P., Molecular genetics of human blood pressure variation, *Science*, 272, 676, 1996.
5. Jeuenmaitre, X., Soubrier, F., Kotelvtsev, Y.V., Lifton, R.P., Williams, C.S., Charru, A., Hunt, S.C., Hopkins, P.N., William, R.R., Lalouel, J.M., and Corvol, P., Molecular basis of human hypertension: role of angiotensinogen, *Cell*, 71, 169–180, 1992.
6. Phillips, M.I. and Kimura, B., Brain angiotensin in the developing spontaneously hypertensive rat, *J. Hypertension*, 6, 607–612, 1988.
7. Phillips, M.I., Mann, J.F.E., Haebara, H., Hoffman, W.E., Dietz, R., Schelling, P., and Ganten, D., Lowering of hypertension by central saralasin in the absence of plasma renin, *Nature*, 270, 445–447, 1977.
8. Wagner, R.W., Gene inhibition using antisense oligodeoxynucleotides, *Nature*, 372, 333–335, 1994.
9. Crooke, S.T., Therapeutic applications of oligonucleotides, *Annu. Rev. Pharmacol. Toxicol.*, 32, 329–376, 1992.
10. Chiasson, B.J., Hooper, M.L., Murphy, P.R., and Robertson, H.A. Antisense oligonucleotide eliminates *in vivo* expression of c-*fos* in mammalian brain, *Eur. J. Pharmacol.*, 277, 451–453, 1992.
11. Wahlestedt, C., Pich, E.M., Koob, G.F., Yee, F., and Heilig, M., Modulation of anxiety and neuropeptide Y-Y1 receptors by antisense oligodeoxynucleotides, *Science*, 259, 528–531, 1993.
12. Weiss, B., Zhou, L.-W., Zhang, S.-P., and Qin, Z.-H., Antisense oligodeoxynucleotide inhibits D_2 dopamine receptor-mediated behavior and D_2 messenger RNA, *Neuroscience*, 55, 607–612, 1993.
13. Zhang, S.-P., Zhou, L.-W., and Weiss, B., Oligodeoxynucleotide antisense to the D_1 dopamine receptor mRNA inhibits D_1 dopamine receptor-mediated behaviors in normal mice and in mice lesioned with 6-hydroxydopamine, *J. Pharmacol. Exp. Ther.*, 271, 1462–1470, 1994.
14. Zhou, L.-W., Zhang, S.-P., Qin, Z.-H., and Weiss, B., *In vivo* administration of an oligodeoxynucleotide antisense to the D_2 dopamine receptor mRNA inhibits D_2 dopamine receptor-mediated behavior and the expression of D_2 dopamine receptors in mouse striatum, *J. Pharmacol. Exp. Ther.*, 268, 1015–1023, 1994.

15. Qin, Z.-H., Zhou, L.-W., Zhang, S.-P., Wang, Y., and Weiss, B., D_2 dopamine receptor antisense oligodeoxynucleotide inhibits the synthesis of a functional pool of D_2 dopamine receptors, *Mol. Pharmacol.*, 48, 730–737, 1995.
16. Wahlestedt, C., Golanov, E., Yamamoto, S., Yee, F., Ericson, H., Yoo, H., Inturrisi, C.E., and Reis, D.J., Antisense oligonucleotides to NMDA-R1 receptor channel protect cortical neurons from excitotoxicity and reduce focal ischemic infarctions, *Nature*, 363, 260–263, 1993.
17. McCarthy, M.M., Masters, D.B., Rimvall, K., Schwartz-Giblin, S., and Pfaff, D.W., Intracerebral administration of antisense oligodeoxynucleotides to GAD65 and GAD67 mRNAs modulates reproductive behavior in the female rat, *Brain Res.*, 636, 209–220, 1994.
18. Gyurko, R., Wielbo, D., and Phillips, M.I., Antisense inhibition of AT_1 receptor mRNA and angiotensinogen mRNA in the brain of spontaneously hypertensive rats reduces hypertension of neurogenic origin, *Regul. Pept.* 49, 167–174, 1993.
19. Simons, R.W., Naturally occurring antisense RNA control — a brief review, *Gene*, 72, 35–44, 1988.
20. Stull, R.A., Taylor, L.A., and Szoka, F.C., Predicting antisense oligonucleotide inhibitory efficacy: a computational approach using histograms and thermodynamic indices, *Nucleic. Acids. Res.*, 20, 3501–3508, 1992.
21. Cowsert, L.M., Fox, M.C., Zon, G., and Mirabelli, C.K., *In vitro* evaluation of phosphorothioate oligonucleotides targeted to the E2 mRNA of papillomavirus: potential treatment for genital warts, *Antimicrob. Agents Chemother.*, 37, 171–177, 1993.
22. Wakita, T. and Wands, J.R., Specific inhibition of hepatitis C virus expression by antisense oligonucleotides. *In vitro* model for selection of target sequence, *J. Biol. Chem.*, 269, 14205–14210, 1994.
23. Lima, W.F., Monia, B.P., Ecker, D.J., and Freier, S.M., Implication of RNA structure on antisense oligonucleotide hybridization kinetics, *Biochemistry*, 31, 12055–12061, 1992.
24. Rittner, K. and Sczakiel, G., Identification and analysis of antisense RNA target regions of the human immunodeficiency virus type 1, *Nucleic. Acid Res.*, 19, 1421–1426, 1991.
25. Jaroszevski, J.W., Syi, J.L., Ghosh, M., Ghosh, K., and Cohen, J.S., Targeting of antisense DNA: comparison of activity of anti-rabbit beta-globin oligodeoxyribonucleoside phosphorothioates with computer predictions of mRNA folding, *Antisense Res. Dev.*, 3, 339–348, 1993.
26. Singer, M. and Berg, P., *Genes and Genomes*, University Science Books, Mill Valley, CA, 54–59, 1991.
27. Iversen, P.L., Zhu, S., Meyer, A., and Zon, G., Cellular uptake and subcellular distribution of phosphorothioate oligonucleotides into cultured cells, *Antisense Res. Dev.*, 2, 211–222, 1992.
28. Colige, A., Sokolov, B.P., Nugent, P., Baserga, R., and Prockop, D.J., Use of an antisense oligonucleotide to inhibit expression of a mutated human procollagen gene (COL1A1) in transfected mouse 3T3 cells, *Biochemistry*, 32, 7–11, 1993.
29. Helene, C., The anti-gene strategy: control of gene expression by triplex-forming-oligonucleotides, *Anticancer Drug Res.*, 6, 569–584, 1991.
30. Bennett, C.F., Condon, T.P., Grimm, S., Chan, H., and Chiang, M.Y., Inhibition of endothelial cell adhesion molecule expression with antisense oligonucleotides, *J. Immunol.*, 152, 3530–3540, 1994.
31. Bacon, T.A. and Wickstrom, E., Walking along human c-myc mRNA with antisense oligonucleotides: maximum efficacy at the 5′ cap region, *Oncogene Res.*, 6, 13–19, 1991.
32. Wahlestedt, C., Antisense oligonucleotide strategies in neuropharmacology, *TIPS*, 15, 42–46, 1994.
33. Li, B., Hughes, J.A., and Phillips, M.I., Uptake and efflux of intact antisense phosphorothioate deoxyoligonucleotide directed against angiotensin receptors in bovine adrenal cells, *Neurochem. Int.*, in press.
34. Campbell, J.M, Bacon, T.A., and Wickstrom, E., Oligodeoxynucleotide phosphorothioate stability in subcellular extracts, culture media, serum and cerebrospinal fluid, *J. Biochem. Biophys. Methods*, 20, 259–267, 1990.
35. Takaku, H., Properties and anti-HIV activity of nicked dumbbell oligonucleotides, *Neurotide*, 15, 519–529, 1996.
36. Loke, S.L., Stein, C.A., Zhang, X.H., Mori, K., Nakanishi, M., Subasinghe, C., Cohen, J.S., and Neckers, L.M., Characterization of oligonucleotide transport into living cells, *Proc. Natl. Acad. Sci. U.S.A.*, 86, 3474–3478, 1989.
37. Rougee, M., Faucon, B., Mergny, J.L., Barcelo, F., Giovannangeli, C., Garestier, T., and Helene, C., Kinetics and thermodynamics of triple-helix formation: effects of ionic strength and mismatches, *Biochemistry*, 31, 9269–9278, 1992.
38. Crooke, R.M., *In vitro* toxicology and pharmacokinetics of antisense oligonucleotides, *Anticancer Drug Res.*, 6, 609–646, 1991.
39. Iversen, P.L., Mata, J., Tracewell, W.G., and Zon, G., Pharmacokinetics of an antisense phosphorothioate oligodeoxynucleotide against rev from human immunodeficiency virus type 1 in the adult male rat following single injections and continuous infusion, *Antisense Res. Dev.*, 4, 43–52, 1994.

40. Ambühl, P., Gyurko, R., and Phillips, M.I., A decrease of angiotensin receptor number in rat brain nuclei by antisense oligonucleotides against the angiotensin AT_{1A} receptor, *Regul. Pept.*, 59, 171–182, 1995.
41. Wielbo, D., Sernia, C., Gyurko, R., and Phillips, M.I., Antisense inhibition of hypertension in the spontaneously hypertensive rat, *Hypertension*, 25, 314–319, 1995.
42. Tomita, N., Morishita, R., Higaki, J., Kaneda, Y., Mikami, H., and Ogihara, T., *In vivo* transfer of antisense oligonucleotide against rat angiotensinogen with HJV-liposome delivery resulted in reduction of blood pressure in SHR, *Hypertension*, 24, 397, 1994.
43. Kaneda, Y., Iwai, K., and Uchida, T., Increased expression of DNA co-introduced with nuclear protein in adult rat liver, *Science*, 243, 375–378, 1989.
44. Wielbo, D., Simon, A., Phillips, M.I., and Toffolo, S., Inhibition of hypertension by peripheral administration of antisense oligodeoxynucleotides, *Hypertension*, 28, 147–151, 1996.
45. Varela, A.E., Galli, S.M., Wilcox, C., and Phillips, M.I., Antisense inhibition shows a role of angiotensin II (Ang II) in chronic hypertension in the 2 kidney-1 clip rat, *Exp. Biol.*, 1917, 1995.
46. Suzuki, S., Pilowsky, P., Minson, J., Arnolda, L., Llewellyn-Smith, I., and Chalmers, J., Antisense to thyrotropin releasing hormone receptor reduces arterial blood pressure in spontaneously hypertensive rats, *Clin. Res.*, 77, 679–683, 1995.
47. Suzuki, S., Pilowsky, P., Minson, J., Arnolda, L., Llewellyn-Smith, I., and Chalmers, J., c-*fos* antisense in rostral ventral medulla reduces arterial blood pressure, *Am. J. Physiol.*, 35, R1418–R1422, 1994.
48. Simons, M., Edelman, E.R., DeKeyser, J.-L., Langer, R., and Rosenberg, R.D., Antisense c-myb oligonucleotides inhibit intimal arterial smooth muscle cell accumulation *in vivo*, *Nature*, 359, 67–70, 1992.
49. Morishita, R., Gibbons, G.H., Kaneda, Y., Ogihara, T., and Dzau, V.J., Pharmacokinetics of antisense oligodeoxyribonucleotides (cyclin B1 and CDC 2 kinase) in the vessel wall *in vivo*: Enhanced therapeutic utility for restenosis by HVJ-liposome delivery, *Gene*, 149, 13–19, 1994.
50. Bennett, M.R., Anglin, S., McEwan, J.R., Jagoe, R., Newby, A.C., and Evan, G.I., Inhibition of vascular smooth muscle cell proliferation *in vitro* and *in vivo* by c-myc antisense oligodeoxynucleotides, *J. Clin. Invest.*, 93, 820–828, 1994.
51. Wang, C., Chao, L., and Chao, J., Direct gene delivery of human tissue kallikrein reduces blood pressure in spontaneously hypertensive rats, *J. Clin. Invest.*, 95, 1710–1716, 1995.
52. Mulligan, R.C., The basic science of gene therapy, *Science*, 260, 926–932, 1993.
53. Katovich, M.J., Lu, D., Lyer, S., and Raizada, M.K., Chronic attenuation of high blood pressure in spontaneously hypertensive rat by retrovirally mediated delivery of antisense cDNA sequence of AT_1 receptor, FASEB Abstr., *Exp. Biol.*, #1588, 1996.
54. Brody, S.L., Jaffe, H.A., Eissa, N.T., and Daniel, C., Administration of an adenovirus containing the human CFTR cDNA to the respiratory tract of individuals with cystic fibrosis, *Natl. Genet.*, 8, 42–51, 1994.
55. Quantin, B., Perricaudet, L.D., Tajbakhsh, S., and Mandel, J.-L., Adenovirus as an expression vector in muscle cells *in vivo*, *Proc. Natl. Acad. Sci. U.S.A.*, 89, 2581–2584, 1992.
56. Le Gal La Salle, G., Robert, J.J., Berrard, S., Ridoux, V., Stratford-Perricaudet, L.D., Perricaudet, M., and Mallet, J., An adenovirus vector for gene transfer into the neurons and glia in the brain, *Science*, 259, 988–990, 1993.
57. Lu, D., Yu, K., and Raizada, M.K., Retrovirus-mediated transfer of an angiotensin type 1 receptor (AT_1-R) antisense sequence decreases AT_1 receptors and angiotensin II action in astroglial and neuronal cells in primary cultures from the brain, *Proc. Natl. Acad. Sci. U.S.A.*, 92, 1162–1166, 1995.
58. Muzyczka, N. and McLaughin, S., Use of adeno-associated virus as a mammalian transduction vector, *Current Communications in Molecular Biology: Viral Vectors*, Gluzman, Y. and Hughes, S.H., Eds., Cold Spring Harbor Laboratory Press, Cold Spring Harbor, NY, 1988, 39–44.
59. Ponnazhagan, S., Nallari, M.L., and Srivastava, A., Suppression of human α-globin gene expression mediated by the recombinant adeno-associated virus 2-based antisense vectors, *J. Exp. Med.*, 179, 733–738, 1994.
60. Chatterjee, S., Johnson, P.R., and Wong, K.K., Dual-target inhibition of HIV-1 *in vitro* by means of an adeno-associated virus antisense vector, *Science*, 258, 1485–1488, 1992.
61. Muzyczka, N., Use of adeno-associated virus as a general transduction vector for mammalian cells, *Current Topics in Microbiology and Immunology*, Vol. 158, Springer-Verlag, Berlin, 97–129, 1992.
62. Samulski, R.J., Zhu, X., Xiao, X., Brook, J.D., Housman, D.E., Epstein, N., and Hunter, L.A., Targeted integration of adeno-associated virus (AAV) into human chromosome 19, *EMBO J.*, 10, 3941–3950, 1991.
63. Lebkowski, J.S., McNally, M.M., Okarma, T.B., and Lerch, B., Adeno-associated virus: a vector system for efficient introduction and integration of DNA into a variety of mammalian cell types, *Mol. Cell. Biol.*, 8, 3988–3996, 1988.

64. Flotte, T.R., Afione, S.A., Solow, R. et al., Stable *in vivo* expression of the cystic fibrosis transmembrane conductance regulator with an adeno-associated virus vector, *Proc. Natl. Acad. Sci. U.S.A*, 90, 10613–10617, 1993.
65. Gyurko, R. and Phillips, M.I., Antisense expression vector decreases angiotensin receptor binding in NG108-15 cells. *Exp. Biol.*, 1915, 1995.
66. Wu, P., Du, B., Phillips, M.I., and Terwilliger, E.F., Efficient and long-term gene delivery into rat brain using adeno-associated viral vectors, *Neuroscience*, 1996.
67. Phillips, M.I., Wielbo, D., and Gyurko, R., Antisense inhibition of hypertension: A new strategy for renin-angiotensin candidate genes, *Kidney Int.*, 46, 1554–1556, 1994.
68. Willard, J.E., Jesse, M.E., Gerard, R.D., and Meidell, R.S., Recombinant adenovirus is an efficient vector for *in vivo* gene transfer and can be preferentially directed at vascular endothelium or smooth muscle cells, *Circulation*, 86, 473, 1992.
69. Mohuczy-Dominiak, D. and Phillips, M.I., Adeno-associated virus vector as a highly efficient transporter of exogenous DNA into cells, *Exp. Biol.*, 2577, 1996.
70. Phillips, M.I., *Hypertension*, 29, 177, 1997.

Chapter **8**

ANTISENSE DNA THERAPY OF BURKITT'S LYMPHOMA IN Eμ-*myc* TRANSGENIC MICE

Eric Wickstrom

CONTENTS

0-8493-8552-0/97/$0.00+$.50

I. INTRODUCTION

A. c-*myc* Oncogene Induction of Lymphoma

One of the most frequent hematological malignancies of childhood is Burkitt's lymphoma.[1] Lymphoma is also a frequent result of HIV infection.[1] This malignancy, like all others, results from a multistep process of oncogene activation or suppressor gene inactivation.[2] Aberrant expression of the viral v-*myc* oncogene, or the mouse or human c-*myc* proto-oncogene has been implicated in a number of leukemias and solid tumors in a variety of avian and mammalian species.[2] In Burkitt's lymphoma, virtually all cases display translocation of chromosomes 8 and 14, placing the c-*myc* proto-oncogene from chromosome 8 under the transcriptional control of the immunoglobulin M heavy chain enhancer from chromosome 14.[3]

Animals can sometimes provide useful therapeutic models for human diseases. To provide an animal model for childhood Burkitt's lymphoma, transgenic mice were created[4] bearing a murine immunoglobulin M enhancer/c-*myc* fusion transgene (Eμ-*myc*) isolated from a mouse plasmacytoma.[5] Mice in these lines, including the Tg(IgH,Myc)Bri157 line used in these studies, develop aggressive multifocal lymphoma/leukemia.[4] Tumors are prominent in 95% of such mice by 16 weeks after birth. It appears that elevated constitutive expression of c-*myc* mRNA and MYC p65 antigen does not directly induce tumor onset, but instead establishes a subpopulation of rapidly proliferating, immature B cells which may be transformed into a malignant phenotype by a subsequent oncogene activation.[6] These transgenic mice provide a well-characterized animal model for studying the role of c-*myc* activation in B-cell lymphoma.

B. Antisense DNA Therapy

In mammalian cells, the c-*myc* oncogene has proved to be a reliable target for antisense DNA inhibition of gene expression.[7-22] The ability of antisense DNA to turn off individual genes in growing cells provides a powerful tool for elucidating the role of a particular gene, and it also provides for therapeutic intervention when that gene is overexpressed or mutated. Antisense DNAs have been applied against a wide variety of target genes in viral, bacterial, plant, and animal systems and both in whole cells[23] and in animal models.[24] It was therefore of interest to determine whether or not antisense DNA therapy could downregulate c-*myc* gene expression in an animal model.[25] Adult mice contain about 2 ml of blood, carrying up to 10^7 lymphocytes/ml.[26]

Thus, for the purpose of studying antisense DNA inhibition of c-*myc* expression, the circulating immature lymphocytes in the bloodstream of a mouse provide a parallel in cell number and volume to cells in a culture dish.

Because normal, unmodified DNA oligomers are rapidly hydrolyzed in the presence of serum nucleases,[27] they are a poor choice for use in animal models. For a test of the effects of a single bolus of antisense DNA, described below, nuclease-resistant methylphosphonate DNAs were administered to Eμ-*myc* transgenic mice by tail vein injection. The methylphosphonates distributed rapidly to the tissues and showed no sign of degradation. This single treatment, at about 50 mg/kg, significantly decreased MYC p65 expression, measured 3 to 4 h after administration.[25] Injection of a scrambled sequence, or saline, had no effect.

Similarly, inhibition of restenosis has been reported in pigs by a single administration of anti-c-*myc* DNA phosphorothioates.[28] Furthermore, significant inhibition of tumorigenesis in nude mice by c-Ha-*ras*-transformed cells was observed previously as a result of pretreatment of the cells with anti-c-Ha-*ras* DNA.[29] Having observed a decrease in MYC antigen in response to a single administration of anti-c-*myc* DNA methylphosphonate,[25] it was logical to hypothesize that prolonged treatment of Eμ-*myc* transgenic mice with anti-c-*myc* DNA, inhibiting c-*myc* expression in the target B cells, might preclude overproliferation of these cells and interdict tumor progression.

To test this hypothesis, DNA was administered by micro-osmotic pumps[30] to Eμ-*myc* mice which were treated continuously for six weeks after weaning, as described below. Due to the limited solubility and antisense activity of methylphosphonates vs. the need for high DNA concentration in the 0.2 ml chamber of the micro-osmotic pumps, phosphorothioates were used for long-term micropump administration. Mice treated with saline or the scrambled control DNA displayed palpable tumors over the usual time course, but 11 of the 12 mice treated with anti-c-*myc* DNA were free of tumors at the age of 9 weeks, when antisense therapy ended. Surprisingly, 75% of the mice treated with antisense DNA were still free of tumors at the age of 26 weeks, implying the establishment of long-term resistance to *myc*-induced lymphoma.

II. MATERIALS AND METHODS

A. Transgenic Mice

Eμ-*myc* transgenic mouse embryos, line Tg(IgH,Myc)Bri157, were the kind gift of Dr. Ralph Brinster.[4] The mouse line is maintained by continually backcrossing Eμ-*myc* positive males with (C57BL/6J X SJL/J)F_1 hybrid females; the hemizygous offspring in each generation is screened for the presence of a ΦX174 marker sequence in the transgene by polymerase chain reaction (PCR) amplification[31] of DNA from toe cells at birth. The reliability of this routine screening method was confirmed by Southern blot, using the c-*myc* probe pRyc7.4,[32] the kind gift of Dr. Maria Luisa Veronese. This investigation was carried out in a specific pathogen-free animal facility accredited by AAALAC, and was reviewed and monitored by the Institutional Animal Care and Use Committee to ensure adherence to NIH guidelines.

B. Oligodeoxynucleotide Synthesis

The anti-c-*myc* DNA methylphosphonate, 5′-dAACGTTGAGGGGCAT-3′, complementary to the initiation codon and the next 4 codons of the human c-*myc* mRNA,[7] and a scrambled sequence control, 5′-dCTGAAGTGGCATGAG-3′, were synthesized[33] on a Biosearch 8750 DNA synthesizer and purified by reversed-phase liquid chromatography.[8] As a normal oligodeoxynucleotide, the anti-c-*myc* DNA sequence has been observed to inhibit MYC protein expression and cellular proliferation in normal peripheral blood lymphocytes[7,10] and in c-*myc*-transformed HL-60 cells,[8,9] and to induce terminal granulocytic differentiation of HL-60 cells.[11,14] The mouse and human sequences differ at the 3′ end of the target sequence,[34] resulting in an A:G mismatch. The scrambled sequence control, as a normal phosphate DNA, did not inhibit c-*myc* expression in human T-lymphocytes.[10]

The anti-c-*myc* DNA phosphorothioate, 5′-dCACGTTGAGGGGCAT-3′, an exact complement to the mouse sequence, and the scrambled DNA phosphorothioate, 5′-dCTGCTGAGAGTCGAG-3′, were synthesized[35] at a scale of 120 and 200 μmol, on a Biosearch 8800 DNA synthesizer. Deprotected oligomers were purified by duplicate precipitation with *n*-butanol,[36] then analyzed to verify purity by high performance liquid chromatography (HPLC),[8] nuclear magnetic resonance spectroscopy,[35] and matrix-assisted laser desorption/ionization mass spectroscopy.[37] Oligomers were sterilized by passage through sterile 0.2-μm pore syringe filter units.

The PCR primers, 5′-dGCAACTTCGGGATGAAAATG-3′ (forward) and 5′-dCGAAGCGCGCATAAATTT-3′ (reverse), for detecting the ΦX174 marker sequence were synthesized as normal phosphate DNAs[38] on an Applied Biosystems 394 DNA synthesizer.

C. Pharmacokinetics

Blood was collected from the retro-orbital sinuses of treated mice at various times after administration of methylphosphonates, and the plasma was isolated by sedimentation. Plasma supernatants were frozen and stored for analysis. For analysis of DNA methylphosphonates, blind coded plasma samples were thawed, and aliquots of 200 μl were mixed with equal volumes of acetonitrile. Insoluble material, mainly precipitated protein, was removed by sedimentation.[39] The supernatant fractions were then lyophilized, redissolved in H_2O, filtered through 0.2-μm filters, and analyzed by reversed-phase liquid chromatography.[8] Oligomers were detected by absorbance at 260 nm; baseline runs were subtracted from sample runs, and peak areas were quantitated by comparison with methylphosphonate standards.

D. Toxicological Analyses

Mice were treated with phosphorothioate DNA administered by prolonged release pellet (Innovative Research of America) at approximately 30 mg/kg/day for 4 weeks, by syringe at approximately 70 mg/kg/day for 5 weeks, and by micropump at approximately 20 mg/kg/day for up to 6 weeks. At the end of each treatment, plasma from each mouse was taken by heart puncture. Some major physiological values such as AST, ALT, BUN, creatinine, glucose, and blood sodium were analyzed on a Kodak 700 chemical analyzer (AMI Town and Country Hospital, Tampa, FL).

E. Detection of MYC p65 Antigen

1. Immunofluorescence

Peripheral lymphocytes were recovered from the blood of mice treated with DNA methylphosphonates, or from untreated nontransgenic mice, by sedimentation on a Percoll density gradient (Pharmacia). Cells were washed twice in Dulbecco's phosphate-buffered saline (DPBS; [Gibco]) supplemented with 0.1% (w/v) bovine serum albumin (Miles Scientific), pelleted, decanted, and resuspended in 900 μl of RPMI 1640 (Gibco), supplemented with 10% fetal calf serum (Gibco), then 100 μl of glycerol was added to each suspension prior to freezing. Blind coded cell samples were brought rapidly to room temperature, washed in 0.5 ml DPBS, and fixed in 1% paraformaldehyde in DPBS for 30 min. The cells were then pelleted, washed with DPBS, and preadsorbed with 1% goat serum (Sigma) in DPBS for 5 min followed by rabbit polyclonal anti-p65 IgG[40] for 1 h. The cells were then washed once in DPBS, preadsorbed with 1% goat serum in DPBS for 5 min, and a fluorescein-conjugated goat polyclonal anti-rabbit IgG (Sigma) was added for 30 min. The cells were then washed twice in DPBS. At least 50 cells were then visualized by light and fluorescence microscopy at ×40, and an average intensity estimated on an arbitrary geometric scale of 0 to 5. The fluorescence intensities from two separate fields were estimated for each sample. For flow cytometry, cell samples were passed through a Becton/Dickinson FACSCAN flow cytometer, and fluorescein fluorescence was quantitated from 10,000 cells. Mean channel fluorescence was linearized by dividing by 64 channels/decade, yielding a quotient that is the logarithm of the fluorescence. The antilog of this number represents the linear fluorescence. Background due to nonspecific binding by preimmume serum was subtracted.

2. *Western Blot*

Total lymphocytes were collected from both spleens and lymph node tumors of mice treated with DNA phosphorothioates or from untreated transgenic mice immediately after sacrifice.[41] Lymphocyte nuclei were isolated,[42] and nuclear protein extracts were prepared.[18] In order to standardize comparison of bands from neighboring lanes, exactly 10 μg of total nuclear protein from each sample, measured with the BCA protein assay Kit (Pierce), were then loaded onto a 4 to 20% polyacrylamide gradient gel, electrophoresed, then blotted onto PVDF membrane (Bio-Rad). Coomassie blue staining of a parallel gel indicated constant intensities of prominent nuclear protein bands in each lane. MYC protein was detected by monoclonal mouse anti-*myc* antibody (Cambridge Research Biochemicals #OM-11-904) and horseradish peroxidase-conjugated anti-mouse IgG (Sigma #A2304) followed by chemiluminescent detection.

F. Detection of c-*myc* mRNA

1. *Solution Hybridization*

Spleens were removed from mice treated with DNA methylphosphonates and homogenized in 1% $NaDodSO_4$, 5 m*M* EDTA, 10 m*M* Tris-HCl, pH 7.4, containing 100 μg/ml proteinase K. Spleen cell total nucleic acid was isolated, and transgene mRNA was measured by solution hybridization[43] using an oligodeoxynucleotide specific for the ΦX174 bacteriophage sequences present in the transgene.[4] Values are reported as pg transgene mRNA/μg total nucleic acid.

2. *Northern Blot*

Total RNA was extracted[44] from about 0.3 g of spleens and lymph node tumors from each mouse treated with DNA phosphorothioates or saline. About 20 μg of total RNA from each sample was electrophoresed on a glyoxal/DMSO gel[45] then blotted onto a nylon membrane and hybridized with two [^{33}P]dCTP-labeled probes: the c-*myc* PstI restriction fragment from pRyc7.4[32] and the pTRI-GAPDH construct (Ambion #7431). The c-*myc* mRNA level was calculated based on the density ratio of the *myc* band compared with the corresponding GAPDH band which was quantitated with a BioImage densitometry system.

G. Statistical Analyses

Tumor onset, Western and Northern blot band densities, and plasma physiological values were analyzed by Kruskal-Wallis one-way analysis of variance on ranks, Dunn's pairwise multiple comparison procedure, and Mann-Whitney rank sum test[46] using the program *SigmaStat*™ (Jandel Scientific). Flow cytometric profiles were compared by the Kolmogorov-Smirnov 2-sample test.[47]

III. RESULTS

A. Intravenous Administration

DNA methylphosphonates were administered i.v. to 4 to 8-week-old Eμ-*myc* transgenic mice, 17 to 25 g each, by injection into the tail vein. In each of the 5 trials, a mouse received 300 nmol of either anti-c-*myc* DNA methylphosphonate or scrambled oligomer in 250 μl DPBS or DPBS alone from blind coded vials. In the fourth trial, a transgenic mouse received no treatment, instead of DPBS. Plasma samples were prepared at 3 min, 1 h, and 3 h. after adminstration, and methylphosphonates were analyzed by reversed-phase liquid chromatography.[8] Plasma from mice treated with DNA methylphosphonates yielded peaks co-eluting with control oligomer (Figure 1). Shorter fragments were not observed, suggesting little or no breakdown of DNA methylphosphonate during 3 h after the injection. Oligomer levels in the bloodstream dropped rapidly during the distribution phase, but they leveled off to a much slower excretion phase during the second and third hours (Figure 2), in agreement with other studies.[48] Changes in MYC levels are described below.

B. Pellet Administration

Four-week prolonged-release pellets (Innovative Research of America), packed with either no drug (placebo) or with 4 μmol of antisense or scrambled phosphorothioate DNAs, were implanted under the skin on the upper back of groups of 3 to 5 Eμ-*myc*-positive mice within two weeks after tumor onset. The total amount of DNA in the pellets and the rate of release from each pellet varied widely and unpredictably. Tumor size, body mass, and lymphocyte differentiation of each mouse were analyzed weekly. Significant percentages of immature lymphocytes were not observed in tail blood smears until late in tumor development, after lymphoid tumors were prevalent throughout the body. Mice with disseminated tumors all displayed blasts and other immature forms, but the extent of peripheral pre-B-cell populations common to these mice varied more from mouse to mouse than from treatment group to treatment group. After four weeks of treatment there were no significant differences in the changes in tumor size increase or body mass increase among the groups of mice treated with placebo, antisense, or scrambled DNA phosphorothioates (data not shown). Methylphosphonate DNAs were similarly ineffective from the prolonged release pellets.

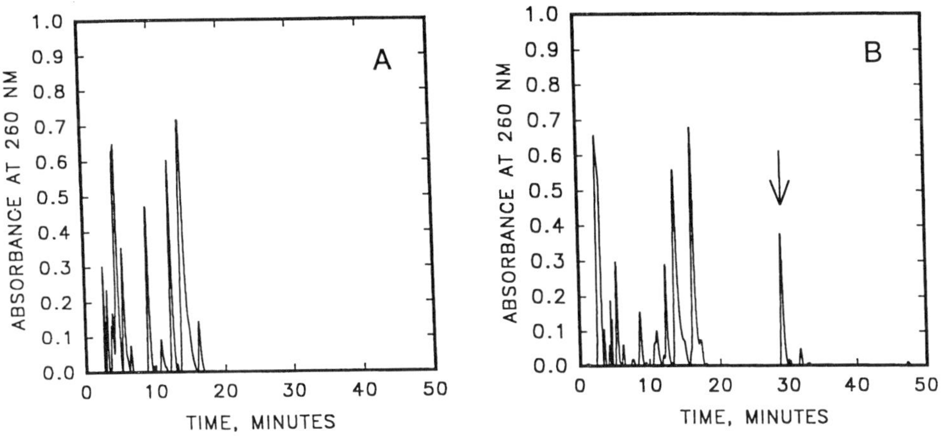

FIGURE 1
Reversed phase liquid chromatograms of DNA methylphosphonates recovered from mouse plasma. (A) Chromatogram of extracted plasma from 250 μl of blood from a mouse treated with DPBS and (B) chromatogram of extracted plasma from a mouse treated with an antisense oligomer for 1 h. Arrow shows normal elution time of the antisense oligomer. (From Wickstrom, E., Bacon, T. A., and Wickstrom, E. L., *Cancer Res.*, 52, 6741, 1992. With permission.)

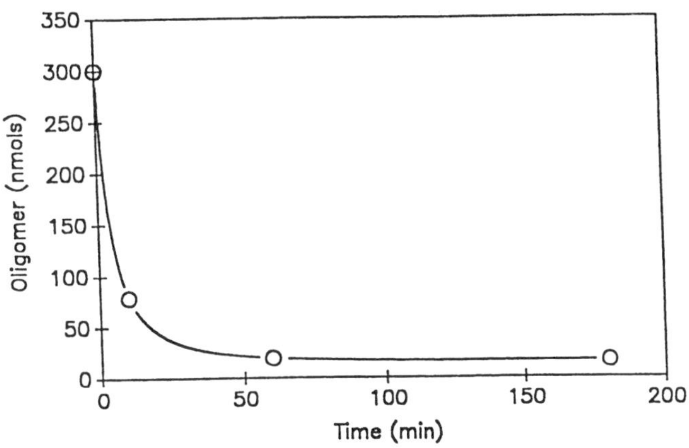

FIGURE 2
Recovery of methylphosphonates from plasma samples of c-*myc* transgenic mice. Samples of 250 μl, removed at 3 min, 1 h, and 3 h, were analyzed by reversed phase liquid chromatography as in Figure 1, quantitated by integrated peak areas, then multiplied by 8 to estimate the number of nanomoles in the entire mouse bloodstream (2 ml). (From Wickstrom, E., Bacon, T. A., and Wickstrom, E. L., *Cancer Res.*, 52, 6741, 1992. With permission.)

C. Subcutaneous Administration

This route was chosen as a simpler and more controllable mode of therapy than pellet implantation. Groups of 3 to 4 Eμ-*myc* transgenic mice were selected at weaning, 3 weeks after birth, based on the criterion of displaying no palpable tumor at that time. Weaning was the earliest age at which DNA could be administered to mice without danger of maternal rejection. Each mouse received normal saline or saline containing 1.0 μmol (5.0 mg) of antisense or scrambled DNA phosphorothioate under the skin of the back, twice weekly for five weeks. At the end of treatment, two out of four mice receiving scrambled DNA displayed tumors, but there were none in the antisense group. In the antisense group, however, epidermal tissues surrounding the site of injection became thick, rigid, and brittle. Therefore, this mode was not pursued further, and methylphosphonates were not used.

D. Micropump Administration

This route was substituted for subcutaneous (s.c.) injection in order to avoid epidermal senescence at the site of injection. Three-week-old Eμ-*myc* transgenic mice with no palpable tumors were randomly distributed into groups of 12. Siblings were assigned into all three treatment groups. Micro-osmotic pumps (Alzet 2002) containing 200 μl of saline, or saline with 5.0 mM scrambled DNA phosphorothioate or anti-c-*myc* DNA phosphorothioate, were implanted s.c. on the upper back of each mouse, which was anesthetized with Avertin (30 mg/kg). Each pump containing DNA therefore dispensed 1.0 μmol (5.0 mg), at 0.5 μl/h, or 2.5 nmol/h, over 14 days. The pumps were replaced at 5 and 7 weeks after birth. Thus, each mouse received a dose of 3.0 μmol of oligomer, or 15 mg, administered continuously at a nearly uniform rate of about 0.36 mg/day over 6 weeks. Because the mass of 3-week-old mice is about 10 g, and the mass of 9-week-old mice is about 30 g, one estimates an initial dose of 36 mg/kg/day, a final dose of 12 mg/kg/day, an average dose of about 20 mg/kg/day, or about 1 mg/kg/h.

The six weeks of therapy represent the longest test of antisense DNA administration in animals to date. During the course of treatment, there were no significant differences in body mass increase or lymphocyte differentiation among the groups of mice treated with either saline, antisense, or scrambled DNA (data not shown). Tumors were detected by palpation twice weekly and confirmed on autopsy. For protein and mRNA measurement from spleens and lymph node tumors, mice with established tumors were treated as above for one week.

E. Tumor Onset

Over several generations of observing the Tg(IgH,Myc)Bri157 line,[4] 57 untreated transgene-positive mice were observed. A few displayed palpable tumors as early as 3 weeks of age, and half of them developed palpable tumors by the age of 8 to 9 weeks (Figure 3). Fifty-five (95%) of the mice developed tumors within 16 weeks.

The cohort of 12 Eμ-*myc* mice treated continuously with scrambled control DNA phosphorothioate, and those treated with saline, displayed tumors over the usual time course (Figure 4). In the saline group, 5 of 12 mice had palpable tumors by 8 weeks of age and 9 of 12 had tumors at 15 weeks. In the scrambled group, 5 of 12 mice had tumors by 10 weeks and 9 of 12 had tumors at 15 weeks. However, in the antisense group only 3 of 12 mice had displayed a tumor by the time of sacrifice at 26 weeks (Figure 4). One of the 3 tumors in the antisense group was already palpable 2 weeks after the beginning of the 6 weeks of therapy; perhaps that tumor was already initiated prior to therapy. The second tumor was detected at 15 weeks and the third at 17 weeks. The tumor-free mice treated with antisense DNA were observed up until sacrifice at 48 weeks.

An overall analysis of variance of the tumor data using the nonparametric Kruskal-Wallis procedure[46] indicated significant effects (H_0, $p = 0.0000851$), and this was followed by multiple pairwise comparisons among the groups using Dunn's nonparametric exact test and the Mann-Whitney rank sum test.[46] By both tests, the antisense treatment group differed significantly from both the saline (H_0, $p < 0.05$)

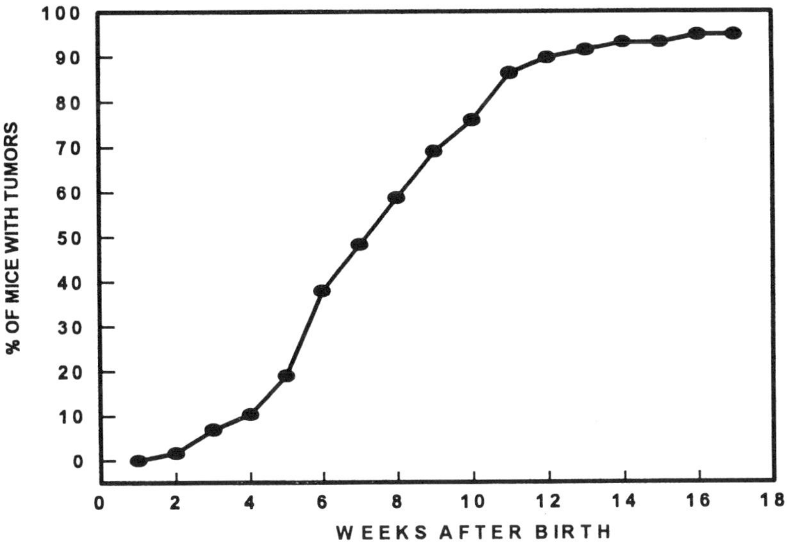

FIGURE 3
Time of onset of lymphoid tumors in untreated Eμ-*myc* transgenic mice from day of birth. The presence of the transgene in these hemizygous mice was detected by PCR analysis of toe tissue at birth. Tumors were detected by palpation twice weekly and confirmed on autopsy. Over several generations, a total of 57 mice were observed. (From Huang, Y., Snyder, R., Kligshteyn, M., and Wickstrom, E., *Mol. Med.*, 1, 647, 1995.With permission.)

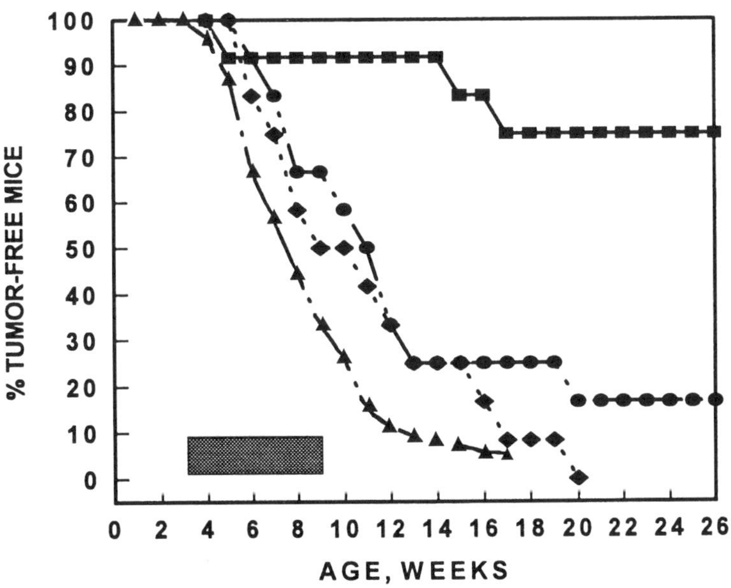

FIGURE 4
Age of onset of lymphoid tumors in Eμ-*myc* transgenic mice treated with saline or scrambled or antisense DNA phosphorothioates. Hatched box shows period of continuous administration of DNA from micro-osmotic pumps. ▲, no treatment (54 mice which were tumor-free at 3 weeks); ♦, saline (12 mice); ●, scrambled DNA phosphorothioate (12 mice); and ■, antisense DNA phosphorothioate (12 mice). (From Huang, Y., Snyder, R., Kligshteyn, M., and Wickstrom, E., *Mol. Med.*, 1, 647, 1995.With permission.)

and scrambled (H_0, p <0.05) groups in tumor onset, while the latter two groups did not differ significantly from each other (H_0, p <0.05). A significant degree of protection by anti-c-*myc* DNA against tumor onset was therefore observed in this trial, continuing until 26 weeks of age. This represents the first demonstration of chemoprevention of tumor onset by prophylactic antisense DNA therapy.

F. Oncogene Expression

Five double-blind studies were conducted to determine the effect of the DNA methylphosphonates on the level of MYC antigen in peripheral lymphocytes. Mice were administered 300 nmol doses of each oligomer, and blood samples were withdrawn 3 to 4 h later. In the first two trials, blood samples were also drawn prior to administration of DNA methylphosphonate in order to check for variability in unperturbed controls. White blood cells were isolated from each sample, and MYC was visualized by indirect immunofluorescence of cells in suspension on slides.[8] In the subsequent trials, blood was not withdrawn prior to treatment in order to maximize the number of cells that could be recovered after administration. In the third and fourth trials, white blood cells collected at 3 to 4 h were sedimented onto slides in order to allow viewing of a large number of cells in a single field. These cells were fixed with cold 95% ethanol prior to blocking.

Averaging MYC immunofluorescence levels among the four methylphosphonate trials above according to the arbitrary geometrically increasing 0 to 5 scale (Figure 5), cells from untreated nontransgenic mice showed faint nuclear fluorescence, in contrast to cells from Eμ-*myc* transgenic mice 3 h after treatment with DPBS, which showed intense nuclear fluorescence. Cells isolated from transgenic mice 3 h after treatment with the scrambled DNA methylphosphonate retained intense nuclear fluorescence. However, cells isolated from mice treated with the antisense oligomer showed nuclear fluorescence equal to or less than that of cells from nontransgenic mice, implying that the antisense DNA methylphosphonate inhibited MYC production. An overall analysis of the data set by the Kruskal-Wallis one-way analysis of variance for ordinal measurements[46] indicated that it was highly unlikely (p <0.01) that all groups came from the same or equivalent populations. Therefore, it is probable that at least one group is statistically different from one other group. Comparisons among individual groups using the Mann-Whitney U test[46] indicated that the DPBS-treated samples were not significantly different from the scrambled-treated samples (p = 0.343). However, the DPBS-treated samples were found unlikely to be equivalent to the antisense-treated samples (p = 0.014), nor were the scrambled-treated samples likely to be equivalent to the antisense-treated samples (p = 0.014). A single trial with 50 nmol of each oligomer yielded no statistically significant dimunition of MYC expression 12 h after administration.

Levels of MYC antigen were quantitated by flow cytometry in one additional 300 nmol trial. Cells were labeled with a fluorescein isothiocyanate-conjugated second antibody only, or with preimmune IgG first, or with polyclonal anti-MYC first, or with polyclonal anti-actin first. No DNA oligomer had any impact on actin levels. When these profiles were compared by the Kolmogorov-Smirnov 2-sample test,[47] each member of each pair of profiles was significantly different from the other member (p <0.001). The linearized MYC fluorescence intensities (Figure 6) further illustrate the correlation of reduced MYC antigen with antisense DNA methylphosphonate treatment.

Levels of c-*myc* mRNA were interpreted by averaging over the first four methylphosphonate trials reported above. Normal mice were negative for the transgene-specific probe. Seven transgenic mice that received no injection displayed 7.16 ± 3.03

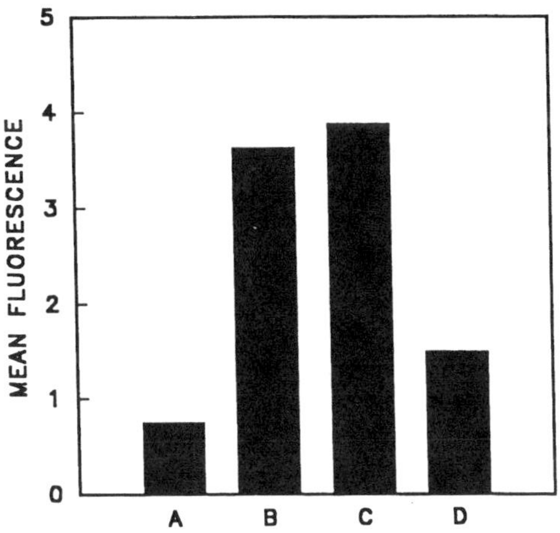

FIGURE 5
Fluorescence measurements of MYC antigen from peripheral blood lymphocytes of mice treated with an i.v. bolus of DNA methylphosphonate. Samples were estimated visually on a geometrically increasing scale from 0 to 5. The bars indicate an average of four experiments. (A) Untreated nontransgenic mouse cells, (B) transgenic mouse cells 3 h after administration of DPBS, (C) transgenic mouse cells 3 h after administration of scrambled DNA methylphosphonate, and (D) transgenic mouse cells 3 h after administration of antisense DNA methylphosphonate. (From Wickstrom, E., Bacon, T. A., and Wickstrom, E. L., *Cancer Res.*, 52, 6741, 1992. With permission.)

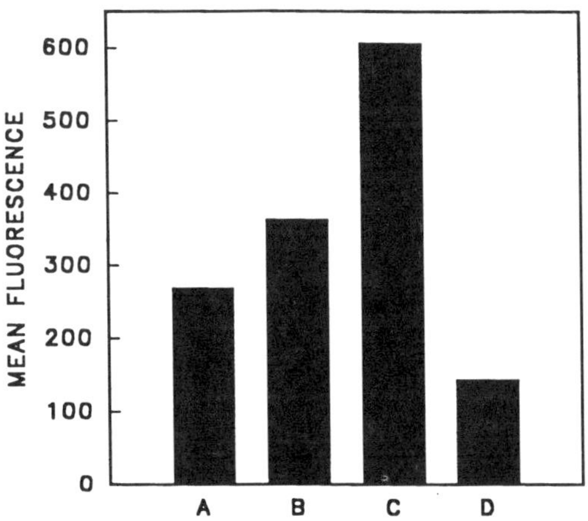

FIGURE 6
Fluorescence measurements of MYC antigen quantitated by flow cytometry of splenic lymphocytes from mice treated with an i.v. bolus of DNA methylphosphonates. Samples were obtained from mice treated as in Figure 5. (A) Untreated nontransgenic mouse cells, (B) transgenic mouse cells 3 h after administration of DPBS, (C) transgenic mouse cells 3 h after administration of scrambled DNA methylphosphonate, and (D) transgenic mouse cells 3 h after administration of antisense DNA methylphosphonate. Fluorescence y-axis is linear. 10,000 cells were measured. Background due to nonspecific binding by preimmume serum was subtracted. (From Wickstrom, E., Bacon, T. A., and Wickstrom, E. L., *Cancer Res.*, 52, 6741, 1992. With permission.)

pg c-*myc* mRNA/μg total nucleic acid in their spleen cells. Three mice that received saline only showed 3.44 ± 0.46 pg/μg, while 4 mice that received the scrambled DNA methylphosphonate had 3.88 ± 1.88 pg/μg, and 4 mice that received the antisense DNA methylphosphonate yielded 2.56 ± 1.20 pg/μg. While the latter value was lower than the others, the difference was not statistically significant.

Next, it was important to determine whether or not antisense DNA therapy could downregulate c-*myc* gene expression in Eμ-*myc* mice over an extended period of therapy that required the use of DNA phosphorothioates. Antigen and messenger measurements, however, were not made on the mice which received long-term therapy from the time of weaning, but on a separate group implanted with micropumps only after tumor onset. In the former group, tumors appeared at arbitrary times in each mouse in each group, and each group included individual mice from different litters born at different times. Thus, it would have been difficult to make comparable protein and RNA measurements after each separate sacrifice of an animal. In the case of antisense DNA treatment, only three mice ever displayed tumors, many weeks apart. In order to maintain the size of the observed cohort, thereby maximizing the statistical reliability of the observations, no mice in the long-term therapy experiment were sacrificed for assay prior to tumor onset.

It was of interest to determine how effectively antisense DNA inhibited *myc* gene expression, both in splenic lymphocytes and in tumor cells of the same animal, at the same time in the middle of a pump cycle for all animals examined. c-*myc* mRNA is expressed at very low levels in splenic lymphocytes of both normal mice and Eμ-*myc* transgenic mice prior to tumor establishment. Therefore, these measurements were carried out in a group of eight mice already displaying palpable tumors. Two micropumps were implanted containing saline vehicle, two with scrambled or four with antisense DNA, at 5.0 m*M* as above. After one week of DNA administration by micropump at about 20 mg/kg/day, c-*myc* mRNA and MYC p65 antigen were measured from each mouse. Nuclear proteins and total RNA were collected from both splenic lymphocytes and lymph node tumors. MYC proteins were detected by Western blots and c-*myc* mRNAs were measured by Northern blots.

MYC protein was virtually undetectable in splenic lymphocytes from all antisense treated mice (Figure 7) as it is in normal mice or Eμ-*myc* mice prior to tumor onset, but prominent bands remained in the splenic lymphocytes of tumor-bearing mice treated with saline or scrambled DNA (Figure 7), and in the lymphoid tumors of mice from all treatment groups (Figure 8). *c-myc* mRNA measured in the same animals, however, was not significantly reduced either in splenic lymphocytes of the mice with the antisense treatment (Figure 9) or in lymphoid tumors, as compared with control groups (Figure 10). The reduction in MYC antigen in the splenic lymphocytes of tumor-bearing mice treated with antisense DNA correlates with treatment with antisense DNA therapy, but the tumors themselves were apparently unaffected. However, this observation made it plausible that prophylactic therapy with antisense DNA prior to tumor establishment might slow the proliferation of the transgenic pre-B-cell population enough to lower the rate of tumor onset in Eμ-*myc* mice.

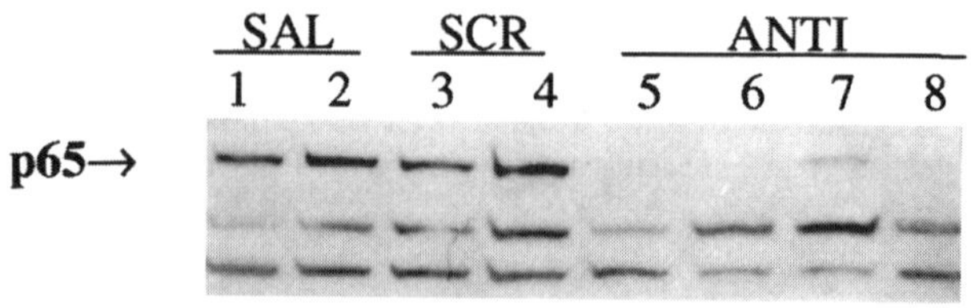

FIGURE 7
Western blot analysis of MYC antigen expression in spleens of Eμ-*myc* transgenic mice. Mice with palpable tumors were treated with saline (SAL) (lanes 1 and 2), or scrambled (SCR) (lanes 3 and 4) or antisense (ANTI) (lanes 5 through 8) DNA phosphorothioates for one week. 10 μg of nuclear protein extract was then applied to each well. p65 indicates the position of the MYC antigen. (From Huang, Y., Snyder, R., Kligshteyn, M., and Wickstrom, E., *Mol. Med.*, 1, 647, 1995. With permission.)

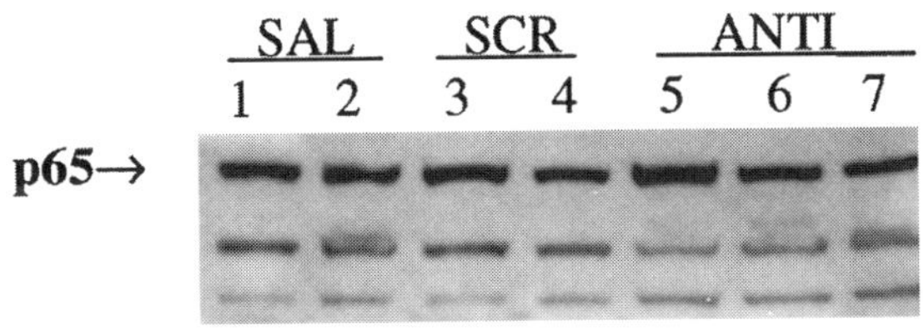

FIGURE 8
Western blot analysis of MYC antigen expression in lymphoid tumors of Eμ-*myc* transgenic mice. Mice with palpable tumors were treated with saline (SAL) (lanes 1 and 2), scrambled (SCR) (lanes 3 and 4) or antisense (ANTI) (lanes 5 through 7) DNA phosphorothioates for one week. 10 μg of nuclear protein extract was then applied to each well. p65 indicates the position of the MYC antigen. (From Huang, Y., Snyder, R., Kligshteyn, M., and Wickstrom, E., *Mol. Med.*, 1, 647, 1995. With permission.)

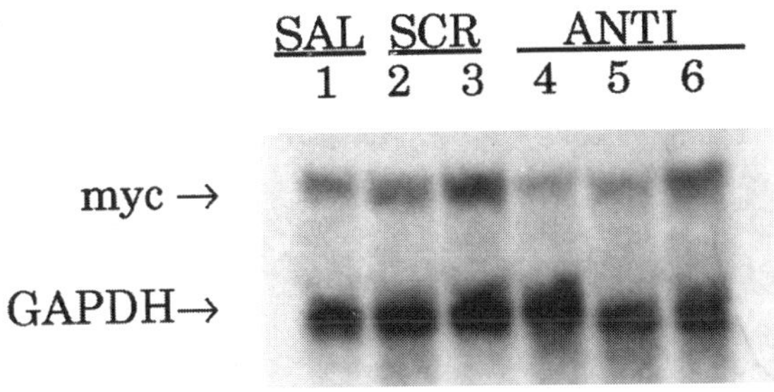

FIGURE 9
Northern blot analysis of c-*myc* and GAPDH (glyceraldehyde phosphate dehydrogenase) mRNA expression in spleens of Eμ-*myc* transgenic mice. Mice with palpable tumors were either untreated (lane 1), or treated with saline (SAL) (lanes 2 through 4), or scrambled (SCR) (lanes 5 through 7) or antisense (ANTI) (lanes 8 through 10) DNA phosphorothioates for one week. Then 20 μg of total cellular RNA was applied to each well. (From Huang, Y., Snyder, R., Kligshteyn, M., and Wickstrom, E., *Mol. Med.*, 1, 647, 1995. With permission.)

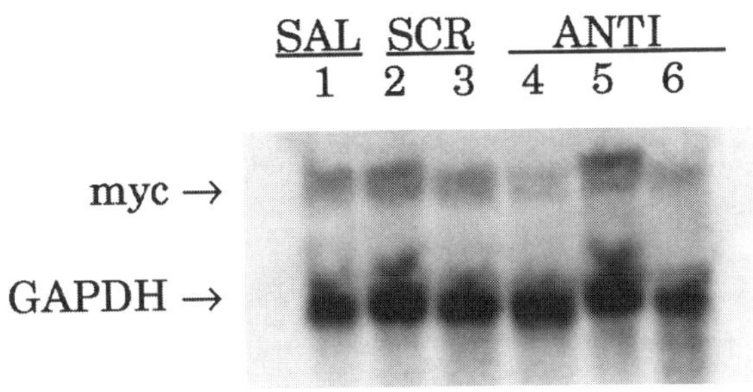

FIGURE 10
Northern blot analysis of c-*myc* and GAPDH mRNA expression in lymphoid tumors of Eμ-*myc* transgenic mice. Mice with palpable tumors were either untreated (lane 1), or treated with saline (lanes 2 through 4), or scrambled (lanes 5 through 7) or antisense (lanes 8 through 10) DNA phosphorothioates for one week. Then 20 μg of total cellular RNA was applied to each well. (From Huang, Y., Snyder, R., Kligshteyn, M., and Wickstrom, E., *Mol. Med.*, 1, 647, 1995. With permission.)

G. Toxicology

In each i.v. trial with methylphosphonates, Eμ-*myc* transgenic mice were administered injections of 300 nmol of either the antisense DNA methylphosphonate or the scrambled methylphosphonate in 250 μl of DPBS or DPBS alone from coded vials. The dose administered corresponded to 50 to 75 mg/kg. Neither the antisense nor scrambled oligomers displayed any observable toxicity in any of the treated mice when compared with untreated or saline-injected control mice, in agreement with others.[49]

Phosphorothioate DNA has been found to be toxic to liver, kidneys, spleen, and some other major organs of mice at intraperitoneal (i.p.) bolus doses above 100 mg/kg, 3 times per week for 2 weeks.[50] At this dose range, serum aspartate aminotransferase (AST) activity doubled or tripled, alanine aminotransferase (ALT) activity doubled, and glucose levels decreased 30%. More than 150 mg/kg in a single bolus induced acute death in some mice.[50] However, among the mice treated with phosphorothioate DNA at the dose rates described in this work, the lack of perturbation of increase in body mass with time provides a general indication of negligible acute toxicity. Furthermore, plasma physiological values were analyzed at the time of sacrifice in normal mice and in transgenic mice which were treated with saline, scrambled, and antisense DNA phosphorothioates. In 8 mice with established tumors, DNA phosphorothioates were administered by pellet at approximately 30 mg/kg/day for 4 weeks. In 4 mice without palpable tumors at 3 weeks, DNAs was administered by s.c. injection at approximately 250 mg/kg twice weekly (70 mg/kg/day) for 5 weeks. In 4 mice without palpable tumors at 3 weeks, DNAs was administered by micropump at 0.36 mg/day, or an average of 20 mg/kg/day, for 6 weeks, or until establishment of large tumors. In contrast to mice treated with i.p. boli of 100 mg/kg,[50] there were no significant differences detected among the three groups in major physiological values such as AST, ALT, creatinine, BUN (blood urea nitrogen), glucose, and blood sodium, indicating the lack of acute toxicity of phosphorothioate DNA at the therapeutic dose (Table 1).

TABLE 1

Major Plasma Physiological Values of Eμ-*myc* Transgenic Mice Treated with DNA Phosphorothioates for 4 to 6 Weeks at Doses up to 70 mg/kg/day

Treatment Group	AST (IU/ℓ)	ALT (IU/ℓ)	BUN (mg/dl)	Blood creatinine (mg/dl)	Blood glucose (mg/dl)	Blood sodium (mEq/dl)
Normal control[a]	438 ± 241 (4)	455 ± 247 (4)	28 ± 14 (4)	0.28 ± 0.15 (4)	202 ± 15 (4)	136 ± 3[c] (4)
Saline only	518 ± 328 (8)	131 ± 120 (8)	31 ± 12 (7)	0.29 ± 0.06 (8)	144 ± 33 (3)	154 ± 14[c] (7)
Scrambled DNA	658 ± 341 (4)	154 ± 72 (4)	35 ± 14 (4)	0.35 ± 0.10 (4)	157 ± 47 (2)	148 ± 11 (2)
Antisense DNA	627 ± 306 (4)	88 ± 10 (4)	38 ± 24 (4)	0.43 ± 0.39 (4)	229 ± 30 (3)	145 ± 0 (3)
ANOVA[b]	No	No	No	No	No	Yes

Note: Numbers in parentheses indicate the number of samples for each measurement.

[a] Eμ-*myc* negative mice.

[b] Nonparametric comparison among groups by Kruskal-Wallis one-way analysis of variance on ranks.

[c] Significant difference between these two groups by Dunn's multiple pairwise comparison method.

(From Huang, Y., Snyder, R., Kligshteyn, M., and Wickstrom, E., *Mol. Med.*, 1, 647, 1995. With permission.)

Splenomegaly has also been reported in mice as a result of phosphorothioate DNA administration.[51] This phenomenon was also observed in the Eμ-*myc* mice treated with antisense or scrambled phosphorothioate DNAs. At an age of 12 to 16 weeks, the mass of spleens from normal mice averaged 0.1 g, while those from Eμ-*myc* mice receiving phosphorothioates averaged 0.3 g. However, the spleens of

Eμ-*myc* mice treated with the placebo averaged 0.25 g, thus the observed splenomegaly may also arise from the stress of bearing tumors and implantation of pellets or micropumps.

Procreation is usually inadvisable during chemotherapy, but three female mice treated with scrambled DNA were mated inadvertently during treatment and gave birth to normal sized healthy litters. A male mouse treated with antisense DNA was mated two weeks after the end of therapy and fathered two normal sized healthy litters. Hence, there was no apparent acute toxicity to the gonads as a result of phosphorothioate therapy at the therapeutic dose.

IV. DISCUSSION

A. Routes of Administration

1. *Intravenous Administration*

For the first attempt at systemic antisense DNA treatment of c-*myc*-induced Burkitt's lymphoma in Eμ-c-*myc* transgenic mice, DNA methylphosphonates were prepared. The neutral methylphosphonate backbone was chosen to avoid nuclease hydrolysis in the blood and to maximize cellular uptake.[52] The DNA methylphosphonates were soluble to >1 m*M* in DPBS, in agreement with partition coefficient measurements showing methylphosphonate preference for water over octanol.[53]

The lack of acute toxicity observed in mice by DNA methylphosphonates at doses that are effective, 50 to 75 mg/kg, implies that further studies *in vivo* are worth pursuing. This observation agrees with an earlier study that reported no signs of toxicity below 140 mg/kg.[49] Similarly, it is encouraging that no breakdown of the DNA methylphosphonates was detected. In a previous study in mice,[48] DNA methylphosphonate undecamers with a normal phosphodiester linkage at the 5′ end were observed to be truncated in the blood to the pure methylphosphonate decamer, which was not further degraded. This report also agrees with the latter work in finding rapid clearance of DNA methylphosphonates from the blood.

The observation of a reduction in the level of c-MYC antigen in lymphocytes of transgenic mice treated with the anti-c-*myc* DNA methylphosphonate, but not with the scrambled sequence, is consistent with previous studies in cells.[7-15] The lack of significant reduction in the level of c-*myc* mRNA in the same cell type agrees with the model that antisense DNA methylphosphonates act by inhibiting ribosomal translation of the targeted mRNA, rather than by inducing the breakdown of mRNA. This observation is consistent with the lack of RNase H degradation of mRNA/DNA methylphosphonate hybrids.[52]

2. *Prolonged Release Pellet*

When long-term antisense DNA administration by pellet was attempted after tumor onset, autopsies revealed numerous tumors in each of the Eμ-*myc* mice, disseminated to most of the lymph nodes, in varying sizes up to several grams. Disease progression was not halted in mice treated by pellet with antisense DNA phosphorothioates or methylphosphonates after tumor establishment. However, the lack of measurable regression may only reflect the pellet mode of administration utilized in the first two trials. Pellet administration was discarded following these unpromising results. Inconsistent, poor delivery of antisense DNA may have resulted in a low effective dose, obscuring any antisense effects. Therefore, another hypothesis to be tested holds that continuous administration of antisense DNA over many weeks might be sufficient to reduce the growth of an established tumor. However, it is apparent from Figure 8 that one week of such therapy failed to depress MYC antigen.

3. *Subcutaneous Adminstration*

One may then hypothesize that inhibition of c-*myc* overexpression early in life, prior to secondary neoplastic transformation, might interdict tumor formation. To test this hypothesis, antisense DNA therapy was initiated at weaning, three weeks of age, the earliest time at which pups could be handled without danger of maternal rejection. Subcutaneous administration was tested, and none of the mice receiving antisense DNA displayed tumors at the age of 8 weeks, when the 5 weeks of therapy ended. However, the senescence of the skin around the site of injection, in the case of antisense DNA, presented an undesirable side effect. Normally, mature epidermis includes a differentiating compartment and a proliferating compartment. MYC protein is one of the crucial factors regulating keratinocyte growth, differentiation, and apoptosis in the mature epidermis.[54] Downregulation of c-*myc* expression directly induces terminal differentiation of keratinocytes and potently initiates apoptosis, as well as inhibits proliferation. Both lead to keratinocyte cell death. Furthermore, keratinocytes efficiently internalize oligodeoxynucleotides.[55] Therefore, the dermal toxicity which occurred in the antisense-treated group was probably a direct effect of a high local concentration of anti-c-*myc* DNA.

4. *Micropump Administration*

The s.c. trial implied that prolonged and frequent administration of antisense DNA under the skin by syringe would be too toxic to use in a longer, larger trial. Prolonged and frequent i.p. administration seemed too traumatic. Envisioning 6 weeks of therapy, we therefore decided to try antisense DNA therapy by implantation of a series of three 14-day micro-osmotic pumps. Following one week of such therapy, MYC antigen was suppressed in the spleens of tumor-bearing mice treated with antisense DNA (Figure 7), although no significant inhibition was observed in the corresponding lymphoid tumors from the same animals (Figure 8). Poor penetration by antisense DNA into the tumors from the blood may be one possible explanation for the lack of MYC ablation in the tumors. In neither spleens nor lymphoid tumors was c-*myc* mRNA reduced (Figures 9 and 10). Perhaps a transcriptional feedback mechanism replenished c-*myc* mRNA presumably ablated by RNase H in the spleens of antisense treated animals. Such a feedback phenomenon has been observed in acute myelogenous leukemia cells treated with antisense DNA against p53, where the antigen level was also depressed, without concomitant reduction of the mRNA band on a Northern blot.[56]

In the micropump trial, anti-c-*myc* DNA therapy dramatically inhibited tumor progression when administered prophylactically, before the appearance of palpable tumors. The dose of racemic antisense DNA phosphorothioate administered corresponds to about 20 mg/kg/day over the six weeks of therapy. The rather high dose which allowed chemoprevention may in principle be reduced. Dose-response experiments which are underway should reveal how low a concentration will be effective. However, one may hypothesize that potency could be elevated significantly by use of stereospecific all-Rp phosphorothioate[57] or all-Rp methylphosphonate[58] oligomers, which display much stronger hybridization than the racemic oligomers used above, or chimeric mixtures of these backbones. For prolonged or chronic therapy, intestinal uptake[59] might even allow oral administration.

B. Sequence Specificity

The question of sequence specificity of antisense DNA inhibition must be addressed, particularly when the antisense sequence includes a G_4 segment.[60] In the case of anti-c-*myc* DNA phosphodiesters used to inhibit proliferation of human promyelocytic HL-60 cells,[7-14] 10 different sites, from the 5′ end to the beginning of the coding domain in the second exon of c-*myc* mRNA, were targeted. All ten antisense DNAs inhibited MYC antigen levels between 40 to 90%, under conditions where our original initiation codon antisense sequence with a G_4 segment induced 70% inhibition. The same sequence failed to inhibit Q8 cells transformed by avian c-*myc* oncogene, with 4 mismatches in the antisense target.[8] In the case of anti-c-*myc* DNA phosphorothioates used to inhibit proliferation of smooth muscle cells involved in restenosis,[17,22,28] our original initiation codon antisense sequence with a G_4 segment and two other antisense sequences were effective inhibitors, but scrambled, sense, reverse, and 4-nt mismatch controls showed no activity. Recently, anti-c-*myb* and anti-c-*myc* DNA phosphorothioates, as well as control sequences, with G_4 segments were observed to inhibit smooth muscle cell proliferation nonspecifically, when the cells were exposed to 30 μ*M* DNA for 24 h.[61] At this toxic dose, however, nonspecific inhibition should be expected.[62] In contrast, typical antisense DNA phosphorothioate concentrations of 0.2 to 2.0 μ*M* result in sequence-specific effects, as in the other studies mentioned above.

Another possibility for nonspecific effects *in vivo* arises from the presence of the 5′-dCACGTT segment of the anti-c-*myc* DNA, a sequence close to the dRRCGYY consensus, which has recently been reported to induce B-cell stimulation in mice 24 h after a bolus of about 25 mg/kg, but not at 5 mg/kg.[63] On the one hand, the micropump dose rate of 1 mg/kg/h may never achieve a threshhold serum level of anti-c-*myc* DNA which might activate B cells. Fluorescence measurements of OliGreen™ bound to anti-c-*myc* DNA in plasma samples from mice treated by micropump as above indicated a steady-state concentration of 0.1 μ*M*.[64] On the other hand, one may hypothesize that elevated B-cell activity in mice over 6 weeks old might contribute to long-term tumor resistance, although no MYC reduction or tumor regression was observed in established tumors (Figure 8).

C. Long-term Tumor Resistance

Another significant question to be addressed concerns the extended tumor-free survival of 9 of the 12 antisense treated mice in the fourth trial (Figure 2). The original hypothesis predicted postponement of tumorigenesis during the course of antisense therapy, i.e., until the end of the sixth week of DNA administration, 9 weeks of age, but not long-term resistance. What mechanism could one then postulate to explain this phenomenon? In the case of Eμ-*myc* mice, it may be that antisense inhibition of the expanded pre-B-cell population limited the opportunities for establishment of tumor clones until the animals were sufficiently mature to eliminate transformed cells by normal immunological processes. In that case, two weeks or four weeks of antisense therapy, up to an age of 7 weeks, might be insufficient to allow long-term resistance. Alternatively, upregulation of c-*myc* expression at the end of therapy in transformed cells may have driven them into apoptosis, as with promyelocytic HL-60 cells.[21] It is also possible that antisense inhibition induced sufficient differentiation of c-*myc* transformed cells[11,14] to expose them to immune surveillance and specific T-cell activation. It will be of great interest to examine and test the hypothetical forms of immunological activation set in motion by antisense DNA therapy.

D. Applications

In view of the positive results of the micropump trial, one could postulate screening of individuals at risk for c-*myc* translocation, such as HIV-infected individuals. Although the 8:14 chromosomal translocation is not frequent enough in children to justify screening of a large population, it does occur frequently in HIV-infected individuals, inducing lymphomas.[1] AIDS-associated non-Hodgkin's lymphomas typically display translocation of c-*myc* to an immunoglobulin locus.[65,66] If c-*myc* translocation precedes onset of lymphoma by any appreciable time, then screening might reveal positive evidence of c-*myc* activation prior to malignancy. Individuals displaying c-*myc* translocation could then be treated with antisense DNA to interdict tumor onset. It may therefore be reasonable to propose prophylactic anti-c-*myc* DNA therapy for HIV-infected individuals who display c-*myc* translocation in peripheral B-cells. Would one not, however, expect to find systemic toxicity upon antisense inhibition of c-*myc* expression in proliferating cells? Fortunately for this prophylactic model, it has been observed in mice that DNA phosphorothioates are preferentially taken up by B cells, particularly when stimulated by a B-cell mitogen,[67] which may possibly include the 5′-dCACGTT segment of the anti-c-*myc* DNA itself.[63] Finally, the downregulation of MYC protein observed in splenic lymphocytes (Figure 7) suggests that anti-c-*myc* therapy might prove beneficial in those hematological malignancies in which cellular proliferation depends upon elevated c-*myc* expression.

ACKNOWLEDGMENTS

The author warmly thanks his associates who have worked on this investigation over several years: Dr. Ye Huang, Erica Wickstrom, and Thomas Bacon. I am most grateful to Dr. Eric P. Sandgren, Dr. Ralph L. Brinster, and Dr. Richard D. Palmiter for their invaluable help at many stages of this investigation, and for their gift of fertilized embryos of the Tg(IgH,Myc)Bri157 Eμ-*myc* transgenic mouse line. The author thanks Dr. Gary Gray for performing the statistical analyses, Dr. Michael Kligshteyn for DNA phosphorothioate synthesis, Ruthanne Snyder for assistance with animal experiments, and Christine O'Connell for flow cytometry analysis. I also thank Dr. Jaspal Khillan and Dr. Tim Manser for their help in establishing the Tg(IgH,Myc)Bri157 line at Jefferson, Dr. Maria Luisa Veronese for a sample of pRyc7.4, and Dr. Grace Ju, Dr. Robert Eisenman, and Dr. Gerard Evan for samples of polyclonal antisera against MYC protein. This work was supported by NIH Grant CA42960 to E.W.

REFERENCES

1. Magrath, I., The pathogenesis of Burkitt's lymphoma, *Adv. Cancer Res.*, 55, 133, 1990.
2. Bishop, J. M., Molecular themes in oncogenesis, *Cell*, 64, 235, 1991.
3. de The, G., The etiology of Burkitt's lymphoma and the history of the shaken dogmas, *Blood Cells*, 19, 667, 1993.
4. Adams, J. M., Harris, A. W., Pinkert, C. A., Corcoran, L. M., Alexander, W. S., Cory, S., Palmiter, R. D., and Brinster, R. L., The c-*myc* oncogene driven by immunoglobulin enhancers induces lymphoid malignancy in transgenic mice, *Nature*, 318, 533, 1985.
5. Corcoran, L. M., Cory, S., and Adams, J. M., Transposition of the immunoglobulin heavy chain enhancer to the *myc* oncogene in a murine plasmacytoma, *Cell*, 40, 71, 1985.

6. Harris, A. W., Pinkert, C. A., Crawford, M., Langdon, W. Y., Brinster, R. L., and Adams, J. M., The Eμ-*myc* transgenic mouse: A model for high-incidence spontaneous lymphoma and leukemia of early B cells, *J. Exp. Med.*, 167, 353, 1988.
7. Heikkila, R., Schwab, G., Wickstrom, E., Loke, S. L., Pluznik, D., Watt, R., and Neckers, L. M., A c-*myc* antisense oligodeoxynucleotide inhibits entry into S phase but not progress from G_0 to G_1, *Nature*, 328, 445, 1987.
8. Wickstrom, E. L., Bacon, T. A., Gonzalez, A., Freeman, D. L., Lyman, G. H., and Wickstrom, E., Human promyelocytic leukemia HL-60 cell proliferation and c-*myc* protein expression are inhibited by an antisense pentadecadeoxynucleotide targeted against c-*myc* mRNA, *Proc. Natl. Acad. Sci. U.S.A.*, 85, 1028, 1988.
9. Holt, J. T., Redner, R. L., and Nienhuis, A. W., An oligomer complementary to c-*myc* mRNA inhibits proliferation of HL-60 promyelocytic cells and induces differentiation, *Mol. Cell. Biol.*, 8, 963, 1988.
10. Haral-Bellan, A., Ferris, D. K., Vinocour, M., Holt, J. T., and Farrar, W. L., Specific inhibition of c-*myc* protein biosynthesis using an antisense synthetic deoxyoligonucleotide in human T lymphocytes, *J. Immunol.*, 140, 2431, 1988.
11. Wickstrom, E. L., Bacon, T. A., Gonzalez, A., Lyman, G. H., and Wickstrom, E., Anti-c-*myc* DNA oligomers increase differentiation and decrease colony formation by HL-60 cells, *In Vitro Cell. Dev. Biol.*, 25, 297, 1989.
12. McManaway, M. E., Neckers, L. M., Loke, S. L., Al-Nasser, A. A., Redner, R. L., Shiramizu, B. T., Goldschmidts, W. L., Huber, B., and Magrath, I. T., Tumour-specific inhibition of lymphoma growth by an antisense oligodeoxynucleotide, *Lancet*, 335, 808, 1990.
13. Bacon, T. A. and Wickstrom, E., Walking along human c-*myc* mRNA with antisense oligonucleotides: maximum efficacy at the 5′ cap region, *Oncogene Res.*, 6, 13, 1991.
14. Bacon, T. A. and Wickstrom, E., Daily addition of an anti-c-*myc* DNA oligomer induces granulocytic differentiation of human promyelocytic leukemia HL-60 cells in both serum-containing and serum-free media, *Oncogene Res.*, 6, 21, 1991.
15. Watson, P. H., Pon, R. T., and Shiu, R. P. C., Inhibition of c-*myc* expression by phosphorothioate antisense oligonucleotide identifies a critical role for c-*myc* in the growth of human breast cancer, *Cancer Res.*, 51, 3996, 1991.
16. Paria, B. C., Dey, S. K., and Andrews, G. K., Antisense c-*myc* effects on preimplantation mouse embryo development, *Proc. Natl. Acad. Sci. U.S.A.*, 89, 10051, 1992.
17. Shi, Y., Hutchinson, H. G., Hall, D. J., and Zalewski, A., Down regulation of c-*myc* expression by antisense oligonucleotides inhibits proliferation of human smooth muscle cells, *Circulation*, 88, 1190, 1993.
18. Biro, S., Fu, Y.-M., Yu, Z.-X., and Epstein, S. E., Inhibitory effects of antisense oligodeoxynucleotides targeting c-*myc* mRNA on smooth muscle cell proliferation and migration, *Proc. Natl. Acad. Sci. U.S.A.*, 90, 654, 1993.
19. Peña, A., Reddy, C. D., Wu, S., Hickok, N. J., Reddy, E. P., Yumet, G., Soprano, D. R., and Soprano, K. J., Regulation of human ornithine decarboxylase expression by the c-Myc·Max protein complex, *J. Biol. Chem.*, 268, 27277, 1993.
20. Cherney, B. W., Bhatia, K., and Tosato, G. A., Role for deregulated c-Myc expression in apoptosis of Epstein-Barr virus-immortalized B cells, *Proc. Natl. Acad. Sci. U.S.A.*, 91, 12967, 1994.
21. Kimura, S., Maekawa, T., Hirakawa, K., Murakami, A., and Abe, T., Alterations of c-*myc* expression by antisense oligodeoxynucleotides enhance the induction of apoptosis in HL-60 cells, *Cancer Res.*, 55, 1379, 1995.
22. Gryaznov, S., Skorski, T., Cucco, C., Nieborowska-Skorska, M., Chiu, C. Y., Lloyd, D., Chen, J., Koziolkiewicz, M., and Calabretta, B., Oligonucleotide N3′→P5′ phosphoramidates as antisense agents, *Nucl. Acid Res.*, 24, 1508, 1996.
23. Wickstrom, E., Ed., *Prospects for Antisense Nucleic Acid Therapy of Cancer and AIDS*, Wiley-Liss, New York, 1991.
24. Agrawal, S., Ed., *Antisense Therapeutics*, Humana Press, Totowa, NJ, 1996.
25. Wickstrom, E., Bacon, T. A., and Wickstrom, E. L., Down-regulation of c-*myc* antigen expression in lymphocytes of Eμ-c-*myc* transgenic mice treated with anti-c-*myc* DNA methylphosphonate, Cancer Res., 52, 6741, 1992.
26. Jacoby, R. O. and Fox, J. G., Biology and diseases of mice. in Fox, J. G., Cohen, B. J., and Loew, F. M., Eds., *Laboratory Animal Medicine*, Academic Press, New York, 1984, chap. 3.
27. Wickstrom, E., Oligodeoxynucleotide stability in subcellular extracts and culture media, *J. Biochem. Biophys. Methods*, 13, 97, 1986.
28. Shi, Y., Fard, A., Galeo, A., Hutchinson, H. G., Vermani, P., Dodge, G. R., Shaheen, F., Hall, D. J., and Zalewski, A., Transcatheter delivery of c-*myc* antisense oligomers reduces neointimal formation in a porcine model of coronary artery balloon injury, *Circulation*, 90, 944, 1994.

29. Gray, G., Hernandez, O., Hebel, D., Pow-Sang, J. M., and Wickstrom, E., Antisense DNA inhibition of tumor growth induced by T24 c-Ha-*ras* oncogene in nude mice, *Cancer Res.*, 53, 577, 1993.
30. Huang, Y., Snyder, R., Kligshteyn, M., and Wickstrom, E., Prevention of tumor formation in a mouse model of Burkitt's lymphoma by six weeks of treatment with anti-c-*myc* DNA phosphorothioate, *Mol. Med.*, 1, 647, 1995.
31. Arita, M., Li, S.-W., Bertolette, D. C., and Khillan, J. S., Quick screening of newborn transgenic mouse pups by polymerase chain reaction (PCR), *Int. J. Anim. Sci.*, 10, 1, 1995.
32. Sun, L. K., Showe, L. C., and Croce, C. M., Analysis of the 3′ flanking region of the human c-*myc* gene in lymphomas with the t(8;22) and t(2;8) chromosomal translocations, *Nucleic Acids Res.*, 14, 4037, 1986.
33. Agrawal, S. and Goodchild, J., Oligodeoxynucleoside methylphosphonates: synthesis and enzymic degradation, *Tetrahedron Lett.*, 28, 3539, 1987.
34. Stanton, L. W., Watt, R., and Marcu, L. B., Translocation, breakage and truncated transcripts of c-*myc* oncogene in murine plasmacytomas, *Nature*, 303, 401, 1983.
35. Iyer, R. P., Phillips, L. R., Egan, W., Regan, J. B., and Beaucage, S. L., The automated synthesis of sulfur-containing oligodeoxyribonucleotides using 3*H*-1,2-benzodithiol-3-one 1,1-dioxide as a sulfur-transfer reagent, *J. Org. Chem.*, 55, 4693, 1990.
36. Sawadogo, M. and Van Dyke, M. W., A rapid method for the purification of deprotected oligodeoxynucleotides, *Nucleic Acids Res.*, 19, 674, 1991.
37. Pieles, U., Zürcher, W., Schär, M., and Moser, H. E., Matrix-assisted laser desorption ionization time-of-flight mass spectrometry: A powerful tool for the mass and sequence analysis of natural and modified oligonucleotides, *Nucleic Acids Res.*, 21, 3191, 1993.
38. Sinha, N. D., Biernat, J., McManus, J., and Köster, H., Polymer support oligonucleotide synthesis XVIII: Use of ß-cyanoethyl-*N,N*-dialkylamino-/*N*-morpholino phosphoramidite of deoxynucleosides for the synthesis of DNA fragments simplifying deprotection and isolation of the final product, *Nucleic Acids Res.*, 11, 4539, 1984.
39. Blanchard, J., Mohammadi, J. D., and Conrad, K. A., Improved liquid-chromatographic determination of caffeine in plasma, *Clin. Chem.*, 26, 1351, 1980.
40. Miyamoto, C., Chizzonite, R., Crowl, R., Rupprecht, K., Kramer, R., Schaber, M., Kumar, G., Poonian, M., and Ju, G., Molecular cloning and regulated expression of the human c-*myc* gene in *Escherichia coli* and *Saccharomyces cerevisiae*: Comparison of the protein products, *Proc. Nat. Acad. Sci. U.S.A.*, 82, 7232, 1985.
41. Mishell, B. B., Shiigi, S. M., Henry, C., Chan, E. L., North, J., Gallily, R., Slomich, M., Miller, K., Marbrood, J., Parks, D., and Good, A. H., Preparation of mouse cell suspensions, *Selected Methods in Cellular Immunology*, Mishell, B. B. and Shiigi, S. M., Eds., W. H. Freeman, San Francisco, 1980, 3.
42. Klempnauer, K. H. and Sippel, A. E., Subnuclear localization of proteins encoded by the oncogene v-*myb* and its cellular homolog c-*myb*, *Mol. Cell. Biol.*, 6, 62, 1986.
43. Durnam, D. M. and Palmiter, R. D., A practical approach for quantitating specific mRNAs by solution hybridization, *Anal. Biochem.*, 131, 385, 1983.
44. Chomczynski, P. and Sacchi, N., Single-step method of RNA isolation by acid guanidinium thiocyanate-phenol-chloroform extraction, *Anal. Biochem.*, 162, 156, 1987.
45. Sambrook, J., Fritsch, E. F., and Maniatis, T., *Molecular Cloning — A Laboratory Manual*, second edition, Cold Spring Harbor Laboratory Press, Cold Spring Harbor, NY, 1989, chap. 7.
46. Siegel, S., *Nonparametric Statistics for the Behavioral Sciences*, McGraw-Hill, New York, 1956.
47. Young, I. T., Proof without prejudice: Use of the Kolmogorov-Smirnov test for the analysis of histograms from flow systems and other sources, *J. Histochem. Cytochem.*, 25, 935, 1977.
48. Chen, T.-L., Miller, P. S., Ts'o, P. O. P., and Colvin, O. M., Disposition and metabolism of oligodeoxynucleoside methylphosphonates following a single IV injection in mice, *Drug Metab. Disp.*, 18, 815, 1990.
49. Sarin, P. S., Agrawal, S., Civeira, M. P., Goodchild, J., Ikeuchi, T., and Zamecnik, P. C., Inhibition of acquired immunodeficiency syndrome virus by oligodeoxynucleoside methylphosphonates, *Proc. Natl. Acad. Sci. U.S.A.*, 85, 7448, 1988.
50. Sarmiento, A. M., Perez, J. R., Becker, J. M., and Narayanan, R., *In vivo* toxicological effects of *rel* A antisense phosphorothioates in CD-1 mice, *Antisense Res. Dev.*, 4, 99, 1994.
51. Branda, R. F., Moore, A. L., Mathews, L., McCormack, J. J., and Zon, G., Immune cell stimulation by antisense oligodeoxynucleotide phosphorothioates complementary to the *rev* gene of HIV-1, *Biochem. Pharmacol.*, 45, 2037, 1993.
52. Miller, P. S. Non-ionic antisense oligonucleotides, *Oligodeoxynucleotides: Antisense Inhibitors of Gene Expression*, Cohen, J. S., Ed., CRC Press, Boca Raton, FL, 1989, 79.
53. Akhtar, S., Basu, S., Wickstrom, E., and Juliano, R. L., Interactions of antisense DNA oligonucleotide analogues with phospholipid membranes (liposomes), *Nucleic Acids Res.*, 19, 5551, 1991.

54. Polakowska, R. R. and Haake, A. R., Apoptosis: The skin from a new perspective, *Cell Death Differentiation*, 1, 19, 1994.
55. Noonberg, S. B., Garovoy, M. R., and Hunt, C. A., Characteristics of oligonucleotide uptake in human keratinocyte cultures, *J. Invest. Dermatol.*, 101, 727, 1993.
56. Bayever, E., Haines, K. M., Copple, B. L., Joshi, S. S., and Iversen, P. L., Interactions between antisense oligonucleotides to p53 mRNA and reactive oxygen in acute myelogenous leukemia, *Proc. Am. Assoc. Cancer Res.*, 36, 411, 1995.
57. Stec, W. J., Grajkowski, A., Koziolkiewicz, M., and Uznanski, B., Novel route to oligo(deoxynucleoside phosphorothioates). Stereocontrolled synthesis of P-chiral oligo(deoxynucleoside phosphorothioates), *Nucleic Acids Res.*, 19, 5883, 1991.
58. Vyazovkina, E. V., Savchenko, E. V., Lokhov, S. G., Engels, J. W., Wickstrom, E., and Lebedev, A. V., Synthesis of specific diastereomers of a DNA methylphosphonate heptamer, d(C*p*C*p*A*p*A*p*A*p*C*p*A), and stability of base pairing with the normal DNA octamer d(TpGpTpTpTpGpGpC), *Nucleic Acids Res.*, 22, 2404, 1994.
59. Hughes, J. A., Avrutskaya, A. V., Brouwer, K., Wickstrom, E., and Juliano, R. L., Radiolabeling of methylphosphonate and phosphorothioate oligonucleotides and evaluation of their transport in everted rat jejunum sacs, *Pharm. Res.*, 12, 817, 1995.
60. Yaswen, P., Stampfer, M. R., Ghosh, K., and Cohen, J. S., Effects of sequence of thioated oligonucleotides on cultured human mammary epithelial cells, *Antisense Res. Dev.*, 3, 67, 1993.
61. Burgess, T. L., Fisher, E. F., Ross, S. L. et al., The antiproliferative activity of c-*myb* and c-*myc* antisense oligonucleotides in smooth muscle cells is caused by a nonantisense mechanism, *Proc. Natl. Acad. Sci. U.S.A.*, 92, 4051, 1993.
62. Ho, P. T. C., Ishiguro, K., Wickstrom, E., and Sartorelli, A. C., Non-sequence-specific inhibition of transferrin receptor expression in HL-60 leukemia cells by phosphorothioate antisense oligodeoxynucleotides, *Antisense Res. Dev.*, 1, 329, 1991.
63. Krieg, A. M., Yi, A.-Y., Matson, S., Waldschmidt, T. J., Bishop, G. A., Teasdale, R., Koretzky, G. A., and Klinman, D. M., CpG motifs in bacterial DNA trigger direct B-cell activation, *Nature*, 374, 546, 1995.
64. Gray, G. D. and Wickstrom, E., Rapid measurement of modified oligonucleotide levels in plasma samples with a fluorophore specific for single-stranded DNA, *Antisense Nucl. Acid Drug Devel.*, 7, in press, 1997.
65. Gaidano, G., Parsa, N. Z., Tassi, V., Della-Latta, P., Chaganti, R. S., Knowles, D. M., and Dalla-Favera, R., *In vitro* establishment of AIDS-related lymphoma cell lines: Phenotypic characterization, oncogene and tumor suppressor gene lesions, and heterogeneity in Epstein-Barr virus infection, *Leukemia*, 7, 1621, 1993.
66. Prevot, S., Raphael, M., Fournier, J. G., and Diebold, J., Detection by *in situ* hybridization of HIV and c-*myc* RNA in tumour cells of AIDS-related B-cell lymphomas, *Histopathology*, 22, 151, 1993.
67. Iversen, P. L., Crouse, D., Zon, G., and Perry, G., Binding of antisense phosphorothioate oligonucleotides to murine lymphocytes is lineage specific and inducible, *Antisense Res. Dev.*, 2, 223, 1992.

Chapter 9

Regulating Genes with Antisense RNA

Jürgen Oberstrass and Wolfgang Nellen

CONTENTS

I. INTRODUCTION

"Antisense techniques" cover a whole range of different methods all aimed at the silencing of genes by introducing into the cell or organism an RNA or a single-stranded DNA (ssDNA) oligonucleotide, which is complementary to a target mRNA of choice. However, the techniques, the mechanisms, and the efficiency of reducing or abolishing gene expression differ widely. One of the most common methods is

0-8493-8552-0/97/$0.00+$.50

the introduction of DNA oligonucleotides modified in various ways. Applications and potential problems with this technique are covered in other chapters of this book.

The other general possibility is the introduction of antisense RNA into cells or organisms. Antisense RNA can be introduced by microinjection, as *in vitro* transcribed RNA, or as a chemically modified oligoribonucleotide. In most cases, an antisense gene construct is either stably or transiently expressed in the cell or organism. The most prominent advantage of this approach is the possibility of modulating gene silencing. In contrast to gene knock outs by homologous recombination, antisense expression can be targeted to specific cell types or specific stages of development. In addition, the level of gene repression may be controlled by using inducible promoters or promoters of different strength to drive antisense expression. Gene expression can thus be reduced instead of completely abolished, and one may be able to detect mutant phenotypes where a gene knock out would be lethal. Lastly, antisense RNA can produce significant effects in diploid or polyploid organisms and can simultaneously downregulate members of a closely related gene family.

The so far unexplained observation of "co-suppression"[1] shows that gene silencing can also be achieved by overexpression of a sense RNA. It remains an open question if this is related to antisense RNA-mediated regulation. A recently discussed model proposed that aberrant and/or excess sense transcripts may be targets for RNA-dependent RNA polymerase (RDRP) and generate antisense transcripts.[2] Co-suppression would thus move back to the realm of true antisense mechanisms. There are, however, clearly other additional mechanisms that can account for co-suppression.[3] Even though co-suppression is an effective way to abolish gene expression in plants and other organisms (for example, see Reference 4), it will not be discussed in this context.

This chapter will mainly focus on antisense RNA transcribed within a cell or a whole organism. The fact that antisense gene silencing occurs in natural as well as in artificial systems implies that similar or identical mechanisms are used. Studying the molecular mechanisms of antisense regulation in natural systems should provide knowledge to construct artificial antisense systems with high efficiency of inhibition.

We will first discuss methods and crucial experimental considerations for antisense experiments and describe specific applications to silence gene expression by antisense RNA. We will then summarize natural antisense systems and examine the mechanisms involved in the regulation.

Derived from the data of artificial and natural antisense-mediated gene silencing, we will propose models which are consistent with the observations and may provide hints for the application of antisense RNA. As investigations on antisense mechanisms are only just beginning, no current model or system can guarantee a successful antisense experiment.

II. ANTISENSE EXPERIMENTS

A. Methods and Experimental Considerations

Various methods are being used to obtain antisense RNA effects:

1. Chemically synthesized antisense RNA or ribozymes with modified bases can be introduced into cultured cells or injected into organisms.
2. *In vitro* synthesized antisense RNA or ribozymes can be applied in *in vitro* systems.

3. *In vitro* synthesized antisense RNA or ribozymes can be microinjected into cells and organisms.
4. Antisense gene constructs can be stably or transiently transfected into cells, and organisms and may direct inducible or tissue-specific transcription of antisense RNA.

With all methods, two crucial considerations have to be taken into account: the size of the antisense RNA and the site of interaction within the target RNA. Both have been addressed by different groups, but no consistent rules have emerged as the available data do not necessarily fit into a general scheme. There are reports that the 3′ and 5′ end, intron-exon junctions and different regions within the translated ORF of an RNA are the best targets for antisense RNA. Similarly, long antisense RNAs may work better than shorter ones and vice versa. It is therefore likely that the local structure of sense and antisense molecules is more important than the site and, above a lower limit, the size of the target. Special precautions on the extent of the hybridizing region are required when ribozymes are applied. This will be discussed later in this section.

Several quite different attempts have been made to choose sites within the target that may provide optimal features for binding to the antisense molecule. The formation of a duplex between sense and antisense strand first requires the resolution of intramolecular structures followed by the formation of an energetically favorable intermolecular structure. A search for sequence regions which are not involved in intramolecular secondary structures may thus help to define efficient target sites. The available computer programs are, however, not very reliable in predicting secondary structures in long molecules and even less when including long range interactions.

Experimental efforts to predict optimal target sites have been aimed at scanning the target with oligonucleotides. A very effective and systematic approach is the synthesis of overlapping oligonucleotides in ordered arrays on a solid support followed by hybridization with the target RNA.[5] "Open" sequences which are readily available for duplex formation will give a stronger hybridization signal with the respective oligonucleotides in the array than sequences which take part in intramolecular base pairing. However, it is not clear whether these data (using DNA oligonucleotides) really reflect the *in vivo* situation where complementary RNAs of potentially different secondary structure and biochemical properties have to anneal.

The method of "kinetic footprinting" was established by Sczakiel and coworkers[6] who investigated the association kinetics of successively 3′ deleted RNA strands to a full length target. By limited alkaline hydrolysis, they generated a pool of 5′ labeled fragments, hybridized these to the unlabeled long chain target, and took samples at different time points during the hybridization process. Single- and double-stranded RNA (dsRNA) were separated on native gels and then run on denaturing polyacrylamide gels. Fast hybridizing molecules first disappeared in the single-strand fraction and appeared in the double-strand fraction, while slowly hybridizing fragments took a longer time to be detected in the hybridized fraction. Regions within an RNA molecule, which were rapidly accessible for hybridization and therefore good targets for antisense RNAs, could thus be determined.[6]

In 1985, Izant and Weintraub[7] showed that an antisense construct directed against 52 nt of the 5′ region of the HSV-TK (thymidine kinase) gene inhibited expression almost as well as a construct covering most of the gene. Furthermore, the 52 nt 5′ construct could, in contrast to the larger antisense transcript, also inhibit the heterologous chicken TK. It appears that shorter transcripts covering highly conserved sequences may be more effective (especially in heterologous systems) than longer ones covering regions with only partial homology. Similar observations have been made by Lichtenstein and co-workers[8] in their attempts to silence replication of related gemini viruses by antisense RNAs.

Target size was examined using HIV-1, as an example, where it was shown that antisense RNA could be shortened from several hundred to 69 nt with even enhanced inhibitory effects.[9] The authors also demonstrated that, similar to prokaryotic systems, inhibition correlated with the association rate of sense and antisense molecules and thus appears to be the rate-limiting step of the reaction.

Not only the target size and target site, but also the developmental or physiological situation of the cell or organism could be important for antisense efficiency.[10] In maturing mouse oocytes, antisense RNAs directed against the 5′ part, the middle portion, or the 3′ part of the tissue plasminogen activator (t-PA) mRNA, all caused reduction in the protein level and generated stable 5′ and 3′ cleavage products. Targeting the 3′ region showed the strongest inhibitory effect. In primary oocytes, only the 3′ region was susceptible to antisense RNA, the effect being an inhibition of translation and polyadenylation and destabilization of t-PA mRNA. This stage-specific antisense activity is reminiscent of the early work by Bass and Weintraub who described successful sense-antisense interaction in *Xenopus* oocytes, but the failure of antisense-mediated gene silencing in early embryos.[11] It may also be similar to the developmentally controlled antisense effects in *Dictyostelium* (see Section III).

In vitro, mRNA splicing can be inhibited by targeting antisense RNA to, or close to, intron-exon boundaries.[12-14] This offers the potential for interfering with nuclear export or to even control splice site choice in alternatively spliced mRNAs. There are, in fact, indications that endogenous antisense transcripts may, in some cases, control splice site choice *in vivo* (see Section III).

The effective localization of antisense transcripts within the cell was examined by using a *cis*-acting ribozyme cleaving close to the 3′ end of the primary transcript.[15,16] The targeted message was no longer polyadenylated and was retained in the nucleus. Compared to conventional antisense RNAs, a significant increase of inhibition was found. These data suggest that a major effect of antisense RNAs can occur in the nucleus. In other cases, there is, however, good evidence that sense-antisense interactions take place preferentially in the cytoplasm.[17]

Usually, antisense RNA has to be expressed in excess over the target. Maximal silencing can be achieved by expression of antisense genes from a strong promoter and by integration of multiple copies of the construct into the genome. Similarly, in antisense microinjection experiments using *in vitro* synthesized RNA, a 50- to 1000-fold excess of antisense RNA has to be applied in order to detect effects.[18]

Modulation of the phenotype caused by antisense RNA injection or expression can be obtained not only by the quantity of antisense molecules generated using promoters of different strength, but also by "masking" the antisense RNA. When located within an unrelated transcript, antisense sequences display reduced efficiency compared to antisense-only transcripts.[19] This may be due to additional secondary structure formation, recruitment of the hybrid transcript to ribosomes, or other interference with sense-antisense hybrid formation. Ribozymes have attracted particular attention for various reasons like the unique property to carry information as well as biochemical activities. In this context, ribozymes are of interest because they can be easily adapted to the experimental requirements and could improve gene silencing by combining antisense effects with the catalytic activity to cleave the target RNA.

Four main groups of ribozymes are in the focus of scientific interest: the *Tetrahymena* group II intron type, the hammerhead ribozyme, the hairpin ribozyme,[20] and the hepatitis delta virus ribozyme.[21] Hairpin and hammerhead ribozymes (Figure 1)

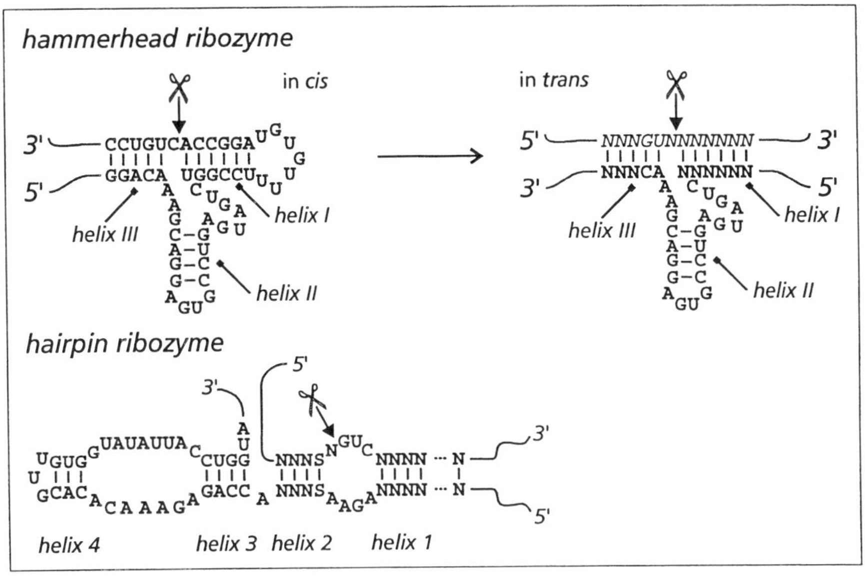

FIGURE 1
Ribozyme structures. On the top left, the structure of the wild-type, *cis*-acting hammerhead ribozyme is shown. The three helices and the cleavage site are indicated. On the right, a derived *trans*-acting hammerhead ribozyme is depicted. The top strand represents the target RNA where only the G and U residues are crucial and the bottom strand represents the ribozyme. The sequences in helix I and helix III are chosen to hybridize with the target. At the bottom the hairpin ribozyme is shown. The top right part of the structure represents the target where only the GUC trinucleotide is crucial. The ribozyme consists of the left and the lower right part of the structure. Sequences in helices 1 and 2 are available for hybrid formation between target and ribozyme.

are small molecules with a well-understood mechanism of action and thus offer the most advantages. Ribozymes usually cleave RNA in *cis*[22] and they are used as *trans*-acting enzymes by separating the catalytic domain from the substrate domain and attaching "recognition" (i.e., antisense) arms to the catalytic center in order to target the molecule to an mRNA of interest. In comparison to the conventional antisense RNAs, ribozymes provide the potential of turnover, with a single molecule being able to degrade multiple target RNAs (Figure 2).

Figure 1 also illustrates how a *trans*-acting ribozyme derives from a natural occurring self-cleaving RNA and shows the alignment of ribozyme and target sequence. The ribozyme hybridizes in two helices, III and I, to the target RNA with helix II being an intramolecular hybrid within the ribozyme. In the 3′ part of helix III, the conserved dinucleotide sequence GU is essential for cleavage after the next 3′ nucleotide. For optimal catalytic activity, the ribozyme has to find and specifically hybridize to the target. The specificity and stability of the resulting hybrid depend on the lengths of helices I and III. However, stable hybrids exhibit low catalytic activity because of slow dissociation from the cleaved substrate.[23] This has been demonstrated *in vivo* as well as *in vitro,* where ribozymes specifically cleave a target mRNA,[24] but the expected increase in efficiency due to ribozyme turnover was less pronounced than anticipated.

Improved dissociation and turnover are observed[25] in asymmetric ribozymes with very short (3nts) left and longer right recognition arms. Homann and co-workers[26] compared antisense and ribozyme approaches for the inhibition of HIV replication. In these experiments, the antisense-ribozyme displayed the strongest inhibition relative to either ribozyme alone or antisense alone.

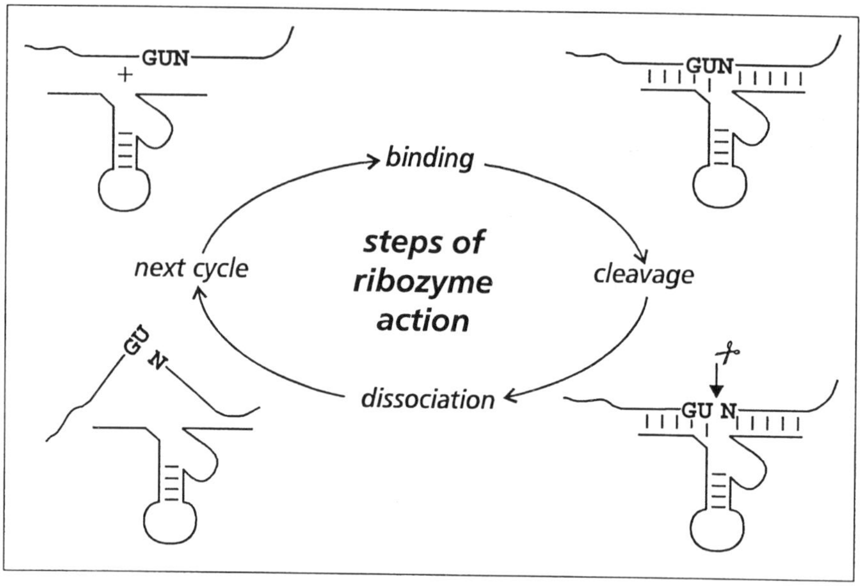

FIGURE 2
Cycle of RNA cleavage by a hammerhead ribozyme. Binding of the substrate (i.e., hybridization of ribozyme and target RNA) results in the catalytically active structure. After cleavage, the two target strands dissociate and the ribozyme strand can go into the next cleavage cycle.

Other efforts to overcome the dissociation problem have been made by the addition of proteins, like hnRNP A1 or the nucleocapsid protein of HIV (NCp7).[27] These proteins increase target binding and improve the dissociation of the ribozyme from the cleaved RNA, depending on the length of the target RNA and the length of the ribozyme. To increase local concentrations, Sullenger and Cech[28] directed a ribozyme to a *lacZ* reporter integrated into a retroviral genome. Localizing the ribozyme by means of a HIV packaging signal enhanced the efficiency of cleavage compared to the conventional ribozyme.

An interesting approach was used by Lisziewicz and co-workers.[29] They applied a combination of a ribozyme directed against the HIV I *gag* region and an RNA decoy consisting of 50 TAR elements in order to titrate out the viral TAT protein. While the decoy alone achieved a 90% inhibition of viral replication, the combination with a ribozyme resulted in >99% inhibition.

In vitro synthesized ribozymes can be applied similarly to antisense oligodeoxynucleotides, thus circumventing the need for stable or transient transformation of the target cells. In contrast to DNA oligonucleotides, they may cause less problems with non-antisense side effects. The dilemma of RNA instability in the cell can be solved by introducing modified deoxyribonucleotides into the antisense arms leaving only the catalytic center in the ribonucleotide conformation.[30,31] In combination with the shortening of the enzymatic core, especially helix II, this has resulted in a ribozyme with improved stability and membrane permeability.

Even though ribozymes do not yet reach their theoretic potential, the combination of ribozymes and other inhibiting strategies can improve gene silencing significantly.

The delivery of antisense gene constructs or antisense RNAs into patients for therapeutic purposes is a demanding problem. One approach is the stable integration of antisense genes into the germline genome.[32] Though effective and important for the understanding of gene silencing mechanisms *in vivo*, this is obviously not applicable to theurapeutic strategies in humans. Adenoviral or retroviral vectors provide ways to introduce antisense gene constructs (mostly transiently) into somatic cells. An advantage of virus-mediated delivery is the production of many antisense molecules by a single virus particle.[33] Delivery by antibody-targeted liposomes provided a more defined localization of *in vitro* transcribed antisense RNA and was successfully used to inhibit expression of the HIV-1 *env* gene.[34] The effective concentration of antisense RNA is, however, limited by the applicable dose and the rather short half-life of the molecules inside a cell.

B. Applications

The methods described above have been used in numerous and diverse applications of antisense RNA:

1. To silence genes which cause diseases or malignant transformation
2. To silence genes in order to abolish undesired traits (e.g., polygalacturonidase in tomatoes)
3. To analyze biochemical mechanisms (e.g., splicing) *in vitro*
4. To obtain insights into the function of unknown gene products (similar to gene knockouts by homologous recombination)
5. To identify new functional genes by transformation with antisense libraries
6. To analyze the mechanisms of antisense-mediated gene silencing

The current areas in antisense applications using RNA are summarized in Table 1. The following selected examples will provide a condensed overview and may also stimulate ideas on new fields of applications.

TABLE 1

Applications of Antisense RNA

Field of research	Problem	Procedure
Tumor biology	Oncogenic potential	Transformation of neoplastic cells
Tumor biology	Analysis of tumor suppressor genes	Transformation of wild type cells
Tumor biology	Relevance of tumor-related genes	Inhibition of tumor-related genes in neoplastic cells
Human therapy	Silencing of disease-causing (mutated) genes	Delivery of antisense gene constructs with viral vectors or liposomes
Developmental genetics	Gene function at defined developmental stages	Use of stage-specific, inducible antisense RNA
Plant biotechnology	Improvement of crop plants	Inhibition of undesired phenotypic properties
Physiology	Physiological role of gene products	Gene inhibition, preferentially inducible
Developmental biology, tumor biology	Identification and isolation of genes causing specific phenotypes	Tagged mutagenesis with antisense expression libraries
Developmental biology, tumor biology	Identification and isolation of genes causing specific phenotypes	Cloning strategy, trapping promoters inserted in antisense orientation into genes

A major field of application is the use of antisense RNA to inactivate mutated or viral genes which cause diseases or malignant transformation of cells. Antisense strategies may determine whether a candidate gene causes a phenotypic alteration or whether a cell transformation is due to a certain part of a viral gene. Investigations on the transforming potential of oncogenes were first performed by silencing the c-*fos* proto-oncogene with an inducible antisense RNA. This demonstrated the importance of c-*fos* for continuous proliferation of fibroblast cells.[35] Since then, there have been numerous investigations on the role of proto-oncogenes (for examples, see References 36-38) and tumor suppressor genes such as p53,[39,40] DCC,[41] and p21[42,43] using antisense RNA.

A therapeutically interesting field includes oncogenes generated by chromosomal translocations, like bcr-abl in chronic myeloid leukemia (CML) or EWS-Fli-1 from Ewing's sarcoma or Askin's tumors. The synthesis of the resulting fusion proteins in the organism is restricted to tumor cells and offers an ideal target for antisense RNA. In the case of Ewing's sarcoma cells, it could be shown that antisense RNA to the transcript of the EWS-Fli-1 fusion protein leads to a loss of tumorigenicity in nude mice.[44] For fusion genes, specificity plays a special role, because the antisense construct has to recognize the fusion mRNA, but not the individual unfused transcripts, generated by the wild-type genes and located on the homologous nontranslocation chromosomes.

The identification of tumor suppressor genes by antisense RNA is based on a different approach, whereas antisense-mediated silencing of an oncogene leads to loss of the transformed phenotype, inactivation of a tumor suppressor gene in a wild-type cell results in oncogenic transformation.

The antisense RNA-mediated decrease in p53 protein in tumor cells and the concomitant reduction in tumor formation led to the incorrect classification of p53 as an oncogene, since it was unknown at that time that mutated p53 is often overexpressed in tumors.[39] In addition to oncogenes and tumor suppressor genes, many tumor-related mRNAs are strongly expressed in transformed cells, though they are not directly affected by mutational events during tumor development. Antisense RNA-mediated inhibition provides an elegant way to investigate the function and potential participation of these genes in tumorigenesis. For example, in glioblastomas, which are genetically very complex tumors, insulin-like growth factor I (IGF-I) accumulates at high levels. Expression of antisense IGF-I led to decreased levels of the factor and reduced tumorigenicity of glioblastoma cells in an *in vivo* assay.[45]

Higgins et al.[46] investigated the function of the transcription factor NF-κB in tumorigenesis. They were the first to demonstrate in cell culture that antisense RNA directed against the NF-κB p65 subunit mRNA restored contact inhibition of transformed cells. The authors then injected tumor cells, which had previously been transfected with a dexamethasone-inducible NF-κB p65 antisense construct into nude mice. After the development of the tumor, p65 antisense expression was induced and resulted in regression of the tumor.

Antisense RNA approaches have significantly contributed to the elucidation of physiological as well as developmental functions of genes. The deletion or disruption of genes by homologous recombination is usually preferred, where applicable, to investigate the function of a gene product *in vivo*. Nevertheless, antisense RNA offers complementary approaches to knock-outs and a whole range of other benefits in certain applications. Antisense RNA is suitable for gene silencing in diploid or polyploid tissues or organisms and effects can be detected in the first, heterozygous generation. Multiple genes of a closely related family[47] or related viruses may be inactivated by a single antisense expression construct. In addition, tissue- or development-specific gene silencing is still more convenient using antisense RNA than conditional knock-outs, which always require time-consuming genetic crosses.

An example is the preferential silencing of the type II glucocorticoid-receptor in the hypothalamus and the cerebral cortex of mice by driving antisense RNA transcription from the neurofilament L promoter.[48] Similarly, Moxham and coworkers[49,50] used the PEPCK promoter to express antisense RNA directed against the G-protein subunit $G_{i\alpha2}$ in transgenic mice. $G_{i\alpha2}$ is an inhibitory G protein for adenylyl cyclase. The PEPCK promoter was specifically induced at birth and was mainly active in adipose tissue and liver. Due to the inhibition of G-protein expression, the antisense mice had higher cAMP levels in the targeted tissues, produced less fat, and had a reduced liver size.

Other targets are components of the cytoskeleton, investigated in different systems such as *Dictyostelium*,[4] *Caenorhabditis elegans*,[51] and human astrocytes.[52] In *Dictyostelium*, antisense-mediated inactivation of myosin II led to the unexpected finding that this protein was not required for cell motility but mainly for cytokinesis. In addition, it was possible to grow these cells under conditions where the antisense promoter was turned off, thus providing an internal control with a wild-type phenotype.

In human astrocytes, the role of the intermediate filament protein GFAP for the interaction of astrocytes with neurons was determined, and it could be shown that GFAP is required for stable astrocytic processes in response to neurons.[52]

An interesting but laborious application is the injection of *in vitro* generated antisense RNAs into cells or organisms in order to elucidate developmental consequences of gene silencing. In *Drosophila*, this technique was used to produce phenocopies of developmental mutants in the early blastoderm stage and to identify isolated genes in a functional assay. However, after the blastoderm stage no antisense effects could be observed upon antisense microinjection.[18]

In plants, antisense RNA expression is the major way to interfere with the expression of endogenous genes. Gene knock-out by homologous recombination is not applicable as a routine method in plants, and antisense oligonucleotides are difficult to introduce through the rigid cell wall. Possibly due to these limitations, antisense technology is particularly advanced in plant systems. The focus of plant antisense research is on the improvement of crop plants, the generation of virus resistance,[53-55] and other commercially useful applications. Nevertheless, valuable information of general importance can be derived from these experiments. In most cases, the strong, tissue-nonspecific cauliflower mosaic virus (CMV) promoter is used to drive expression of the antisense gene construct, which is integrated into the genome as one or a few copies. Similar to other systems, no clear preference can be given to the expression of antisense 5′, 3′, or central parts of a gene. Gene silencing is usually, but not always, correlated with a loss of the corresponding mRNA, indicating antisense-mediated mRNA degradation in most cases.

Examples of successful applications are the silencing of the polygalacturonase gene in tomato plants which leads to a delay in fruit decay (for review see Reference 56), the inhibition of granule-bound starch synthase (GBSS) in potato-generating tubers which produce predominantly amylopektin as a starch component,[57] and resistance against the tobacco golden mosaic virus (TGMV) by a viral antisense gene transcript which also provides resistance against a related gemini virus.[55]

As a technique to elucidate gene function and to identify genes involved in specific pathways, two methods have recently been developed. Gomer and colleagues[58] used shot gun transformation with antisense expression libraries to identify genes required for development in *Dictyostelium*. As in other antisense experiments, there is the advantage that families of sufficiently related genes may be silenced by a single, highly expressed antisense construct.

A similar approach was used by Li and Cohen[59] who randomly inserted promoters into the genome of a cell line and screened for transformed cells. The integration could cause disruption of a gene on one chromosomal complement and, if inserted in the opposite orientation to a disrupted open reading frame, generate antisense transcripts that can interfere with the wild-type mRNA transcribed from the other complement. They could, thus, directly select a clone which had the tumor susceptible gene tsg101 disrupted in one of the chromosomes and the transcripts from the other chromosome inactivated by antisense expression.

Of all organisms examined to date, the yeast *Saccharomyces cerevisiae* appears to be a remarkable exception in that it has resisted numerous attempts of antisense experiments. To our knowledge there is not a single reported case where an endogenous gene has been successfully silenced by antisense RNA in *S. cerevisiae*. The review by Atkins[60] provides a valuable summary of many, mostly unpublished efforts.

III. NATURAL ANTISENSE SYSTEMS

If one uses the term "antisense" *in sensu latu*, several molecular mechanisms can be placed into the category of "natural antisense systems."

mRNA splicing in eukaryotes requires a complex assembly of proteins and RNAs. An essential part is U1-snRNA, which specifically binds to the 5′ splice junction by base pairing. Essentially, U1 is a small antisense RNA that mediates specific cleavage of mRNA. In addition, the spliceosome contains proteins which support or specify the annealing process. They have been termed "hybrid-promoting-proteins" and belong to a growing family of ssRNA binding proteins. We have previously proposed that proteins of this family also participate in conventional antisense mechanisms.[61]

RNA editing in *Trypanosome* mitochondria is controlled by guide RNAs, which are, in part, complementary to the unedited transcript and, after the editing process, complementary to the entire region they edited. Guide RNAs may be regarded as short antisense transcripts which also mediate specific cleavage of the target RNA for the insertion or deletion of uridine residues. The removal of the antisense RNA from the target is essential to avoid the conventional antisense effect of target hydrolysis. In fact, it has recently been found that a highly specific RNA helicase of the DEAD-box family is part of the editosome and appears to facilitate the dissociation of both RNAs.[62-64] Intramolecular base pairing may be regarded as sense and antisense transcripts in one molecule. Several bacterial RNAs, e.g., the ribosomal 30S RNA precursor, are folded to form intramolecular structures which are then targets for processing by RNase III. Interestingly, RNase III homologs have recently been detected in various eukaryotes (*Schizosaccharomyces pombe*,[65] *Arabidopsis thaliana*,[66] and *Caenothabditis elegans*[67]), but their targets, which are most likely dsRNAs, are not known.

Taken together, there are many examples from ubiquitous cellular processes which are similar to antisense mechanisms. Moreover, these processes appear to be facilitated and regulated by proteins like RNA helicases, dsRNases, and hybrid-promoting proteins. Reports on natural antisense systems, which regulate gene expression by means of an endogenous transcript complementary to an mRNA, are rare. This is mainly due to the difficulty in screening specifically for sequences transcribed in both directions and then proving that the antisense transcript really has a regulatory function. Consequently, natural antisense systems have usually been detected by accident and in most cases, a regulatory function has not been proven. The examples range from the mere description of divergent transcripts (e.g., References 68 and 69) to circumstantial evidence for antisense function,[70] with only a few cases of genuine regulatory antisense RNA.

Some examples of naturally occurring antisense RNAs and implications on the underlying mechanisms will be discussed. The existence of antisense transcripts complementary to human and murine c-*myc* has been reported in several papers[71-74] and regulatory functions have been suggested. In addition, Celano and co-workers[75] have characterized a transcript, designated ASM-1, which displays 85% identity to the antisense strand of the second intron of the human c-*myc* gene and high homology to other growth- and differentiation-related genes like N-*myc*, p53, and TK. Notably, the identity extends over stretches of 20 or more nucleotides without interruption and could, thus, be a target for many dsRNA binding proteins.

Antisense-mediated deamination, and, thus, inactivation of mRNAs, has been extensively discussed after the discovery of the dsRAD enzyme.[11] There is recent evidence that dsRAD may participate in polyoma virus gene regulation by deamination of a sense-antisense RNA hybrid.[76] Unfortunately, the observation that the endogenous bFGF sense and antisense RNA complex was deaminated by dsRAD[77] was mainly due to experimental conditions and did not truly reflect the *in vivo* situation.[78] Nevertheless, comparison of *in situ* hybridization with bFGF sense and antisense transcripts with bFGF protein levels provided circumstantial evidence that the antisense RNA may increase the turnover of the mRNA.[79]

The murine Hoxa-11[70] and Hoxd-3[80] genes are differentially transcribed in both orientations. Both antisense transcripts are processed and contain large open reading frames. In the case of Hoxa-11 antisense RNA, a regulatory role has been suggested. Similarly, Adelman et al.[68] reported divergent transcription of the murine gonadotropin-releasing hormone (GnRH) gene. The antisense RNA (SH) is also processed and gives rise to 4 different RNAs, one of which potentially encodes a polypeptide of 106 amino acids.[68] The observation that in all three cases both complementary RNAs could co-exist in certain tissues and could be translated, may indicate that coding antisense transcripts do not serve regulatory functions but are recruited to ribosomes and thus not available for interaction with their sense counterpart in the cytoplasm.

The best studied examples are the plasmid copy number systems in bacteria (see Reference 81). Small, intrinsically unstable antisense RNAs transcribed from the same genetic locus as the corresponding sense transcript anneal close to the 5′ end of the sense RNA. In most cases, hybridization occurs via highly ordered secondary structures which have been termed kissing complexes. The effect is mainly the inhibition of further secondary structures or the promotion of alternative structures further downstream from the kissing complex. These structural alterations can, for example, prevent the generation of RNA primers for plasmid replication or the translation of a protein essential for replication. At the site of sense and antisense RNA interaction, usually no further changes are observed except for secondary structure formation. In some cases RNase III cleavage has been found, but this appears to be a nonessential secondary effect. The *rom* protein binds to and stabilizes a secondary structure intermediate of the RNA I/RNA II hybrid from colEI plasmids, but again this seems not to be essential. Overall, no proteins seem to be strictly required for antisense activity in plasmid copy number control, but structural changes appear to be crucial. This is well documented by the observation that small mutations in the stem-loop structures of copA/copT (plasmid R1 copy number control), which do not impair the complementarity of sense and antisense RNA, have substantial consequences on the function of the antisense system.[82] Another surprising observation is that the copA/copT hybrid seems to remain incomplete. After the initial hybridization of the loops in the kissing complex, the intermolecular hybrid does not extend into the stems of the hybridization partners.[83] The three-dimensional structure and function of this unexpected mixture of inter- and intramolecular hybrids remains to be elucidated. The stem-loop formation of copA/copT as well as of other plasmid copy number control RNAs is essential for hybrid formation and may provide clues for the use of antisense strategies in other organisms. As an example, the copA/copT antisense system is shown in Figure 3.

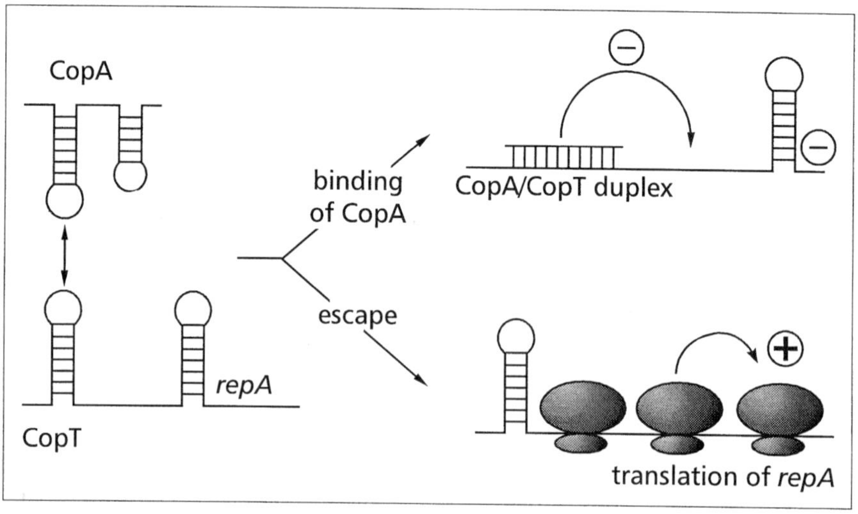

FIGURE 3
Changes in secondary structure by antisense RNA: the copA/copT system. Duplex formation between copA and copT is mediated by the stem-loop structures of the kissing complex. With high concentrations of copA, hybridization to copT takes place and the formation of a secondary structure required for translation of the repA protein is impaired. At low concentrations of copA, translation is initiated and repA is produced. (Modified from Wagner, E. G. and Simons, R. W., *Annu. Rev. Microbiol.*, 48, 713, 1994. With permission.)

In *C. elegans*, a quite different antisense system has been detected. Here, short antisense RNAs are transcribed from the *lin*-4 locus (Figure 4). These are partially complementary to the 3′ end of the *lin*-14 mRNA which is encoded by a gene at a different locus in the genome. While the mRNA is more or less constitutively transcribed, the antisense RNAs are under transcriptional control. They appear to hybridize to the 3′ untranslated region of the mRNA and block translation. Interestingly, the incomplete hybrid contains bulged G residues, which appear to be conserved not only in the seven different targets on the mRNA but also in other nematode species. Furthermore, a mutant with impaired antisense regulation has been found which disrupts one of the G bulges. It is suggested that these structures provide a binding site for a regulatory protein.[84,85] The *lin*-4/*lin*-14 system is reminiscent of the tcRNAs, the first translational control antisense RNAs described in 1975.[86] They are also short and can form bulged hybrids with the 5′ end of chicken myosin heavy chain mRNA.[87,88]

In *Dictyostelium*, the late developmental gene PSV-A (formerly EB4) is constitutively transcribed but silenced in early development by an endogenous antisense transcript generated from the same locus in the genome.[17] PSV-A protein is expressed only in prespore cells but not in prestalk cells. Preliminary evidence suggests that

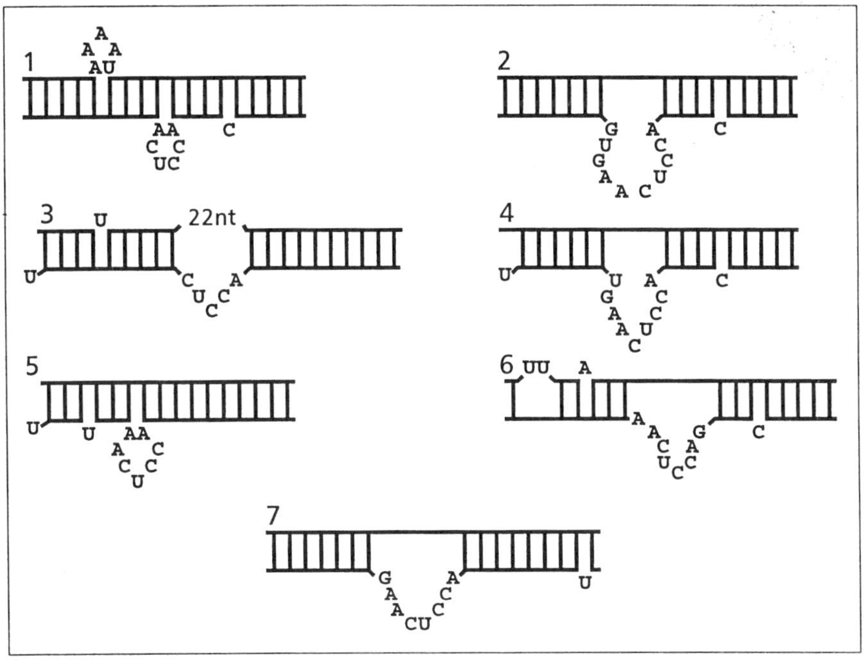

FIGURE 4
Translational control by antisense RNA: Predicted hybrids of *lin*-14/*lin*-4 RNAs. The seven conserved sequence elements within the *lin*-14 3′ UTR are shown as hybrids with the regulatory *lin*-4 transcripts. The *lin*-14 strand is shown on top and the *lin*-4 strand at the bottom of each duplex. The bulged C in elements 1, 2, 4, and 6 and the stacked GC base pairs in the right arm of all elements (not shown) suggest sites for protein binding. (Modified from Wightman, B., Ha, I., and Ruvkun, G., *Cell*, 75, 855, 1993. With permission.)

not only the developmental regulation, but the cell-type specific regulation is also mediated by the antisense transcript; prestalk but not prespore cells display activity of the antisense promoter.[89]

Pharmacological treatment of developing cells causes a partial dedifferentiation resulting in a rapid induction of antisense transcription and a rapid decay of the mostly cytoplasmic PSV-A mRNA. Antisense transcripts are intrinsically unstable and never accumulate to high levels. Run-on transcription assays have shown, however, that, under activating conditions, the antisense promoter is at least ten times stronger than the sense promoter.

Interestingly, antisense-mediated downregulation of PSV-A mRNA appears to be regulated by the cell. In late development, under certain pharmacologically modified conditions, and in some developmental mutants, the interaction between sense and antisense RNA is impaired and the mRNA is not degraded. Similar observations have been made in cells transformed with artificial antisense gene constructs. While complete downregulation of the message was seen in growing cells and in early development, inhibition was strongly reduced in later development.[90]

Further investigations on the *Dictyostelium* PSV-A gene have suggested that even though antisense RNA predominantly caused mRNA degradation, there are also effects on translation. Under conditions when sense and antisense transcripts did not engage in degradative interaction, a significant reduction in PSV-A protein was observed.[91]

In human T cells, the expression of the translation initiation factor eIF-2α is strongly induced by stimulating cells to proliferate. While there is only a minor increase in transcriptional activity, nuclear precursors and cytoplasmic eIF-2α mRNA accumulate significantly. Safer and co-workers[92] detected an antisense promoter within the first intron of the gene. Apparently, the antisense transcript destabilizes nuclear precursors but not cytoplasmic eIF-2α mRNA. This appears to be one of the few cases where antisense function can be directly localized to the nucleus.

An intriguing twist in eIF-2α regulation is the functional inactivation of the translation initiation factor by phosphorylation. Phosphorylation is specifically carried out by PKR, a protein kinase which is activated by dsRNA. Though this may only be coincidence, it suggests that eIF-2α sense-antisense hybrids could serve two functions: first, to decrease the nuclear half-life of the mRNA precursor and, second, to indirectly inactivate the eIF-2α protein pool by stimulating PKR.

Munroe and co-workers[12] showed that antisense RNA directed against splice junctions and exon sequences downstream of the splice site could efficiently inhibit RNA processing *in vitro*. They also demonstrated that antisense-mediated splice site choice is likely to be an endogenous mechanism for alternative splicing of the erbAα precursor, which is differentially processed to erbAα1 and erbAα2 mRNAs. An antisense transcript Rev-ErbAα appears to block the splicing required for erbAα2 mRNA formation. Consistent with this observation, increased expression of Rev-ErbAα correlates with the accumulation of erbAα1 mRNA.[93]

IV. MODELS FOR GENE REGULATION BY NATURAL OR ARTIFICIAL ANTISENSE GENES

The mechanisms of antisense-mediated gene silencing are diverse, and different mechanisms may be found in one organism. They may inhibit translocation of the sense RNA from the nucleus to the cytoplasm,[94] interfere with mRNA splicing,[93] lead to degradation of nuclear[92] or cytoplasmic RNA,[17] impair translation,[85,88,95] or all of the above. Why apparently similar molecules can elicit different responses in a given cell is unknown.

In *C. elegans*, translation of *lin*-14 mRNA is inhibited by short endogenous transcripts generated from a different chromosomal locus. In addition, the secondary structure of the proposed hybrid seems to be of importance, and the participation of proteins binding to these structures is suggested.[85] Similarly, inhibition of translation was observed with artificially introduced antisense constructs.[96,97]

In contrast, the endogenous *Dictyostelium* antisense system is based on a transcript from the same chromosomal locus as the mRNA. Because the antisense transcript is not processed, a potential hybrid would contain an unpaired loop (corresponding to the nonspliced antisense intron) of approximately 100 nucleotides. PSV-A antisense transcripts lead to the degradation of predominantly processed, cytoplasmic mRNA. Nevertheless, when mRNA degradation is impaired, a less pronounced inhibitory effect on translation is observed.[91]

Similarly, in the case of eIF2α, the antisense transcript is encoded at the same locus but decreases the half-life of nuclear pre-mRNA instead of cytoplasmic transcripts. Artificially introduced antisense constructs may also cause degradation of mRNA.[7,98] For the erbAα transcript, antisense RNA inhibits splicing of a specific intron, resulting in a strong bias of splice site choice.[93] Similar interference with splicing has been observed with artificially introduced antisense constructs.[12-14,99] The bacterial plasmid copy number control systems are mainly based on antisense-mediated alterations in RNA secondary structures which can lead to the inhibition of replication-primer generation or translation. The types of sense-antisense hybrids are listed in Table 2 and the mechanisms of antisense action are compiled in Table 3.

TABLE 2

Types of Sense-Antisense Hybrids

Type of hybrid	Locus of transcription	Origin of antisense	Ref.
Completely base-paired dsRNA	Antisense and sense from same locus	Endogenous	17, 92
Completely base-paired dsRNA	Antisense and sense from different loci	Artificially introduced antisense constructs	75, 94
Incomplete double strands due to stable secondary structures	Antisense and sense from same locus	Endogenous	83
Incomplete double strands with loops and/or bulges	Antisense and sense from different loci	Endogenous and artificially introduced antisense constructs	84

TABLE 3

Mechanisms of Antisense Action

Mechanism	Ref.
Interference with translation	95
Interference with nuclear export	94
Cytoplasmic mRNA degradation	17
Nuclear precursor degradation	92
Interference with functional secondary structures	108
Inhibition of RNA processing	93

In addition to this diversity, several observations create further problems. Most models postulate the formation of extended sense-antisense hybrids, but these have only been detected in a few specialized cases.[94,100] For antisense-mediated mRNA destabilization, this suggests that the dsRNA intermediate is rapidly degraded. A double-stranded, specific RNase (dsRNase) would be required for this reaction (see below).

In *Dictyostelium,* sense and antisense RNAs are sometimes found as apparently separate, reasonably stable molecules in the same cell, and no or only minor antisense effects are observed.[90] Similarly, Volloch et al.[101] show the occurrence of endogenous globin antisense RNA in mouse erythroid tissues and provide indirect evidence that it may originate from transcription of an mRNA template by RDRP (RNA dependent RNA polymerase). This implies a double-stranded intermediate, which is not degraded by dsRNase but instead generates a stable, single-stranded cytoplasmic antisense transcript. It is unclear why this antisense RNA does not participate in gene silencing. Both examples suggest that hybrid formation is a regulated and reversible process.

In several experiments, we and others have observed that antisense effects in *Dictyostelium* elicited by artificially introduced antisense constructs were not detected, even though large amounts of antisense RNA were expressed.[102] Similarly, antisense effects were sometimes lost after prolonged growth of the cell culture, even though high levels of antisense RNA were still expressed. Cells may therefore be able to activate mechanisms to evade antisense effects or to "deliberately" target sense and antisense transcripts to different compartments and thus abolish interaction.

Taken together, these available data demonstrate that antisense RNA can function at different levels and by different mechanisms which are not necessarily mutually exclusive. Furthermore, one or more cellular machineries (regulatory pathways) are involved, which control the efficiency of antisense RNA-mediated gene silencing. Figure 5 summarizes the pathways by which antisense RNAs may act in the nucleus (Figure 5A) and in the cytoplasm (Figure 5B).

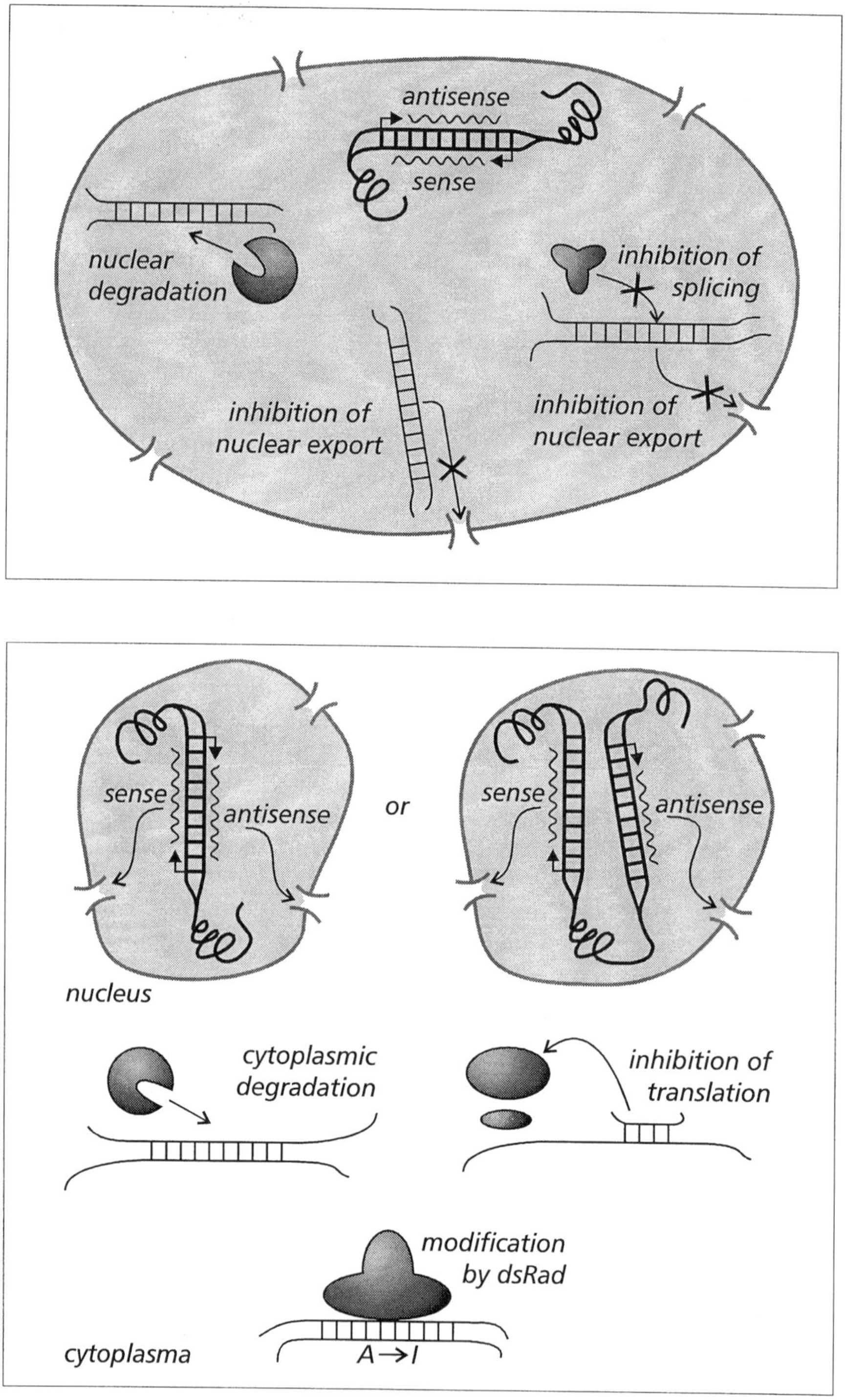

FIGURE 5
Nuclear mRNA inactivation. Antisense-mediated inactivation of mRNA may occur in the nucleus by degradation of hybrids (dsRNase), inhibition of splicing (masking assembly sites for spliceosomes), and inhibition of export to the cytoplasm. (B) Cytoplasmic mRNA inactivation. Sense and antisense RNA transcribed from the same (left) or different (right) chromosomal locations are transported to the cytoplasm if the mechanisms shown in Figure 5A do not take place. In the cytoplasm, degradation by dsRNase, the inhibition of translation or modification by dsRAD (resulting in a nonfunctional mRNA) can occur.

V. PROTEINS AND OTHER FACTORS POTENTIALLY INVOLVED IN ANTISENSE RNA-MEDIATED GENE REGULATION

Inactivation of gene expression by antisense transcripts may, at first glance, appear obvious and straightforward, but the contrary is the case. This is best documented by the many failures to use antisense strategies in yeast (for review see References 60,103).We believe that the controlled formation of hybrids and their degradation is not a trivial reaction but requires a well-designed enzymatic setup and regulatory pathways.

What are the potential components of such an antisense machinery? Hybrid formation may require proteins to dissolve intramolecular secondary structures and support the formation of intermolecular hybrids. Good candidates are single-strand RNA-binding proteins (RBP) of the RNP A1 family. Binding of RBPs can extend the duration of microcollisions of individual RNAs and thus increase the probability of productive hybridization by a factor of 1000 or more (reviewed in Reference 104). We propose that such "hybrid promoting proteins" participate in the formation of sense-antisense hybrids. RBPs are mostly localized in the nucleus, and for some (e.g., hnRNP protein A1) their participation in splice site selection has been demonstrated.[105] They are, however, not restricted to the nucleus and can shuttle back and forth to the cytoplasm.[106] In *Dictyostelium* we have seen the constitutive expression of the RBP DdRBP1 in the cytoplasm and a developmentally regulated accumulation in the nucleus.[107] If these proteins are involved in sense-antisense RNA annealing, they could do so in both cellular compartments.

In prokaryotes, hybridization of RNAs strongly depends on the secondary structure of the kissing complex. Wagner and co-workers[108] have shown that mutations in the copA/copT system which conserve complementarity but change the secondary structure, cause an impairment in the plasmid copy number control system. In eukaryotes, the different antisense effects of distinct parts of a gene may be due to secondary structures, but to our knowledge, no systematic evaluation of secondary structure requirements has been done for eukaryotic sense-antisense RNA interaction.

Another possibility to enhance and/or regulate RNA hybridization could be by RNA helicases. These enzymes mainly unwind RNA duplexes in an ATP-dependent reaction in order to separate guide RNAs from edited transcripts in *Trypanosomes*.[64] In addition, RNA helicases "trans-wind" a given hybrid if an energetically favorable structure is possible (e.g., by addition of a third, competing transcript which can form longer double helical regions).[109] Theoretically, RNA helicases may dissolve intramolecular structures in favor of intermolecular hybrids of sense and antisense RNA.

The consequence of hybrid formation is in some cases the inhibition of RNA processing. Most likely, the masking of splice sites interferes with the assembly of the spliceosome. Even if processing is not impaired or not required for a particular mRNA, a partially double-stranded molecule may not be exported to the cytoplasm. Unprocessed or retained RNAs will either be degraded or accumulated in the nucleus. Examples, where antisense activity is observed in the cytoplasm in the inhibition of translation, can be explained by masking of the ribosome entry site, particularly since in most reports on translation inhibition, antisense transcripts cover the 5′ part of the message. Translation inhibition by antisense RNA annealing to the 3′ end of the message could be due to functional interactions between 5′ and 3′ ends which appear to be required for translational initiation.

The most common effect of antisense RNA is the partial or complete loss of the message. Except for a few cases, intermediates of the degradation have not been found. It is therefore assumed that the duplex is specifically degraded by an enzymatic activity which recognizes dsRNA. Several dsRNases have been described in the literature,[110-114] but no molecular analysis of their function has been done. Table 4 lists the protein factors which are potentially involved in antisense mechanisms.

TABLE 4

Proteins Potentially Involved in Antisense Mechanisms

Protein	Potential function	Known function
dsRNase	Degradation of dsRNA	Processing of RNA, cuts at double-stranded sites (RNase III)
PKR	Signaling in response to the formation of dsRNA to other components of the system	eIF2α phosphorylation
dsRAD	Inactivation of mRNA in hybrids by deamination	RNA editing, deamination of sense-antisense hybrids.
Hybrid promoting proteins	Facilitation of hybrid formation	Facilitation of assembly of splicing components
from-related proteins	Facilitation of hybrid formation	Stabilization of hybrid-intermediates by rom
dsRNA binding proteins	Impairment of translation or processing	dsRNA binding in PKR, RNA localization by staufen protein in *Drosophila*
RDRP	Generate antisense RNA from sense transcripts	Probably virus replication
RNA helicases	Unwinding dsRNA hybrids, inactivating targets for RNA degradation	Unwinding editing complexes, part of spliceosome

All of the proteins proposed to participate in antisense mechanisms could be subject to differential regulation and thus explain the variations in the efficiency of antisense-mediated gene silencing. We have partially purified a predominantly cytoplasmic RNase from *Dictyostelium,* which specifically cleaves dsRNA and which may be subject to post-translational modification affecting its activity.[115] The dsRNase from tobacco anthers[114] is developmentally regulated and could potentially account for different activities of antisense approaches in different developmental stages. It is an attractive speculation that the dsRNA-dependent protein kinase (PKR, formerly DAI kinase, reviewed in Reference 116) is a modifier of these proteins; upon formation of sense-antisense hybrids, the extremely sensitive kinase could be induced and activate components of the antisense machinery (or inactivate proteins which impair antisense mechanisms).

Nevertheless, the diversity of cellular responses to antisense RNA makes it difficult to develop a general model for the mechanisms. Based on a previous proposal,[61] we present here an extended model which is in agreement with most of the available information (Figure 6). The model's value could be twofold: it can help with the rational design of antisense experiments, and it can generate testable ideas on the mechanisms and components of the antisense machinery. For example, a cellular machinery that is set to inactivate antisense mechanisms may be circumvented by a combination of antisense RNA and ribozymes or by the 2-5A system developed by the group of Silverman.[117] In both cases, mRNA cleavage is performed by an activity that is not usually involved in antisense-mediated RNA degradation. If the lack of antisense function was due to an inactive dsRNase, it could be bypassed. However, if compartmentalization, unwinding, or an inactive hybrid promoting protein was the reason for nonfunctional antisense RNA, this would not solve the problem.

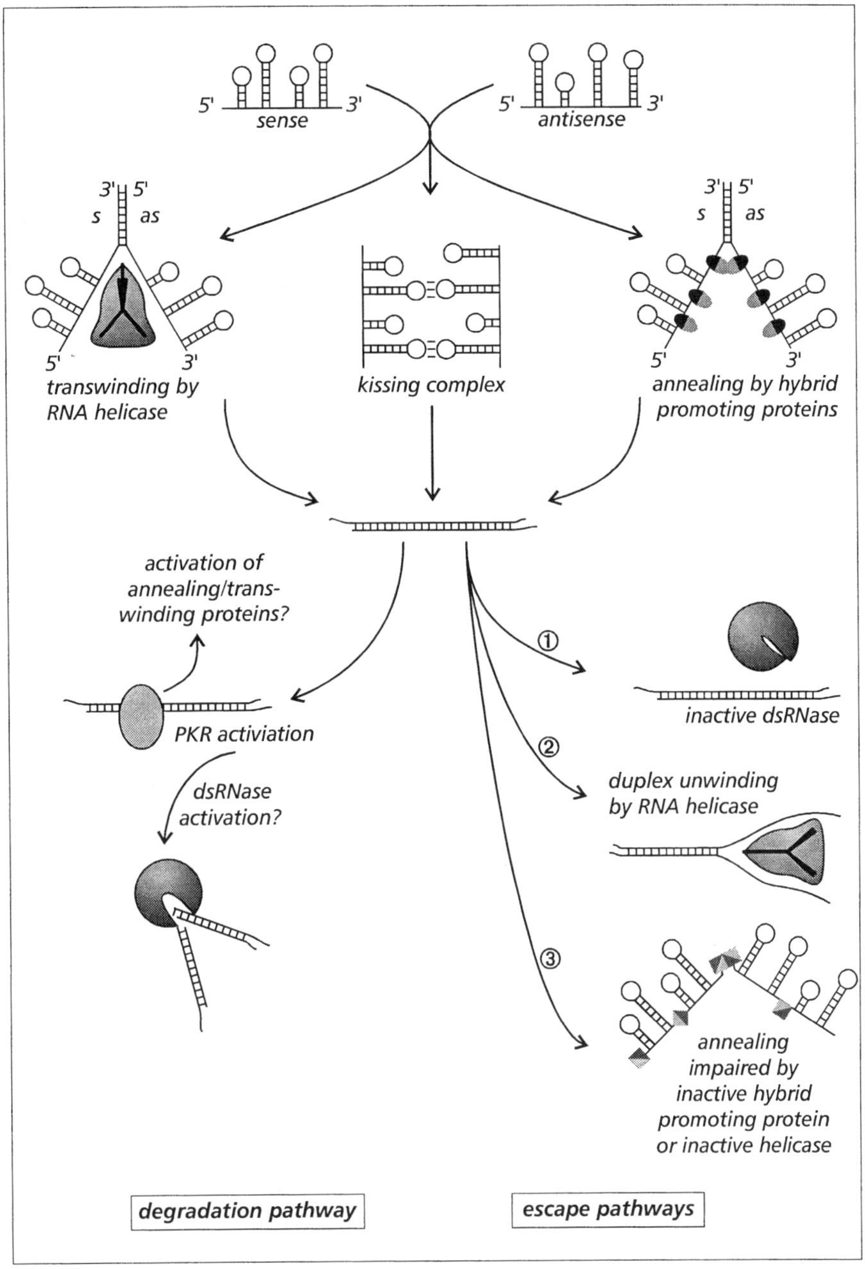

FIGURE 6
Model for modulating antisense-mediated mRNA degradation. Annealing of sense and antisense RNA may be facilitated by RNA helicases, which can unwind intramolecular secondary structures and promote intermolecular hybrid formation (top left). Similarly, hybrid promoting proteins may increase the time of microcollisions between RNA molecules and thus enhance hybrid formation (top right). Intramolecular secondary structures may initiate hybridization by formation of kissing complexes (top middle). The resulting dsRNA can activate PKR, which may, in turn, modulate the activity of dsRNase (left) or hybrid facilitating proteins (top) in the degradation pathway. On the right, different possibilities are depicted which may allow an mRNA to escape from degradation: (1) dsRNase may be inactive; (2) RNA helicases may unwind a sense-antisense hybrid; and (3) inactivation of the transwinding activity or of hybrid promoting proteins may impair hybrid formation. Pathways proposed in this model are consistent with experimental data but not proven facts.

Overexpression of dsRNase or hybrid promoting proteins may improve antisense mechanisms and potentially make organisms like *S. cerevisiae* amenable for antisense approaches.

The participation of PKR, helicases, and hybrid promoting proteins can be tested in cell lines depleted of these enzymes, and the involvement of secondary structures can be easily examined by using appropriate sequences in combination with a tester gene. There are, with certainty, other components involved; for example, the suggested proteins binding to the *lin*-4/*lin*-14 hybrids. Understanding the properties and characteristics of the components of antisense machineries may open up new routes in antisense applications.

VI. PERSPECTIVES AND CONCLUSIONS

One of the most important issues for regulating genes in transgenic organisms by antisense approaches is probably to learn more about the mechanisms by which antisense-mediated gene silencing may occur. To date, the compilation of data suggests that various pathways may be used in different tissues and under different conditions. Thus, the approaches should be adapted to the respective situation. This requires a careful evaluation and dissection of the different pathways in the respective cells. As a result, gene silencing by artificially introduced antisense RNA could not only become more efficient, but the approaches would be more focused than the current experiments, which are more or less carried out by trial and error. Surprisingly, investigations on antisense mechanisms are mainly focused on prokaryotic systems (reviewed in Reference 81). A first systematic attempt in this direction could be performed by the elegant method of Volloch and co-workers[101] to specifically identify endogenous antisense transcripts in eukaryotic cells. This would provide a broader basis to study cellular pathways of antisense effects. In addition, there should be more emphasis on the potential components of the antisense machinery as an initial approach to understand the mechanisms at a molecular level.

New methods using antisense techniques are being developed, not only for applied, but also for basic science. One of the most prominent examples is the combination of oligonucleotides with 2-5A which activates the 2-5A-dependent ribonuclease and acts similarly to the ribozyme-targeted mRNA cleavage.[118] New applications like antisense libraries open up exciting ways to generate mutants and identify the respective genes.[59]

Antisense techniques have branched into various subdisciplines, each having strong advantages in different areas. The current focus on antisense oligonucleotides covers just a small section of a much wider range of applications. The elucidation of mechanisms that mediate gene silencing by antisense RNA is only just beginning. In the near future, a better understanding of the molecular pathways and the identification of the participating cellular components will substantially enhance the power of this fascinating technique.

ACKNOWLEDGMENTS

We thank B. Schnell for critical reading of the manuscript and C. Bartke for preparing the figures. This work was supported by a grant of the Deutsche Forschungsgemeinschaft to W.N. and by the Zentrale Forschungsförderung Hessen to J.O.

REFERENCES

1. Metzlaff, M., O'Dell, M., and Flavell, R. B., Suppression of chalcone synthase A activities in Petunia by the addition of a transgene encoding chalcone synthase A, in *Mechanisms and Applications of Gene Silencing*, Grierson, D., Lycette, G. W., and Tucker, G. A., Eds., Nottingham University Press, Nottingham, 1996, chap. 3.
2. Flavell, R. B., Inactivation of gene expression in plants as a consequence of specific sequence duplication, *Proc. Natl. Acad. Sci. U.S.A.*, 91, 3490, 1994.
3. Matzke, A. J. M. and Matzke, M. A., Trans-inactivation of homologous sequences in *Nicotiana tabacum, Gene Silencing in Higher Plants and Related Phenomena in Other Eukaryotes*, Peter Meyer, Ed., Springer-Verlag, Heidelberg, 1995, chap. 1.
4. Scherczinger, C. A. and Knecht, D. A., Co-suppression of *Dictyostelium discoideum* myosin II heavy-chain gene expression by a sense orientation transcript, *Antisense Res. Dev.*, 3, 207, 1993.
5. Southern, E. M., Maskos, U., and Elder, K., Analysing and comparing nucleic acid sequences by hybridization to arrays of oligonucleotides: evaluation using experimental models, *Genomics*, 13, 1008, 1992.
6. Rittner, K., Burmester, C., and Sczakiel, G., *In vitro* selection of fast hybridizing antisense RNAs directed against the human immunodeficiency virus type 1, *Nucleic Acids Res.*, 21, 1381, 1993.
7. Izant, J. G. and Weintraub, H., Constitutive and conditional suppression of exogenous and endogenous genes by anti-sense RNA, *Science*, 229, 345, 1985.
8. Bejarano, E. R. and Lichtenstein, C. P., Expression of TGMV antisense RNA in transgenic tobacco inhibits replication of BCTV but not ACMV geminiviruses, *Plant Mol. Biol.*, 24, 241, 1994.
9. Homann, M., Rittner, K., and Sczakiel, G., Complementary large loops determine the rate of RNA duplex formation *in vitro* in the case of an effective antisense RNA directed against the human immunodeficiency virus type 1, *J. Mol. Biol.*, 233, 7, 1993.
10. Strickland, S., Huarte, J., Belin, D., Vassalli, A., Rickles, R. J., and Vassalli, J.-D., Antisense RNA directed against the 3′ noncoding region prevents dormant mRNA activation in mouse oocytes, *Science*, 241, 680, 1988.
11. Bass, B. L. and Weintraub, H., A developmentally regulated activity that unwinds RNA duplexes, *Cell*, 48, 607, 1987.
12. Munroe, S. H., Antisense RNA inhibits splicing of pre-mRNA *in vitro, EMBO J.*, 7, 2523, 1988.
13. Volloch, V., Schweitzer, B., and Ritts, S., Inhibition of pre-mRNA splicing *in vitro:* effect of RNA containing sequences complementary to exons, *Biochem. Biophys. Res. Commun.*, 179, 1593, 1991.
14. Volloch, V., Schweitzer, B., and Ritts, S., Inhibition of pre-mRNA splicing *in vitro:* effect of RNA containing sequences complementary to introns, *Biochem. Biophys. Res. Commun.*, 179, 1600, 1991.
15. Liu, Z. and Carmichael, G. G., Nuclear antisense RNA. An efficient new method to inhibit gene expression, *Mol. Biotechnol.*, 2, 107, 1994.
16. Liu, Z., Batt, D. B., and Carmichael, G. G., Targeted nuclear antisense RNA mimics natural antisense-induced degradation of polyoma virus early RNA, *Proc. Natl. Acad. Sci. U.S.A.*, 91, 4258, 1994.
17. Hildebrandt, M. and Nellen, W., Differential antisense transcription from the *Dictyostelium* EB4 gene locus: implications on antisense-mediated regulation of mRNA stability, *Cell*, 69, 197, 1992.
18. Nauber, U., Schuh, R., and Jaeckle, H., Application of antisense nucleic acids in Developmental biology: *Drosophila, Antisense Nucleic Acids and Proteins, Fundamentals and Applications*, Mol, J. N. M. and van der Krol., A. R., Eds., Marcel Dekker, New York, 1990.
19. Maniak, M. and Nellen, W., Evidence for a feedback regulated back-up promoter which controls permanent expression of a *Dictyostelium* gene, *Nucleic Acids Res.*, 18, 5375, 1990.
20. von Ahsen, U. and Schroeder, R., RNA as a catalyst: Natural and designed ribozymes, *Bioessays*, 15, 299, 1993.
21. Been, M. D., *Cis*- and *trans*-acting ribozymes from a human pathogen, hepatitis delta virus, *Trends Biochem. Sci.*, 19, 251, 1994.
22. Symons, R. H., Self-cleavage of RNA in the replication of small pathogens of plants and animals, *Trends Biochem. Sci.*, 14, 445, 1989.
23. Bertrand, E., Pictet, R., and Grange, T., Can hammerhead ribozymes be efficient tools to inactivate gene function?, *Nucleic Acids Res.*, 22, 293, 1994.
24. Heinrich, J.-C., Tabler, M., and Louis, C., Attenuation of white gene expression in transgenic *Drosophila melanogaster:* possible role of a catalytic antisense RNA, *Dev. Gen.*, 14, 258, 1993.
25. Tabler, M., Homann, M., Tzortzakaki, S., and Sczakiel, G., A three-nucleotide helix I is sufficient for full activity of a hammerhead ribozyme: advantages of an asymmetric design, *Nucleic Acids Res.*, 22, 3958, 1994.
26. Homann, M., Tzortzakaki, S., Rittner, K., Sczakiel, G., and Tabler, M., Incorporation of the catalytic domain of a hammerhead ribozyme into antisense RNA enhances its inhibitory effect on the replication of human immunodeficiency virus type 1, *Nucleic Acids Res.*, 21, 2809, 1993.

27. Bertrand, E. L. and Rossi, J. J., Facilitation of hammerhead ribozyme catalysis by the nucleocapsid protein of HIV-1 and the heterogeneous nuclear ribonucleoprotein A1, *EMBO J.*, 13, 2904, 1994.
28. Sullenger, B. A. and Cech, T. R., Tethering ribozymes to a retroviral packaging signal for destruction of viral RNA, *Science*, 262, 1566, 1993.
29. Lisziewicz, J., Sun, D., Smythe, J., Lusso, P., Lori, F., Louie, A., Markham, P., Rossi, J., Reitz, M., and Gallo, R., Inhibition of human immunodeficiency virus type 1 replication by regulated expression of a polymeric Tat activation response RNA decoy as a strategy for gene therapy in AIDS, *Proc. Natl. Acad. Sci. U.S.A.*, 90, 8000, 1993.
30. McCall, M. J., Hendry, P., and Jennings, P. A., Minimal sequence requirements for ribozyme activity, *Proc. Natl. Acad. Sci. U.S.A.*, 89, 5710, 1992.
31. Thomson, J. B., Tuschl, T., and Eckstein, F., Activity of hammerhead ribozymes containing non-nucleotidic linkers, *Nucleic Acids Res.*, 21, 5600, 1993.
32. Han, L., Yun, J. S., and Wagner, T. E., Inhibition of Moloney murine leukemia virus-induced leukemia in transgenic mice expressing antisense RNA complementary to the retroviral packaging sequences, *Proc. Natl. Acad. Sci. U.S.A.*, 88, 4313, 1991.
33. Chatterjee, S., Johnson, P. R., and Wong, K. K., Dual target inhibition of HIV-1 *in vitro* by means of adeno-associated virus antisense vector, *Science*, 258, 1485, 1991.
34. Renneisen, K., Leserman, L., Matthes, E., Schröder, H. C., and Müller, W. E. G., Inhibition of expression of human deficiency virus-1 *in vitro* by antibody-targeted liposomes containing antisense RNA to the *env* region, *J. Biol. Chem.*, 265, 16337, 1990.
35. Holt, J. T., Gopal, T. V., Moulton, A. D., and Nienhuis, A. W., Inducible production of c-*fos* antisense RNA inhibits 3T3 cell proliferation, *Proc. Natl. Acad. Sci. U.S.A.*, 83, 4794, 1986.
36. Levi, B. Z. and Ozato, K., Constitutive expression of c-*fos* antisense RNA blocks c-fos gene induction by interferon and by phorbol ester and reduces c-*myc* expression in F9 embryonal carcinoma cells, *Genes Dev.*, 2, 554, 1988.
37. Zhang, Y., Mukhopadhyay, T., Donehower, L. A., Georges, R. N., and Roth, J. A., Retroviral vector-mediated transduction of k-*ras* antisense RNA into human lung cancer cells inhibit expression of the malignant phenotype, *Human Gene Therapy*, 4, 451, 1993.
38. Hunts, J., Merlino, G., Pastan, I., and Shimizu, N., Reduction of EGF receptor synthesis by antisense RNA vectors, *FEBS Lett.*, 206, 319, 1986.
39. Shohat, O., Greenberg, M., Reisman, D., Oren, M., and Rotter, V., Inhibition of cell growth mediated by plasmids encoding p53 anti-sense, *Oncogene*, 1, 277, 1987.
40. Mukhopadhyay, T. and Roth, J. A., A codon 248 p53 mutation retains tumor suppressor function as shown by enhancement of tumor growth by antisense p53, *Cancer Res.*, 53, 4362, 1993.
41. Narayanan, R., Lawlor, K. G., Schaapveld, R. Q., Cho, K. R., Vogelstein, B., Bui-Vinh Tran, P., Osborne, M. P., and Telang, N. T., Antisense RNA to the putative tumor-suppressor gene DCC transforms Rat-1 fibroblasts, *Oncogene*, 7, 553, 1992.
42. Nakanishi, M., Adami, G. R., Robetorye, R. S., Noda, A., Venable, S. F., Dimitrov, D., Pereira-Smith, O. M., and Smith, J. R., Exit from G_0 and entry into cell cycle of cells expressing $p21^{Sdi1}$ antisense RNA, *Proc. Natl. Acad. Sci. U.S.A.*, 92, 4352, 1995.
43. Del Sal, G., Murphy, M., Ruaro, E., Lazarevic, D., Levine, A. J., and Schneider, C., Cyclin D1 and p21/wafl are both involved in p53 growth suppression, *Oncogene*, 12, 177, 1996.
44. Ouchida, M., Takatoshi, O., Fujimura, Y., Rao, V. N., and Reddy, E. S. P., Loss of tumorigenicity of Ewing's sarcoma cells expressing antisense RNA to EWS-fusion transcripts, *Oncogene*, 11, 1049, 1995.
45. Trojan, J., Blossey, B. K., Johnson, T. R., Rudin, S. D., Tykocinski, M., Ilan, J., and Ilan, J., Loss of tumorigenicity of rat glioblastoma directed by episome-based antisense cDNA transcription of insulin-like growth factor I., *Proc. Natl. Acad. Sci. U.S.A.*, 89, 4874, 1992.
46. Higgins, K. A., Perez, J. R., Coleman, T. A., Dorshkind, K., McComas, W. A., Sarmiento, U. M., Rosen, C. A., and Narayanan, R., Antisense inhibition of the p65 subunit of NF-kappa B blocks tumorigenicity and causes tumor regression, *Proc. Natl. Acad. Sci. U.S.A.*, 90, 9901, 1993.
47. Crowley, T., Nellen, W., Gomer, R., and Firtel, R. A., Phenocopy of discoidin I-minus mutants by antisense transformation in *Dictyostelium*, *Cell*, 43, 633, 1985.
48. Pepin, M.-C., Pothier, F., and Barden, N., Impaired type II glucocorticoid-receptor function in mice bearing antisense RNA transgene, *Nature*, 355, 725, 1992.
49. Moxham, C. M., Hod, Y., and Malbon, C. C., $G_{i\alpha2}$ mediates the inhibitory regulation of adenelyl cyclase *in vivo*: analysis in transgenic mice with Gi α2 suppressed by inducible antisense RNA, *Dev. Gen.*, 14, 266, 1993.
50. Moxham, C. M., Hod, Y., and Malbon, C. C., Induction of G alpha-specific antisense RNA *in vivo* inhibits neonatal growth, *Science*, 260, 991, 1993.

51. Fire, A., Albertson, D., Harrison, S. W., and Moerman, D. G., Production of antisense RNA leads to effective and specific inhibition of gene expression in *C. elegans* muscle, *Development*, 113, 503, 1991.
52. Weinstein, D. E., Shelanski, M. L., and Liem, R. K. H., Suppression by antisense mRNA demonstrates a requirement for the glial fibrillary acidic protein in the formation of stable astrocytic processes in response to neurons, *J. Cell Biol.*, 112, 1205, 1991.
53. Powell, P. A., Stark, D. M., Sanders, P. R., and Beachy, R. N., Protection against tobacco mosaic virus in transgenic plants that express tobacco mosaic virus antisense RNA, *Proc. Natl. Acad. Sci. U.S.A.*, 86, 6949, 1989.
54. Nelson, A., Roth, D. A., and Johnson, J. D., Tobacco mosaic virus infection of transgenic *Nicotiana tabacum* plants is inhibited by antisense constructs at the 5′ region of viral RNA, *Gene*, 127, 227, 1993.
55. Bejarano, E. R. and Lichtenstein, C. P., Prospects for engineering virus resistance in plants with antisense RNA, *Trends Biotechnol.*, 10, 383, 1992.
56. Hamilton, A. J., Fray, R. G., and Grierson, D., Sense and antisense inactivation of fruit ripening genes in tomato, *Gene Silencing in Higher Plants and Related Phenomena in Other Eukaryotes*, Meyer, P., Ed., Springer-Verlag, Berlin, 1995, chap. 6.
57. Visser, R. G. F., Kuipers, A. G. J., and Jacobsen, E. (1996): Antisense granule-bound starch synthase effects in potato, *Mechanisms and Applications of Gene Silencing*, Grierson, D., Lycett, G. W., and Tucker, G. A., Eds., Nottingham University Press, 1996, chap. 10.
58. Spann, T. P., Brock, D. A., Lindsey, D. F., Wood, S. A., and Gomer, R. H., Mutagenesis and gene identification in *Dictyostelium* by shsotgun antisense, *Proc. Natl. Acad. Sci. U.S.A.*, 93, 5003, 1996.
59. Li, L. and Cohen, S. N., tsg101: A novel tumor susceptible gene isolated by controlled homozygous functional knockout of allelic loci in mammalian cells, *Cell*, 85, 319, 1996.
60. Atkins, D., Arndt, G. M., and Izant, J. G., Antisense gene expression in yeast, *Biol. Chem. Hoppe Seyler*, 375, 721, 1994.
61. Nellen, W. and Lichtenstein, C., What makes an mRNA anti-sense-itive?, *Trends Biochem. Sci.*, 18, 419, 1993.
62. Missel, A. and Goeringer, H. U., *Trypanosoma brucei* mitochondria contain RNA helicase activity, *Nucleic Acids Res.*, 22, 4050, 1994.
63. Missel, A., Noerskau, G., Shu, H. H., and Goeringer, H. U., A putative RNA helicase of the DEAD box family from *Trypanosoma brucei*, *Mol. Biochem. Parasitol.*, 75, 123, 1995.
64. Missel, A. and Goeringer, H. U., Personal communication, 1996.
65. Iino, Y., Sugimoto, A., and Yamamoto, M., *S. pombe* pac1+, whose overexpression inhibits sexual development, encodes a ribonuclease III-like RNase, *EMBO J.*, 10, 221, 1991.
66. Jacobsen, S., Personal communication, 1995.
67. Wilson, R., Ainscough, R., Anderson, K., Baynes, C., Berks, M., Bonfield, J., Burton, J., Connel, M., Copsey, T., and Cooper, J., 2.2 Mb of contiguous nucleotide sequence from chromosome III of *C. elegans*, *Nature*, 368, 32, 1994.
68. Adelman, J. P., Bond, C. T., Douglass, J., and Herbert, E., Two mammalian genes transcribed from opposite strands of the same DNA locus, *Science*, 235, 1514, 1987.
69. Spencer, C. A., Gietz, R. D., and Hodgetts, R. B., Overlapping transcriptions units in the dopa decarboxylase of *Drosophila*, *Nature*, 322, 279, 1986.
70. Hsieh-Li, H. M., Witte, D. P., Weinstein, M., Branford, W., Li, H., Small, K., and Potter, S. S., Hoxa 11 structure, extensive antisense transcription, and function in male and female fertility, *Development*, 121, 1373, 1995.
71. Bentley, D. L. and Groudine, M., A block to elongation is largely responsible for decreased transcription of c-*myc* in differentiated HL60 cells, *Nature*, 321, 702, 11986.
72. Bentley, D. L. and Groudine, M., Novel promoter upstream of the human c-*myc* gene and regulation of c-*myc* expression in B-cell lymphomas, *Mol. Cell. Biol.*, 6, 3481, 1986.
73. Kindy, M. S., McCormack, J. E., Buckler, A. J., Levine, R. A., and Sonenshein, G. E., Independent regulation of transcription of the two strands of the c-*myc* gene, *Mol. Cell. Biol.*, 7, 2857, 1987.
74. Nepveu, A. and Marcu, K. B., Intragenic pausing and anti-sense transcription within the murine c-*myc* locus, *EMBO J.*, 5, 2859, 1986.
75. Celano, P., Berchtold, C. M., Kizer, D. L., Weeraratna, A., Nelkin, B. D., Baylin, S. B., and Casero, R. A., Jr., Characterization of an endogenous RNA transcript with homology to the antisense strand of the human c-*myc* gene, *J. Biol. Chem.*, 267, 15092, 1992.
76. Carmichael, G. G., Personal communications, 1995.
77. Kimelman, D. and Kirschner, M. W., An antisense mRNA directs the covalent modification of the transcript encoding fibroblast growth factor in *Xenopus* oocytes, *Cell*, 59, 687, 1989.
78. Saccomanno, L. and Bass, B. L., The cytoplasm of *Xenopus* oocytes contains a factor that protects double-stranded RNA from adenosine-to-inosine modification, *Mol. Cell. Biol.*, 14, 5425, 1994.

79. Savage, M. P. and Fallon, J. F., FGF-2 mRNA and its antisense message are expressed in a developmentally specific manner in the chick limb bud and mesonephros, *Dev. Dyn.*, 202, 343, 1995.
80. Bedford, M., Arman, E., Orr-Urtreger, A., and Lonai, P., Analysis of the Hoxd-3 gene: structure and localization of its sense and natural antisense transcripts, *DNA Cell Biol.*, 14, 295, 1995.
81. Wagner, E. G. and Simons, R. W., Antisense RNA control in bacteria, phages, and plasmids, *Annu. Rev. Microbiol.*, 48, 713, 1994.
82. Hjalt, T. and Wagner, E. G., The effect of loop size in antisense and target RNAs on the efficiency of antisense RNA control, *Nucleic Acids Res.*, 20, 6723, 1992.
83. Romby, P. and Wager, G., Personal communication, 1996.
84. Ruvkun, G., Ambros, V., Coulson, A., Waterson, R., Sulston, J., and Horvitz, H. R., Molecular genetics of the Caenorhabditis elegans heterochronic gene *lin*-14, *Genetics*, 121, 501, 1989.
85. Lee, R. C., Feinbaum, R. L., and Ambros, V., The *C. elegans* heterochronic gene *lin*-4 encodes small RNAs with antisense complementarity to *lin*-14, *Cell*, 75, 843, 1993.
86. Bester, A. J., Kennedy, D. S., and Heywood, S. M., Two classes of translational control RNA: their role in the regulation of protein synthesis, *Proc. Nat. Acad. Sci. U.S.A.*, 72, 1523, 1975.
87. Heywood, S. M., tcRNA as a naturally occurring antisense RNA in eukaryotes, *Nucleic Acids Res.*, 14, 6771, 1986.
88. Zezza, D. J. and Heywood, S. M., Analysis of tcRNA 102 associated with myosin heavy chain mRNPs in control and dystrophic chick pectoralis muscle, *J. Biol. Chem.*, 261, 7461, 1986.
89. Oberosler, P. and Nellen, W., Unpublished data, 1995.
90. Sadiq, M., Hildebrandt, M., Maniak, M., and Nellen, W., Development regulation of antisense-mediated gene silencing in *Dictyostelium*, *Antisense Res. Dev.*, 4, 263, 1994.
91. Hildebrandt, M. and Nellen, W., Effects of antisense transcripts on translation and mRNA stability, *Mechanisms and Applications of Gene Silencing*, Grierson, D., Lycette, G. W., and Tucker, G. A., Eds., Nottingham University Press, Nottingham, 1995, chap. 2.
92. Noguchi, M., Silverman, T. A., and Safer, B., Characterization of an antisense Inr element in the eIF-2 alpha gene, *J. Biol. Chem.*, 269, 29161, 1993.
93. Munroe, S. H. and Lazar, M. A., Inhibition of c-erb mRNA splicing by a naturally occurring antisense RNA, *J. Biol. Chem.*, 266, 22083, 1991.
94. Kim, S. K. and Wold, B. J., Stable reduction of thymidine kinase activity in cells expressing high levels of anti-sense RNA, *Cell*, 42, 129, 1985.
95. Wightman, B., Ha, I., and Ruvkun, G., Posttranscriptional regulation of the heterochronic gene *lin*-14 and *lin*-4 mediates temporal pattern formation in *C. elegans*, *Cell*, 75, 855, 1993.
96. Melton, D. A., Injected anti-sense RNAs specifically block messenger RNA translation *in vivo*, *Proc. Natl. Acad. Sci. U.S.A.*, 82, 144, 1985.
97. Stephenson, M. L. and Zamecnik, P. C., Inhibition of Rous sarcoma viral RNA translation by a specific oligodeoxyribonucleotide, *Proc. Natl. Acad. Sci. U.S.A.*, 75, 285, 1978.
98. Izant, J. G. and Weintraub, H., Inhibition of thymidine kinase gene expression by anti-sense RNA: A molecular approach to genetic analysis, *Cell*, 36, 1007, 1984.
99. Temsamani, J., Agrawal, S., and Pederson, T., Biotinylated antisense methylphosphonate oligodeoxynucleotides: inhibition of spliceosome assembly and affinity selection of U1 and U2 small nuclear RNPs, *J. Biol. Chem.*, 266, 468, 1991.
100. Lukacs, N., Detection of sense-antisense duplexes by structure-specific anti-RNA antibodies, Antisense Regulation: A Practical Approach, IRL Press Oxford, Lichtenstein, C. P., Nellen, W., Eds., in preparation.
101. Volloch, V., Schweitzer, B., and Ritts, S., Antisense globin RNA in mouse erythoid tissues: Structure, origin and possible function, *Proc. Natl. Acad. U.S.A.*, 93, 2476, 1996.
102. Hildebrandt, M. and Nellen, W., Unpublished data, 1995.
103. Atkins, D. and Gerlach, W. L., Artificial ribozyme and antisense gene expression in *Saccharomyces cerevisiae*, *Antisense Res. Dev.*, 4, 109, 1994.
104. Nellen, W. and Sczakiel, G., *In vitro* and *in vivo* action of antisense RNA, *Mol. Biotechnol.*, 6, 7, 1996..
105. Mayeda, A. and Krainer, A. R., Regulation of alternative pre-mRNA splicing by hnRNP A1 and splicing factor SF2, *Cell*, 68, 365, 1992.
106. Pinol-Roma, S. and Dreyfuss, G., Shuttling of pre-mRNA binding proteins between nucleus and cystoplasm, *Nature*, 355, 730, 1992.
107. Oberosler, P. and Nellen, W., manuscript in preparation.
108. Hjalt, T. A. and Wagner, E. G., Bulged-out nucleotides in an antisense RNA are required for rapid target RNA binding *in vitro* and inhibition *in vivo*, *Nucleic Acids Res.*, 23, 580, 1995.
109. Stahl, H., Personal communication, 1995.
110. D'Alessio, G., Parente, A., Guida, C., and Leone, E., Dimeric structure of seminal ribonuclease, *FEBS Lett.*, 27, 285, 1972.

111. Hall, S. H. and Crouch, R. J., Isolation and characterization of two enzymatic activities from chick embryos which degrade double-stranded RNA, *J. Biol. Chem.*, 252, 4092, 1977.
112. Rech, J., Cathala, G., and Jeanteur, P., Partial purification of a double-stranded RNA specific ribonuclease (RNase D) from Krebs II ascites cells, *Nucleic Acids Res.*, 3, 2055, 1978.
113. Meegan, J. M. and Marcus, P. I., Double-stranded ribonuclease coinduced with interferon, *Science*, 244, 1089, 1989.
114. Matousek, J., Trnena, L., Oberhauser, R., Lichtenstein, C. P., and Nellen, W., dsRNA degrading nucleases are differentially expressed in tobacco anthers, *Biol. Chem. Hoppe-Seyler*, 375, 261, 1994.
115. Hildebrandt, M., Schirmacher, H., and Nellen, W., Unpublished data, 1995.
116. Proud, C. G., PKR: A new name and new roles, *Trends Biochem. Sci.*, 20, 241, 1995.
117. Maran, A., Maitra, R. K., Kumar, A., Dong, B., Xiao, W., Li, G., Williams, B. R., Torrence, P. F., and Silverman, R. H., Blockage of NF-kappa B signaling by selective ablation of an mRNA target by 2-5A antisense chimeras, *Science*, 265, 789, 1994.
118. Zhou, A., Hassel, B. A., and Silverman, R. H., Expression cloning of 2-5A-dependent RNase: a uniquely regulated mediator of interferon action, *Cell*, 72, 753, 1993.

Chapter 10

Development of Retroviral Vectors Expressing Antisense RNA to Inhibit Replication of the Human Immunodeficiency Virus

Bruce A. Bunnell and Richard A. Morgan

CONTENTS

I. INTRODUCTION

Acquired immune deficiency syndrome (AIDS) is a rapidly expanding global pandemic. Approximately 15 million people worldwide are infected with HIV-1, the causative agent of AIDS. Despite a decade of intense research efforts aimed at understanding the HIV-1 virus and developing an effective therapy for AIDS, HIV-1 infection remains an incurable and fatal disease. The high rate of mutation in the viral genome and the generation of drug-resistant strains of HIV-1 are the major factors that prevent the development of an effective drug-based therapy. The inability of traditional drug-based therapies to effectively inhibit the HIV-1 replication has made it vital to develop new and innovative therapies for this deadly disease.

Gene therapy is defined as the introduction of new genetic material into the cells of an individual that results in a therapeutic benefit.[1,2] Gene therapy holds considerable potential for the treatment of both hereditary and acquired genetic diseases. Because in its normal life cycle the HIV-1 virus integrates into the host cell's genome, AIDS can be regarded as an acquired genetic disease. Therefore, AIDS may be amenable to treatment by gene therapy approaches.

Gene therapy for HIV-1 infection requires the introduction of genes that will effectively inhibit HIV-1 replication by efficiently inhibiting expression of HIV-1 viral genes or altering the normal function of HIV-1-associated proteins. This concept was denoted as "intracellular immunization" by Baltimore.[3] The ultimate goal of HIV-1 gene therapy is to inhibit viral replication at a molecular level and, in turn, limit or prevent progression to AIDS. Anti-HIV-1 gene therapy approaches can be divided into three broad categories: (1) gene therapies based on nucleic acid moieties, including gene vaccines, antisense DNA/RNA, RNA decoys that function by competition for the binding of proteins essential for HIV-1 replication, and catalytic RNA moieties (ribozymes) that inhibit HIV-1 gene expression by cleaving the viral RNA; (2) protein approaches (transdominant negative proteins and single chain antibodies) that are based on the intracellular expression of protein moieties which interfere or inhibit normal viral replication or function; and (3) immunotherapeutic approaches in which new or enhanced HIV-1-specific lymphocytes are generated and used to attack HIV-1-infected cells.

This review will focus solely on the development of retroviral vectors for the expression of antisense sequences for gene therapy of HIV-1 infection. The extent to which antisense-mediated gene therapy will be effective against HIV-1 is the direct result of several key factors: (1) selection of the appropriate target cell or tissue for gene therapy; (2) the efficiency of the gene delivery system; (3) appropriate expression, regulation, and stability of the antisense gene product(s); and (4) the efficiency of the inhibition of viral replication by the anti-HIV-1 antisense entity.

II. LIFE-CYCLE OF HIV-1

The HIV-1 virus is a member of the lentivirus family of retroviruses. The viral genome encodes three sets of viral proteins: the structural proteins (Gag, Pol, and Env), the regulatory proteins (Tat, Rev, and Nef), and the maturation proteins (Vif, Vpu, and Vpr; Figure 1). The life cycle of the virus is diagrammed in Figure 2. The initial stage of infection (the early phase) begins with the binding of the viral envelope protein gp120 to its cell-surface receptor, the CD4 molecule. The gp 41 protein then mediates fusion of the virus with the host cell plasma membrane. The HIV-1 nucleocapsid is internalized into the cytoplasm where the viral genome is uncoated. The RNA genome is reverse transcribed into DNA by the reverse transcriptase (RT)

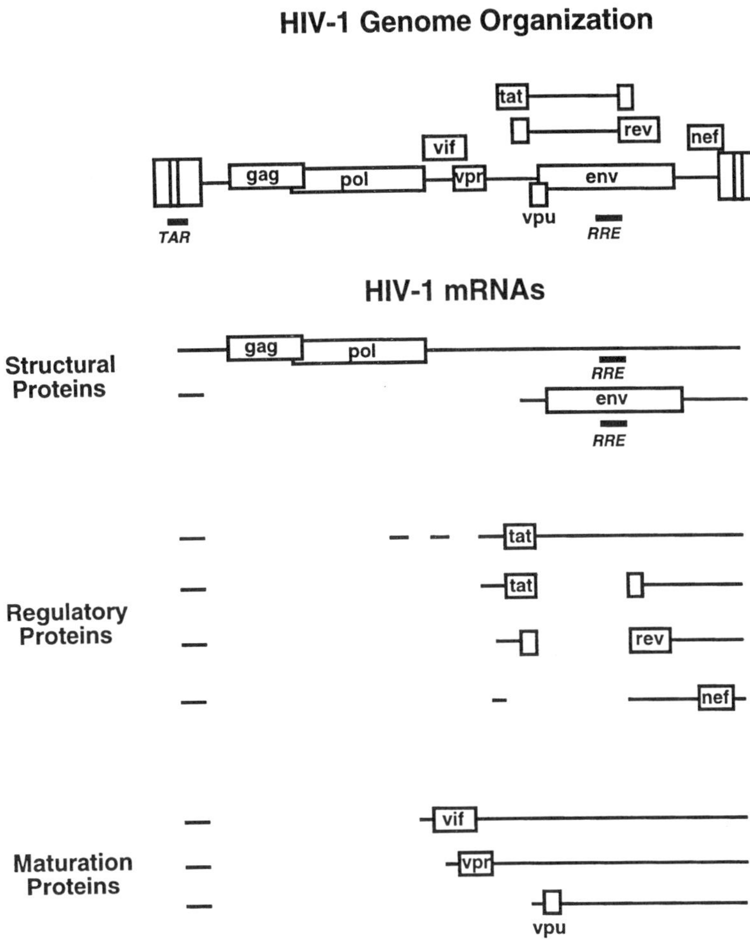

FIGURE 1
The genomic organization and mRNA expression pattern of HIV-1. This diagram depicts the organization of the nine predominant genes of HIV-1. The diagram below represents the major RNAs derived from the HIV-1 genome by alternative splicing of the HIV-1 genome. Three distinct classes of viral proteins are generated from these mRNAs: structural proteins, regulatory proteins, and maturation proteins. The structural proteins include the viral envelope protein (gp 120, gp 41), which is encoded by the *env* gene, and the core proteins (p6, p9, p17, and p24), which are encoded by the *gag* gene. The *pol* gene generates the viral-associated reverse transcriptase, integrase, RNase H, and protease enzyme activities. The viral associated regulatory proteins are encoded by the *tat*, *rev*, and *nef* genes, respectively. The Tat and Rev proteins are powerful regulatory proteins. The Tat protein interacts with the TAR (tat responsive) element, which leads to a strong transactivation of viral gene expression, while the Rev protein interacts with the RRE (rev response element), which enhances the nuclear export of unspliced and single-spliced viral mRNA. The third class of viral proteins are the maturation proteins, which are encoded by the *vif*, *vpr*, and *vpu* genes.

protein encoded by the pol sequences. The newly synthesized viral DNA genome then randomly integrates into the host cell genome; this integrated form of the virus is denoted as the provirus. The provirus can remain latent for extended periods of time and, in so doing, is passed along to all progeny cells derived from the original infected cell.

Although the mechanism of proviral activation is unclear, once the provirus is activated the intermediate stage of viral infection begins. Activation induces transcription of multiply spliced viral RNAs that are utilized to produce the Tat and Rev proteins which act as powerful regulatory proteins during virus replication. The Tat

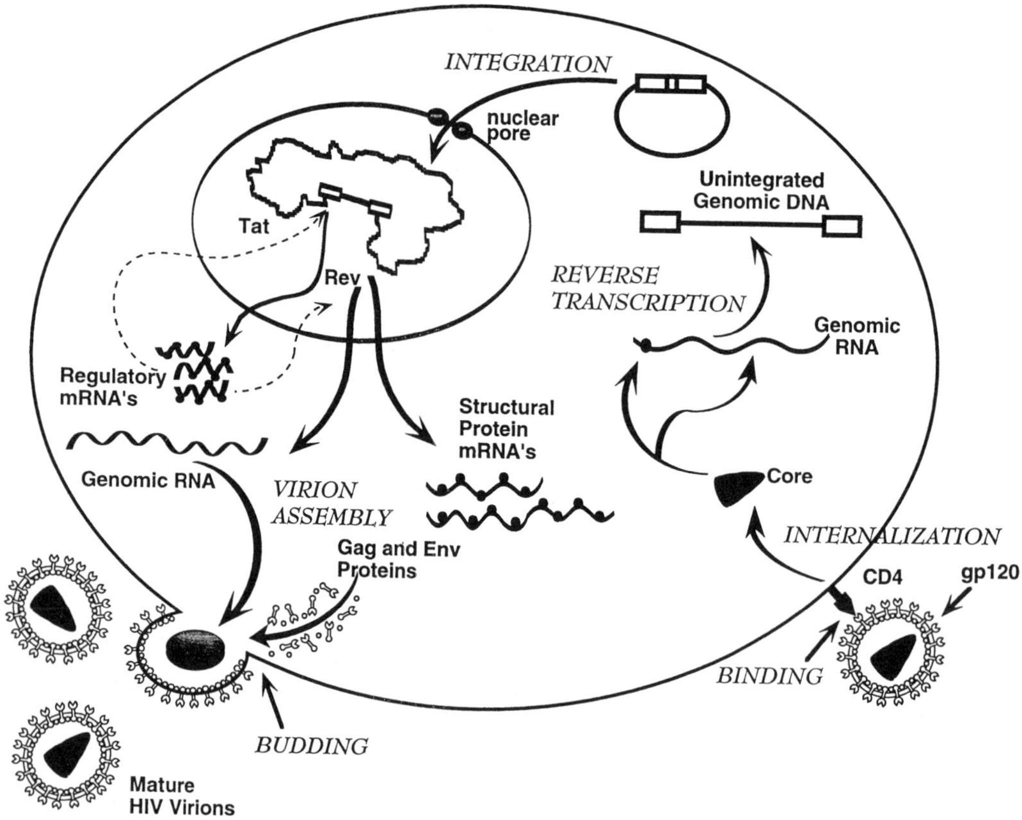

FIGURE 2
The life cycle of the HIV-1 virus.

protein is a strong transactivator of viral gene expression. The Rev protein markedly enhances nuclear export of single-spliced and nonspliced viral mRNAs from the nucleus and these RNAs encode the viral structural proteins.

The late phase of HIV-1 infection begins upon the accumulation of significant amounts of structural protein. The late phase consists of the assembly of virus particles containing two copies of the viral RNA genome. The assembled particles are transported to the cell membrane where the mature virus particles bud off from the plasma membrane. In theory, the life cycle of the HIV-1 virus can be interrupted by blocking or inhibiting the function of one or more or the key viral proteins or their *cis*-acting regulatory elements.

III. ANTISENSE GENE TRANSFER SYSTEMS

In order for antisense gene therapy to be effective, it is vital to efficiently deliver genes into the target cells. A variety of gene delivery systems including viral vectors based on retrovirus, adenovirus, and adeno-associated virus (AAV), as well as non-viral-based gene transfer techniques are currently being evaluated for their effectiveness for gene delivery.[4-13] The viral-derived gene transfer systems have been extensively tested on both hematopoietic stem cells (HSCs) and CD4+ lymphocytes. Only the retroviral vector system has been repeatedly demonstrated to effectively deliver genes into these target cells, albeit at low levels in HSCs. Thus, retroviral-mediated gene transfer is currently the optimal gene transfer system available for use in HIV-1 gene therapy.

A. Retroviral Vectors

Recombinant retroviral vector particles are obtained by transfection of a recombinant retroviral vector plasmid DNA into a mouse fibroblast packaging cell line. Several distinct packaging cell lines have been developed, such as PA317 and PG13.[14-16] The recombinant retroviral vector contains the therapeutic gene and the *cis*-acting regulatory sequences required for encapsidation (Ψ+ region) and replication of the retroviral genome. The packaging cell line harbors a helper provirus that produces all of the retroviral structural proteins (Gag, Pol, and Env) necessary for retroviral assembly. The recombinant provirus contained within the packaging cell cannot be incorporated into retrovirus virions because it does not contain the necessary Ψ+ element. Thus, only the recombinant retroviral genomes containing the therapeutic gene and Ψ+ element are packaged into retrovirus particles. The recombinant retrovirus particles produced by packaging cells are replication defective because they do not harbor any of the retroviral structural proteins required for replication and production of the retrovirus. The packaging cells release the recombinant retrovirus particles into the culture medium where they can be harvested and used for gene transfer into target cells. The retrovirus particles achieve gene transfer by infection of the target cell and incorporation into the host cell's genome.

The most commonly used retroviral vectors are derived from the Moloney murine leukemia virus (Mo-MLV). Mo-MLV-derived retroviral vectors are capable of gene transfer into a wide variety of cell types. The current design of retroviral vectors express either single genes or multiple genes. The current retroviral vectors improved on the design of previous vectors by incorporating a series of mutations into the 5′ end and packaging signal (Ψ+) regions.[17] An additional improvement for vector design was created by deletion of the Neo^R gene 3′ untranslated region and all sequences derived from the Mo-MLV env gene.[18] Recently, vectors containing multiple cloning sites for gene insertion have been described.[19,20] In some vectors, the retroviral splice donor sequence is retained. The importance of retaining the splice donor (SD) sequence in the vectors has been investigated by two groups.[21,22] In these reports, it was demonstrated that while some SD mutations do not affect viral titer or gene expression, some other SD alterations can adversely influence titer. Additional vectors designed to express individual genes by a spliced mRNA have been developed.[23,24]

An alternative to expression of inserted genes from the retroviral long terminal repeat (LTR) is to drive the expression from an internal promoter. The potential advantage to this design is that nonviral promoter/enhancer elements may permit tissue-specific gene expression. One theoretical reason to avoid using the retroviral LTR as a promoter is that, in certain cell types, the viral LTR can either have limited activity or is turned off by cellular functions.[25,26] An alternative to the use of internal promoters is to use a modified LTR. Several groups have reported that transcriptional silencing may be overcome by either using natural variants of the retroviral LTR or by making chimeric enhancer elements within the context of the normal LTR enhancer.[27-29]

In the majority of applications it is often advantageous to have more than one gene expressed from a retroviral vector. Of obvious utility is to have a selectable marker gene co-expressed in the same cell as the investigational gene, which permits enrichment for gene-containing cells. The first vector to drive the expression of two independent genes was an alternative splicing vector, where the retroviral LTR is used to directly promote the expression of a gene of interest while a selectable marker gene (in this case the Neo^R gene) is produced via splicing.[30]

The most common design for the construction of multi-gene retroviral vectors, is to use an internal promoter element. Variations on this theme are extensive and include the use of internal promoters (including HIV-1) derived from strong viral promoters, the use of cellular promoters, and the use of intact (intron-containing) cellular genes. As with splicing vectors, most internal promoter vectors express a selectable marker as one of the two genes.[21,22,31]

A new class of retroviral vectors has recently been reported that can be used to express multiple genes without the use of internal promoters or alternative splicing.[32,33] These vectors use internal ribosome entry sites (IRES) to facilitate the internal translation initiation of multiple protein coding domains. The IRES elements used in these vectors are naturally occurring sequences found in the 5′ untranslated regions of picornaviruses (e.g., the human poliovirus or the mouse encephalomyocarditis virus). Insertion of an IRES between protein coding sequences (between the stop codon of the first gene and the start codon of the second gene) produces a bicistronic mRNA. In our experience with these vectors, we have found them to be useful for expression of multiple genes. Furthermore, constructs containing up to three genes can easily be assembled.

A final category of vectors that can be used to express multiple genes are the double-copy vectors.[34-36] It was demonstrated that manipulation in the U3 region of the 3′ LTR is transferred to both LTRs following transduction. In addition to deletions, insertions into the U3 region are also propagated to both LTRs. The site of these insertions is in the extreme 5′ part of the U3 region, upstream of the enhancer. This insertion site places the double-copy promoter outside of the retroviral transcription unit, leaving the normal LTR promoter intact and functional.

The limitation of retroviral vectors is the inability to infect nondividing cells due to the requirement for DNA replication in order to efficiently integrate into the host cell genome. However, the recent development of a retroviral vector system derived from HIV-1 has been demonstrated to be capable of transduction of nondividing cell types both *in vitro* and *in vivo*.[37] This new system involves a three plasmid expression system. The plasmid used for packaging of retroviral particles contains the human cytomegalovirus immediate-early promoter to drive the expression of all HIV-1 viral proteins required for packaging. The packaging plasmid contains mutations that inactivate expression of both the HIV-1 env gene and vpu gene. Also, the HIV-1 packaging signal (ψ) has been deleted. To increase the tropism of the virus, a second plasmid is used, encoding either a Mo-MLV amphotropic or vesicular stomatitis virus (VSV) G-protein envelope sequence. The last plasmid contains the HIV-1 *cis*-acting signals required for packaging, reverse transcription, and integration. The vector system has been demonstrated to transduce nondividing cells *in vitro* and *in vivo*. Although this vector system needs to be studied in greater detail, the HIV-1-derived retroviral vectors may significantly increase the applicability of retroviral vectors in gene therapy.

IV. ANTISENSE RNA

Antisense nucleic acids utilize Watson-Crick nucleic acid base pairing to block gene expression in a sequence-specific fashion. Antisense transcripts can be designed to target various regions of the HIV-1 genome. In general, antisense strategies should be targeted against highly conserved regions of the genome or against genes that are essential for HIV-1 replication. Although the mechanism of antisense-mediated inhibition of gene expression is not completely understood, it is hypothesized that RNA duplexes (antisense RNA and target RNA) are degraded by RNase H or otherwise functionally inactivated, thereby blocking subsequent translation of the mRNA. Synthetic antisense DNA oligonucleotides have been designed that effectively inhibit the replication of HIV-1.[38-43] However, their use for the inhibition of HIV-1 has been limited because uptake of free oligonucleotides from the extracellular environment is extremely inefficient and an efficient oligonucleotide delivery system has not yet been devised. Also, the oligonucleotides taken up by cells are rapidly degraded such that any inhibitory activity is transient, and the gene inhibition that is observed is often nonspecific.

Stable intracellular expression of antisense HIV-1 sequences is currently the most efficient method by which antisense technology can be utilized to inhibit HIV-1 gene expression. Preliminary studies demonstrated limited antiviral activity with antisense transcripts to the viral genes *tat, rev, vpu,* and *gag,* as well as the primer binding site.[44-49] An in-depth analysis of potential HIV-1 antisense gene sequences was performed in which various antisense RNAs targeted to ten different regions of the HIV-1 genome were compared for their antiviral effects.[50] The antisense gene sequences with the greatest antiviral activity were those that targeted a 1-kb region within the *gag* gene and a sequence specific for a 562-bp genomic fragment encompassing the *tat* and *rev* genes. Further analysis of the antiviral effects of the antisense *tat/rev* gene fragment has demonstrated a strong inhibition of HIV-1 replication in the Jurkat cell line and primary CD4+ peripheral blood lymphocytes (PBL), but breakthrough was observed as the multiplicity of infection was increased.[51]

The *trans*-activating response (TAR) element is found in the 5′ untranslated region of all HIV-1 transcripts and is the sequence where the TAT protein binds to enhance HIV-1 RNA transcription (see above). An antisense sequence encompassing bases +15 to +75 of the 5′ untranslated region of HIV-1 (spanning the TAR element) was cloned into an AAV vector and tested in human hematopoietic and non-hematopoietic cell lines.[52] The antisense TAR expressing cell lines demonstrated a 99% inhibition of infectious virus production. Our group tested this potent antisense to the TAR region in the context of a retroviral vector in both T-cell lines and primary PBL. We determined that the antisense TAR alone or antisense TAR expressed with the Rev transdominant negative protein effectively inhibited HIV-1 replication.[53,54]

Additional regions of HIV-1 targeted by our laboratory include the *tat* and *rev* genes because expression of both the Tat and Rev proteins are absolutely essential for HIV-1 replication. We have developed retroviral vectors expressing an antisense gene that encompasses the entire *rev* gene and the 3′ half of the *tat* gene. The antisense *Tat/Rev* gene has been demonstrated to inhibit HIV-1 replication in both T-cell lines and primary PBL.[55,54] Other investigators have focused on inhibiting the *tat* gene. One group has developed a retroviral vector that expresses a polymeric RNA decoy for the TAR element in combination with an antisense fragment to the *tat* gene.[56-58] This dual function anti-*tat* gene therapy has been demonstrated to inhibit virus replication in T-cell lines and primary PBL from HIV-1-infected individuals. An antisense sequence to the HIV-1 *gag* gene has been shown to inhibit virus replication in combination with the TAR decoy.[59] Recently, a chimeric RNA polymerase III transcript derived from the adenovirus VA1 gene containing a short antisense RNA sequence, complementary to a conserved region of the HIV-1 rev transcript, was demonstrated to inhibit HIV-1 replication in the CEM cells.[60] The potential advantages of a pol III-based transcription system are discussed below.

A major limitation to the use of stable expression of antisense sequences as a therapy for HIV-1 infection is that long-term high levels of antisense expression are required in order to effectively inhibit viral replication. The mechanism through which antisense moieties inhibit gene expression requires that one antisense molecule efficiently bind to one target molecule. The stoichiometry of antisense sequences to target sequences must be at a minimum 1:1 antisense to target, but ratios of 5:1 or 10:1 lead to more effective inhibition of viral replication. Thus, the antisense gene expression must be much higher than the levels of HIV-1 expression for an antisense gene therapy strategy to be effective. Standard gene therapy vectors containing pol II promoters often do not produce sufficient levels of antisense sequence to inhibit viral replication. To overcome this problem, vectors containing alternative promoter systems have been developed. A retroviral vector containing a pol III promoter in the context of a double-copy expression cassette (the pol III promoter and antisense gene of interest are contained within each of the two retroviral vector LTRs) potentially could be utilized to achieve high levels of expression.[35,61,62] Our group successfully used a pol III retroviral vector expressing an antisense to the TAR sequence to inhibit HIV-1 *in vitro*. Another retroviral vector in which the HIV-1 LTR is used as a promoter for the expression of therapeutic genes has also been developed.[63] This vector would allow for the efficient expression of antisense sequences upon infection of a CD4 lymphocyte by HIV-1.

V. RIBOZYMES (CATALYTIC ANTISENSE RNA)

Ribozymes are antisense RNA molecules that have catalytic activity. The initial description of RNA-mediated catalysis was made in *Tetrahymena thermophilia*.[64,65] They function by binding to the target moiety through Watson-Crick base pairing and inactivate it by cleaving the phosphodiester backbone at a specific target site. Five classes of ribozymes have been described based on their unique three-dimensional conformations. The classes are denoted as follows: (1) the group I intron, (2) RNase P, (3) the hammerhead ribozyme, (4) the hairpin ribozyme, and (5) the hepatitis delta virus ribozyme.[66] Both the hairpin and hammerhead classes of catalytic RNAs have been successfully adapted for use in HIV-1 gene therapy. A distinct advantage of ribozymes over antisense RNA is that they are not consumed during the target cleavage reaction and, therefore, a single ribozyme can inactivate multiple targets. Due to their unique catalytic properties, ribozymes have the potential to be highly efficient inhibitors of gene expression, even at low concentrations. Ribozymes also have greater sequence specificity than antisense RNA because the substrate must have the correct target sequence to allow binding, and the cleavage sight must be present in the right position. Each type of ribozyme requires ten base pairs or more of flanking sequence surrounding the cleavage site to allow for specificity for the desired target. For the cleavage site for hammerhead ribozymes the nucleotide sequence is N-U-X (N = any nucleotide and X = A, C, or U) , while the cleavage site for the hairpin ribozymes is N-G-U-C.[67-69] However, because ribozymes are short single-stranded RNA moieties with a simple secondary structure, it is possible that their use for gene therapy could be limited because they could be highly susceptible to cellular nucleases, and they may lose of activity when expressed in the context of a longer RNA.

The hairpin ribozyme motif has been utilized for the development of anti-HIV-1 gene therapies. A hairpin ribozyme targeted to the leader sequence of HIV-1 was demonstrated to efficiently inhibit virus replication, but also to inactivate incoming viral RNAs prior to integration into the genome, thereby inhibiting the establishment of infection.[70,71] This ribozyme has further been demonstrated to provide long-term protection from HIV-1 infection in T-cell lines and human PBL *in vitro*.[72,73] A significant limitation to the use of hairpin ribozymes in HIV-1 gene therapy strategies is the highly specific sequence requirements necessary to direct cleavage of the target RNA. Due to the high rate of mutation associated with HIV-1 replication, any disruption of the binding or cleavage sites within the target sequence required by the hairpin ribozyme for activity could render it totally inactive.[74]

The majority of studies aimed at inhibiting HIV-1 replication with ribozymes have utilized the hammerhead motif. Because hammerhead ribozymes only require the three-nucleotide sequence N-U-X, the number of potential cleavage sites within the HIV-1 RNA is significantly greater than the number of potential sites for the hairpin ribozyme. The small size and standard composition of the catalytic domain have allowed for the hammerhead ribozymes to be generated as nuclease-resistant RNA oligonucleotides that can be delivered exogenously.[75] However, the hammerhead ribozymes are subject to the same concerns regarding nuclease sensitivity and stability as the hairpin ribozymes.

The initial report of ribozymes designed to inhibit HIV-1 was performed by transfecting a hammerhead ribozyme targeted to the viral gag sequence under the control of a β-actin promoter into CD4+ HeLa cells.[76] Upon challenge with HIV-1, the cells were demonstrated to express reduced levels of full-length gag RNA molecules and markedly reduced levels of the gag-derived protein p24. Another hammerhead ribozyme developed to target the 5′ leader sequence of HIV-1 expressed in a variety of retroviral vectors was demonstrated to significantly inhibit HIV-1 replication in T-cell lines.[77] This ribozyme has the potential to globally inhibit viral gene expression because the leader sequence is contained within all of the HIV-1 derived RNAs. A hammerhead ribozyme targeted to the *tat* gene of the HIV-1 genome has been demonstrated to inhibit HIV-1 replication in primary PBLs.[78,79] Multi-target ribozymes have been developed recently that cleave the target RNA at as many as nine highly conserved regions within the HIV-1 env RNA.[80] Two hammerhead ribozymes designed to cleave HIV-1 RNA in the *tat* gene or in the common exon for *tat* and *rev* were tested for their ability to inhibit HIV-1 replication in primary human T lymphocytes in the context of retroviral vectors.[81] In this study, it was determined that ribozymes can efficiently inhibit HIV-1 replication even in the context of long retrovirus-derived transcripts.

Ribozyme transcriptional units are small enough so that several ribozymes could be incorporated into a single vector; thus, ribozymes targeted to several regions of the HIV-1 genome can be delivered within the same cell. The development of ribozymes that co-localize with their HIV-1 target RNA to the same subcellular compartment may increase their effectiveness as anti-HIV-1 agents. A ribozyme that contained the retroviral packaging signal was demonstrated to efficiently inactivate newly synthesized HIV-1 genomic RNA prior to particle assembly, resulting in the release of noninfectious HIV-1 particles.[82] The ability to prevent the establishment of infection by HIV-1 may allow uninfected cells to become permanently resistant to HIV-1 infection.

VI. CELLULAR TARGETS FOR GENE THERAPY

The dominant sites of HIV-1 infection and replication are the cells of lymphoid and myeloid origin. In order for HIV-1 gene therapy to be effective, it is vital that cells derived from these lineages be utilized as recipients for anti-HIV-1 gene therapeutics. The pluripotent HSCs generate all cells of lymphoid and myeloid origin; therefore, these cells are the ideal candidates for use in gene therapy. In theory, permanent protection from HIV-1 infection could be achieved through the introduction of anti-HIV-1 genes into HSCs because these cells are self-regenerating. It is not currently possible to isolate pure HSC populations, but several enrichment techniques based on selection for CD34+ cells have been developed. The CD34+ enriched cells isolated from bone marrow, mobilized PBLs, or umbilical cord blood have been used for *in vitro* analysis of HIV-1 gene therapies.[83-85] Unfortunately, the post-transplant levels of gene transfer obtained with these cells is very low (1 to 10%) and in the cells that express the introduced gene, expression may be silenced over time.[86,87] Improvements in the gene transfer technology may eventually make HSCs viable candidates for use in gene therapy.

Due to the inefficiency of gene transfer into HSCs, investigators have turned to the major host cell of HIV-1, the mature CD4+ T cell, as an alternative target for gene therapy. Using CD4+ cells, high levels of transduction can be achieved, and cells can be selected for during expansion in tissue culture prior to reinfusion into the patient.[88] The questions surrounding the use of CD4+ lymphocytes for gene therapy deal with the survival and life span of the cells *in vivo*. Preliminary investigations using non-human primates revealed that a small number of transduced autologous T cells could be recovered from the peripheral blood of rhesus monkeys two years after a single injection of gene-marked cells.[89] Studies in cancer patients suggest that the life span of a mature lymphocyte may be as long as two years.[90] Studies using gene-marked tumor-infiltrating lymphocytes (TIL) demonstrated that reinfused transduced TIL cells survived several weeks.[91] Recent primate studies in which autologous CD4+ lymphocytes were transduced with an anti-HIV-1 retroviral vector indicate that a low level of transduced lymphocytes survive for as long as 21 weeks in the peripheral blood and lymph nodes of these animals.[92] A gene-marking clinical protocol involving identical twins suggests that gene-marked lymphocytes survive at low levels for up to 14 weeks in HIV-1-infected individuals.[93] Results from the adenosine deaminase (ADA-SCID) human gene therapy trial indicate that the infused lymphocytes survive and divide for up to four years post-infusion.[94] The transduced lymphocytes used in the ADA clinical trial are hypothesized to have a survival advantage over nontransduced lymphocytes due to the presence of the ADA gene product. Taken together, this evidence indicates that long-term persistence of mature lymphocytes can be achieved in some experimental settings.

VII. ANTI-HIV-1 ANTISENSE GENE THERAPY CLINICAL TRIALS

The clinical protocols designed for HIV-1-infected individuals can be divided into three categories: (1) gene marking studies; (2) immunotherapy (these gene therapy strategies are aimed at stimulating an anti-HIV-1 immune response); and (3) inhibition of virus replication (these anti-HIV-1 strategies are aimed at the intracellular inhibition of virus replication). This review will only focus on the two approved clinical trials that will attempt to inhibit HIV-1 replication through the use of antisense RNA. One protocol uses the expression of an antisense gene to the TAR region of the HIV-1 genome in combination with a Rev transdominant negative protein, while the other clinical trial utilizes a ribozyme that cleaves within the HIV-1 leader sequence.

A. *Trans*-Dominant Rev in Combination with Antisense-TAR

Activation of the HIV-1 provirus initiates the transcription of multiply spliced RNAs early in the HIV-1 life cycle, and these produce the two key HIV-1 regulatory proteins Tat and Rev.[95] The HIV-1 Tat and Rev proteins are essential, conserved regulatory proteins that are powerful *trans*-activators of HIV-1 viral gene expression. Inhibition of Tat and/or Rev function may preclude HIV-1 gene expression and replication. We, therefore, developed anti-HIV gene therapy strategies aimed at specifically inhibiting the function of Tat and Rev by *trans*-dominant mutant Rev protein and antisense TAR, respectively.

To specifically inhibit the function of Rev, we have generated a new *trans*-dominant Rev mutant (RevTD) based on the previously described Rev M10 mutant, and we showed that the presence of just one point mutation in the activator domain (Leu78 to Asp78) was sufficient to confer a dominant negative phenotype. To inhibit Tat function, we developed an antisense strategy targeted at the HIV-1 TAR element. The TAR element corresponds to an RNA stem-loop structure present within the untranslated leader sequence of all HIV-1 transcripts, including the RNA genome, and is required for HIV-1 Tat function.[96] The interaction between Tat and TAR can lead to a potent transactivation (increasing expression by 20 -to 100-fold) by inducing transcriptional initiation and/or elongation.[97-99] We constructed a retroviral vector that expresses a chimeric $tRNA_i$-Met-antisense TAR fusion transcript complementary to the HIV-1 TAR region.[54] Using transient and stable transfection assays, we showed that antisense-TAR inhibited Tat-mediated transactivation of HIV-1 LTR-CAT in a dose-dependent fashion. The exact mechanism involved in this inhibition is not fully understood, but it may involve inhibition of Tat binding on the TAR element or RNase degradation of the RNA duplex between the antisense TAR and its complementary target sequence. This RNA duplex may also inhibit ribosome binding and consequently inhibit translation.

We have proposed a clinical protocol for AIDS gene therapy using retroviral-mediated gene transfer to deliver antisense-TAR and RevTD genes to syngeneic lymphocytes in identical twins discordant for HIV-1 infection. This phase I pilot study is based on the preclinical data obtained with the antisense-TAR and RevTD retroviral vectors and on the adoptive transfer of NeoR-marked syngeneic CD4+ T-cell in HIV-1 discordant identical twins.[100] In this clinical trial we will evaluate the safety, survival, and potential efficacy of the adoptive transfer of genetically engineered syngeneic lymphocytes obtained from HIV-seronegative identical twins on the functional immune status of HIV-infected twin recipients.[101]

B. Anti-HIV-1 Ribozyme

A clinical protocol for AIDS gene therapy using the HIV-1 leader-specific hairpin ribozyme has been proposed by Wong-Staal and co-workers.[71] In this phase I clinical trial, the safety and efficacy of ribozyme gene therapy will be evaluated in HIV-1-infected patients (CD4 counts between 250 to 500) by reinfusing autologous CD4+ T cells that have been transduced *ex vivo* with a retroviral vector that expresses the HIV-1 leader sequence ribozyme. Transduction of HIV-1-infected cells *in vitro* will require culture conditions that inhibit the spread of endogenous HIV-1 (100 m*M* nevirapine + 10 m*M* CD4-PE40). The *in vivo* kinetics and survival of ribozyme-transduced cells will be compared by limiting dilution PCR with those of a separate aliquot of cells transduced with a control vector (identical except for the ribozyme cassette). The level and persistence of ribozyme expression will also be assessed. The results will determine whether this ribozyme can protect CD4+ T cells in patients with HIV-1 infection and will aid in the design of future trials of hematopoietic stem cell gene therapy for AIDS.

VIII. CONCLUSIONS

A large variety of anti-HIV-1 antisense gene therapy strategies have been developed that effectively inhibit HIV-1 *in vitro*. Significant progress has recently been made in demonstrating that primary CD4+ T lymphocytes can be protected from infection with HIV-1, including primary patient isolates, using gene therapy approaches based on antisense and ribozymes.[27,42] Based on these preclinical findings, two anti-HIV-1 antisense gene therapy strategies have received RAC/FDA approval for testing in HIV-1-infected individuals. It is hoped that these clinical trials will be able to address the question of whether rendering a cell resistant to HIV-1 infection by gene therapy will have a therapeutic benefit to the patient.

REFERENCES

1. Anderson, W. F., Human gene therapy, *Science*, 256, 808, 1992.
2. Cournoyer, D. and Caskey, C. T., Gene therapy of the immune system, *Annu. Rev. Immunol.*, 11, 297, 1993.
3. Baltimore, D., Intracellular immunization, *Nature*, 335, 395, 1988.
4. Miller, A. D., Retroviral vectors, *Curr. Top. Microbiol. Immunol.*, 158, 1, 1992.
5. Morgan, R. A., Retroviral vectors in human gene therapy, *Human Viruses in Gene Therapy*, Vos, J.-M. H., Ed., Academic Press, Durham, NC, 1994, 77.
6. Mulligan, R. C., The basic science of gene therapy, *Science*, 260, 926, 1993.
7. Perricaudet, M. and Stratford-Perricaudet, L. D., Adenovirus-mediated *in vivo* gene therapy, *Human Viruses in Gene Therapy*, Vos, J.-M. H., Ed., Academic Press, Durham, NC, 1994, 1.
8. Rosenfeld, M. A., Siegfried, W., Yoshimura, K., Yonegama, K., Fukayama, M., Steir, L. E., Paakko, P. K., Gilardi, P., Stratford-Perricaudet, L. D., Perricaudet, M., Jallat, S., Pavirani, A., Lecocq, J.-P., and Crystal, R. G., Adenovirus-mediated transfer of a recombinant alpha 1-antitrypsin gene to the lung epithelium *in vivo*, *Science*, 252, 431, 1991.
9. Rosenfeld, M. A., Yoshimura, K., Trapnell, B., Yonegama, K., Rosenthal, E. R., Dalemans, W., Fukayama, M., Bargon, J., Stier, L., Stratford-Perricaudet, L., Perricaudet, M., Guggino, W. B., Pavirani, A., Lecocq, J.-P., and Crystal, R. G., *In vivo* transfer of the human cystic fibrosis transmembrane conductance regulator gene to the airway epithelium, *Cell*, 65, 143, 1992.
10. Muzyczka, N., Use of adeno-associated virus as a general transduction vector for mammalian cells, *Curr. Top. Microbiol. Immunol.*,158, 97, 1992.
11. Samulski, R. J., Parvoviruses, *Human Viruses in Gene Therapy*, Vos, J.-M. H., Ed., Academic Press, Durham, NC, 1994, 53.
12. Felgner, P. L., Gadek, T. R., and Holm, M., Lipofection: A highly efficient, lipid-mediated DNA-transfection procedure, *Proc. Natl. Acad. Sci. U.S.A.*, 84, 7413, 1987.
13. Wu, G. Y., Wilson, J. M., and Shalaby, F., Receptor-mediated gene delivery *in vivo*: Partial correction of genetic analbuminemia in Nagase rats, *J. Biol. Chem.*, 266, 14338, 1991.
14. Miller, A. D. and Buttimore, C., Redesign of retrovirus packaging cell lines to avoid recombination leading to helper virus production, *Mol. Cell. Biol.*, 6, 2895, 1986.
15. Miller, A. D., Garcia, J. V., von Suhr, N., Lynch, C. M., Wilson, C., and Eiden, M., Construction and properties of retrovirus packaging cells based on gibbon ape leukemia virus, *J. Virol.*, 65, 2220, 1991.
16. Miller, A. D., Miller, D. G., Garcia, J. V., and Lynch, C. M, Use of retroviral vectors for gene transfer and expression, *Methods Enzymol.*, 217, 581, 1993.
17. Bender, M. A., Palmer, T. D., Gelinas, R. E., and Miller, A. D., Evidence that the packaging signal of Moloney murine leukemia virus extends into the gag region, *J. Virol.*, 61, 1639, 1987.
18. Miller, A. D. and Roseman, G. J., Improved retroviral vectors for gene transfer and expression, *BioTechniques*, 7, 980, 1989.
19. McLachlin, J. R., Mittereder, N., Daucher, M. B., Kadan, M., and Eglitis, M. A., Factors affecting retroviral vector function and structural integrity, *Virology*, 195, 1, 1993.
20. Faustinella, F., Kwon, H., Serrano, F., Belmont, J. W., Caskey, C. T., and Aguilar-Cordova, E., A new family of murine retroviral vectors with extended multiple cloning sites for gene insertion, *Hum. Gene Ther.*, 5, 307, 1994.

21. Morgenstern, J. P. and Land, H., Advanced mammalian gene transfer: High titre retroviral vectors with multiple drug selection markers and a complementary helper-free packaging cell line, *Nucleic Acids Res.*, 18, 3587, 1990.
22. Miller, A. D. and Roseman, G. J., Improved retroviral vectors for gene transfer and expression, *BioTechniques*, 7, 980, 1989.
23. Ohashi, T., Boggs, S., Robbins, P., Bahnson, A., Patrene, K., Wei, F.-S., Wei, J.-F., Li, J., Lucht, L., Fei, Y., Clark, S., Kimak, M., He, H., Mowery-Rushton, P., and Barranger, J. A., Efficient transfer and sustained high expression of the human glucocerebrosidase gene in mice and their functional macrophages following transplantation of bone marrow transduced by a retroviral vector, *Proc. Natl. Acad. Sci. U.S.A.*, 89, 11332, 1992.
24. Jaffee, E. M., Dranoff, G., Cohen, L. K., Hauda, K. M., Mulligan, R. C., and Pardol, D., High efficiency gene transfer into primary human tumor explants, *Cancer Res.*, 53, 2221, 1993.
25. Hoeben, R. C., Migchielsen, A. A. J., vander Jagt, R. C. M., van Ormondt, H., and Vander Eb, A. J., Inactivation of the Moloney murine leukemia virus long terminal repeat in murine fibroblast cell lines is associated with methylation and dependent on its chromosomal position, *J. Virol.*, 65, 904, 1991.
26. Palmer, T. D., Rosman, G. J., Osborne, W. R. A., and Miller, A. D., Genetically modified skin fibroblasts persist long after transplantation but inactivate introduced genes, *Proc. Natl. Acad. Sci. U.S.A.*, 88, 1330, 1991.
27. Couture, L. A., Mullen, C. A., and Morgan, R. A., Retroviral vectors containing chimeric promoter/enhancer elements exhibit cell-type-specific gene expression, *Hum. Gene Ther.*, 5, 667, 1994.
28. Moore, K. A., Scarpa, M., Kooyer, S., Utter, A., Caskey, C. T., and Belmont, J. W., Evaluation of lymphoid specific enhancer addition or substitution on a basic retroviral vector, *Hum. Gene Ther.*, 2, 307, 1991.
29. Valerio, D., Einerhard, M. P. W., Wamsley, P. M., Bakx, T. A., Li, C. L., and Verma, I. M., Retrovirus-mediated gene transfer into embryonal carcinoma and hematopoietic stem cells: Expression from a hybrid long terminal repeat, *Gene*, 84, 419, 1989.
30. Cepko, C. L., Roberts, B. E., and Mulligan, R. C., Construction and applications of a highly transmissable murine retrovirus shuttle vector, *Cell*, 37, 1053, 1984.
31. Korman, A. J., Frantz, J. D., Strominger, J. L., and Mulligan, R. C., Expression of human class II major histocompatability complex antigens using retrovirus vectors, *Proc. Natl. Acad. Sci. U.S.A.*, 84, 2150, 1987.
32. Adam, M. A., Ramesh, N., Miller, A. D., and Osborne, W. R. A., Internal initiation of translation in retroviral vectors carrying picornavirus 5′ nontranslated regions, *J. Virol.*, 65, 4985, 1991.
33. Morgan, R. A., Couture, L., Elroy-Stein, O., Ragheb, J., Moss, B., and Anderson, W. F., Retroviral vectors containing putative internal ribosome entry sites: development of a polycistronic gene transfer system and applications to human gene therapy, *Nucleic Acids Res.*, 20, 1293, 1992.
34. Hantzopolous, P. A., Sullenger, B. A., Ungers, G., and Gilboa, E., Improved gene expression upon transfer of the adenosine deaminase minigene outside the transcriptional unit of a retroviral vector, *Proc. Natl. Acad. Sci. U.S.A.*, 86, 3519, 1989.
35. Sullenger, B. A., Gallardo, H. F., Ungers, G. E., and Gilboa, E., Analysis of trans-acting response decoy RNA-mediated inhibition of human immunodeficiency virus type 1 transactivation, *J. Virol.*, 65, 6811, 1991.
36. Sullenger, B. A., Lee, T. C., Smith, C. A., Ungers, G. E., and Gilboa, E., *Mol. Cell. Biol.*, 10, 6512, 1990.
37. Naldini, L., Blomer, U., Gallay, P., Ory, D., Mulligan, R. C., Gage, F. H., Verma, I. M., and Trono, D., *In vivo* gene delivery and stable transduction of nondividing cells by a lentiviral vector, *Science*, 272, 263, 1996.
38. Kinchington, D., Galpin, S., Jaroszewski, J., Ghosh, K., Subasinghe, C., and Cohen, J. S., A comparison of gag, pol and rev antisense oligodeoxynucleotides as inhibitors of HIV-1, *Antiviral Res.*, 17, 53, 1992.
39. Morvan, F., Porumb, H., Degols, G., Lefebvre, I., Pompon, A., Sproat, B. A., Raynor, B., Malvy, C., Lebleu, B., and Imbach, J.-L., Comparative evaluation of seven oligonucleotide analogues as potential antisense agents, *J. Med. Chem.*, 36, 280, 1993.
40. Lisziewicz, J., Sun, D., Klotman, M., Agrawal, S., Zamencik, P., and Gallo, R., Specific inhibition of human immunodeficiency virus type 1 replication by antisense oligonucleotides: An *in vitro* model for treatment, *Proc. Natl. Acad. Sci. U.S.A.*, 89, 11209, 1992.
41. Lisziewicz, J., Sun, D., Metelev, V., Zamencik, P., Gallo, R. C., and Agrawal, S., Long-term treatment of human immunodeficiency virus-infected cells with antisense oligonucleotide phosphorothioates, *Proc. Natl. Acad. Sci. U.S.A.*, 90, 3860, 1993.
42. Bordier, B., Helene, C., Barr, P. J., Litvak, S., and Sarih-Cottin, L., *In vitro* effect of antisense oligonucleotides on human immunodeficiency virus type 1 reverse transcription, *Nucleic Acids Res.*, 20, 5999, 1992.

43. Agrawal, S. and Tang, J. Y., GEM 91 — An antisense oligonucleotide phosphorothioate as a therapeutic agent for AIDS, *Antisense Res. Dev.*, 2, 261, 1992.
44. Rhodes, A. and James, W., Inhibition of heterologous strains of HIV by antisense RNA, *AIDS*, 5, 145, 1991.
45. Sczakiel, G. and Pawlita, M., Inhibition of human immunodeficiency virus type 1 replication in human T cells stably expressing antisense RNA, *J. Virol.*, 1991, 65, 468, 1991.
46. Rhodes, A. and James, W., Inhibition of human immunodeficiency virus replication in cell culture by endogenously synthesized antisense RNA, *J. Gen. Virol.*, 71, 1965, 1990.
47. Joshi, S., Van Brunschot, A., Asad, S., Van Der Elst, I., Read, S. E., and Bernstein, A., Inhibition of human immunodeficiency virus type 1 multiplication by antisense and sense RNA expression, *J. Virol.*, 65, 5524, 1991.
48. Rittner, K., Burmester, C., and Sczakiel, J., *In vitro* selection of fast-hybridizing and effective antisense RNAs directed against the human immunodeficiency virus type 1, *Nucleic Acids Res.*, 21, 1381, 1993.
49. Gyotoko, J.-I., El-Farrash, M. A., Fujimoto, S., Gemeraad, W. T., Watanabe, Y., Teshigawara, K., Harada, S., and Katsura, Y., Inhibition of human immunodeficiency virus replication in a human T cell line by antisense RNA expressed in the cell, *Virus Genes*, 5, 189, 1991.
50. Rittner, K. and Sczakiel, J., Identification and analysis of antisense RNA target regions of the human immunodeficiency virus type 1, *Nucleic Acids Res.*, 19, 1421, 1991.
51. Sczakiel, G., Oppenlander, M., Rittner, K., and Pawlita, M., Tat- and rev-directed antisense RNA expression inhibits and abolishes replication of human immunodeficiency virus type 1: A temporal analysis, *J. Virol.*, 66, 5576, 1992.
52. Chatterjee, S., Johnson, P. R., and Wong, K. K., Dual-target inhibition of HIV-1 *in vitro* by means of an adeno-associated virus antisense vector, *Science*, 258, 1485, 1992.
53. Chuah, M. K. L., VandenDriessche, T., Chang, H., Ensoli, B., and Morgan, R. A., Inhibition of human immunodeficiency virus type-1 by retroviral vectors expressing antisense TAR, *Hum. Gene Ther.*, 5, 1467, 1994.
54. VandenDriessche, T., Chuah, M. K. L., Chiang, L., Chang, H.-K., Ensoli, B., and Morgan, R. A., Inhibition of clinical human immunodeficiency virus (HIV) type 1 isolates in primary CD4+ T lymphocytes by retroviral vectors expressing anti-HIV genes, *J. Virol.*, 69, 4045, 1995.
55. Chang, H.-K., VandenDriessche, T., Chuah, M. K. L., Morgan, R. A., Gallo, R. C., and Ensoli, B., Inhibition of HIV-1 replication by simultaneously blocking Tat and Rev function with vectors expressing an antisense tat/rev RNA, *AIDS Res. Hum. Retrov.*, in press.
56. Chang, H-K., Gendelman, R., Lisziewicz, J., Gallo, R. C., and Ensoli, B., Block of HIV-1 infection by a combination of antisense tat RNA and TAR decoys: a strategy for control of HIV-1, *Gene Ther.*, 1, 208, 1994.
57. Lisziewicz, J, Sun, D., Trapnell, B., Thomson, M., Chang, H.-K., Ensoli, B., and Peng, B., An autoregulated dual function antitat gene for human immunodeficiency virus type 1 gene therapy, *J. Virol.*, 69, 206, 1995.
58. Lisziewicz, J., Sun, D., Liszciewicz, A., and Gallo, R. C., Antitat gene therapy: A candidate for late-stage AIDS patients, *Gene Ther.*, 2, 218, 1995.
59. Lori, F., Lisziewicz, J., Smythe, J., Cara, A., Bunnag, T. A., Curiel, D., and Gallo, R. C., Rapid protection against human immunodeficiency virus type 1 (HIV-1) replication by high efficiency non-retroviral delivery of genes interfering with HIV-1 tat and gag, *Gene Ther.*, 1, 27, 1994.
60. Cagnon, L., Cucchiarini, M., Lefebvre, J.-C., and Doglio, A., Protection of a T-cell line from human immunodeficiency virus replication by the stable expression of a short antisense RNA sequence carried by a shuttle RNA molecule, *J. AIDS Hum. Retrov.*, 9, 349, 1995.
61. Sullenger, B. A., Gallardo, H. F., Ungers, G. E., and Gilboa, E., Overexpression of TAR sequences renders cells resistant to human immunodeficiency virus replication, *Cell*, 63, 601, 1990.
62. Lee, S.-W., Gallardo, H. F., Gilboa, E., and Smith, C., Inhibition of human immunodeficiency virus in human T cells by a potent Rev response element decoy consisting of the 13-nucleotide minimal rev-binding domain, *J. Virol.*, 68, 8254, 1994.
63. Lisziewicz, J., Rappaport, J., and Dhar, R., Tat-regulated production of multimerized TAR RNA inhibits HIV-1 gene expression, *New Biol.*, 1991, 3, 82, 1991.
64. Cech, T. R., Zaug, A. J., and Grabowski, P. J., *In vitro* splicing of the ribosomal RNA precursor of Tetrahymena: Involvement of a guanosine nucleotide in the excision of the intervening sequence, *Cell*, 27, 487, 1981.
65. Cech, T. R., Self-splicing group I introns, *Annu. Rev. Biochem.*, 59, 543, 1990.
66. Campbell, T. B. and Sullenger, B. A., Alternative approaches for the application of ribozymes as gene therapies for retroviral infections, *Adv. Pharmacol.*, 33, 143, 1995.
67. Koizumi, M., Iwai, S., and Ohtsuka, E., Construction of a series of several self-cleaving RNA duplexes using synthetic 21-mers, *FEBS Lett.*, 228, 228, 1988.

68. Ruffner, D. E., Stormo, G. D., and Uhlenbeck, O. C., Studies on the requirements of the hammerhead RNA self-cleavage reaction, *Biochemistry,* 29, 10695, 1990.
69. Chowrira, B. M., Berzal-Herranz, A., and Burke, J. M., Novel guanosine requirement for catalysis by the hairpin ribozyme, *Nature,* 354, 320, 1991.
70. Dropulic, B., Lin, N. H., Martin, M. A., and Jeang, K. T., Functional characterization of a U5 ribozyme: Intracellular suppression of human immunodeficiency virus type 1 expression, *J. Virol.,* 66, 1432, 1992.
71. Wong-Staal, F., Yu, M., Yamada, O., Leavitt, M., Marwyama, M., and Ho, A., Development of ribozyme gene therapy against HIV, *J. Cell. Biochem. Suppl.,* 18A, 221, 1994.
72. Yamada, O., Yu, M., Yee, J. K., Kraus, G., Looney, D., and Wong-Staal, F., Intracellular immunization of human cells with a hairpin ribozyme against human immunodeficiency virus type 1, *Gene Ther.,* 1, 38, 1994.
73. Leavitt, M. C., Yu, M., Yamada, O., Kraus, G., Looney, D., Poeschla, E., and Wong-Staal, F., Transfer of an anti-HIV-1 ribozyme gene into primary human lymphocytes. *Hum. Gene Ther.,* 5, 1115, 1994.
74. Richman, D. D., HIV drug resistance, *Annu. Rev. Pharmacol. Toxicol.,* 33, 149, 1993.
75. Pieken, W. A., Olsen, D. B., Benseler, F., Aurup, H., and Eckstein, F., Kinetic characterization of ribonuclease-resistant 2′-modified hammerhead ribozymes, *Science,* 253, 314, 1991.
76. Sarver, N., Cantin, E. M., Chang, P. S., Zaia, J. A., Ladne, P. A., Stephens, D. A., and Rossi, J. J., Ribozymes as potential anti-HIV-1 therapeutic agents, *Science,* 247, 1222, 1990.
77. Weerasinghe, M., Liem, S. E., Asad, S., Read, S. E., and Joshi, S., Resistance to human immunodeficiency virus type 1 (HIV-1) infection in human CD4+ lymphocyte-derived cell lines conferred by using retroviral vectors expressing an HIV-1 RNA-specific ribozyme, *J. Virol.,* 65, 5531, 1991.
78. Sun, L. Q., Wang, L., Gerlach, W. L., and Symonds, G., Target sequence-specific inhibition of HIV-1 replication by ribozymes directed to tat RNA, *Nucleic Acids Res.,* 23, 2909, 1995.
79. Sun, L. Q., Pyati, J., Smythie, J., Wang, L, Macpherson, J., Gerlach, W., and Symonds, G., Resistance to human immunodeficiency virus type 1 infection conferred by transduction with ribozyme, antisense, or polymeric trans-activation response element constructs, *Proc. Natl. Acad. Sci. U.S.A.,* 92, 7272, 1995.
80. Chen, C. J., Banerjea, A. C., Harrison, G. G., Haglund, K., and Schubert, M., Multitarget-ribozyme directed to cleave at up to nine highly conserved HIV-1 env RNA regions inhibits HIV-1 replication-potential effectiveness against most presently sequenced HIV-1 isolates, *Nucleic Acids Res.,* 20, 4581, 1992.
81. Zhou, C., Bahner, I. C., Larson, G. P., Zaia, J. A., Rossi, J. J., and Kohn D. B., Inhibition of HIV-1 in human T-lymphocytes by retrovirally transduced anti-tat and rev ribozymes, *Gene,* 149, 33, 1994.
82. Sullenger, B. A. and Cech, T. R., Tethering ribozymes to a retroviral packaging signal for destruction of viral RNA, *Science,* 262, 1566, 1993.
83. Rill, D. R., Moen, R. C., Buschle, M., Bartholomew, C., Foreman, N. K., Mirro, Jr., J., Krance, R. A., Ihle, J. N., and Brenner, M. K., An approach for the analysis of relapse and marrow reconstitution after autologous marrow transplantation using retrovirus-mediated gene transfer, *Blood,* 15, 2694, 1992.
84. Van Beusechem, V. W., Kukler, A., Heidt, P. J., and Valerio, D., Long-term expression of human adenosine deaminase in rhesus monkeys transplanted with retrovirus-infected bone-marrow cells. *Proc. Natl. Acad. Sci. U.S.A.,* 89, 7640, 1992.
85. Kohn, D. B., Weinberg, K. I., Nolta, J., Heiss, L. N., Lenarsky, C., Crooks, G. M., Hanley, M., Annett, G., Brooks, J. S., El-Khoureiy, A., Lawrence, K., Wells, S., Moen, R. C., Bastian, J., Williams-Herman, D. E., Elder, M., Wara, D., Bowen, T., Hershfield, M. S., Mullen, C. A., Blaese, R. M., and Parkman, R., Engraftment of gene-modified umbilical cord blood cells in neonates with adenosine deaminase deficiency, *Natl. Med.,* 1, 1017, 1995.
86. Apperly, J. F., Luskey, B. D., and Williams, D. A., Retroviral gene transfer of human adenosine deaminase in murine hematopoietic cells: Effect of selectable marker sequences on long-term expression, *Blood,* 78, 310, 1991.
87. Challita, P.-M. and Kohn, D. B., Lack of expression from a retroviral vector after transduction of murine hematopoietic stem cells is associated with methylation *in vivo, Proc. Natl. Acad. Sci. U.S.A.,* 91, 2567, 1994.
88. Culver, K., Cornetta, K., Morgan, R., Morecki, S., Aebersold, P., Kasid, A., Lotze, M., Rosenberg, S. A., Anderson, W. F., and Blaese, R. M., Lymphocytes as cellular vehicles for gene therapy in mouse and man. *Proc. Natl. Acad. Sci. U.S.A .,* 88, 3155, 1991.
89. Culver, K. C., Morgan, R. A., Osborne, W. R., Lee, R. T., Lenschow, D., Able, C., Cornetta, K., Anderson, W. F., and Blaese, R. M., In vivo expression and survival of gene-modified T lymphocytes in rhesus monkeys, *Hum. Gene Ther.,* 1, 399, 1990.
90. Michie, C. A., McLean, A., Alcock, C., and Beverley, P. C. L., Lifespan of human lymphocyte subsets defined by CD45 idoforms, *Nature,* 360, 264, 1992.

91. Rosenberg, S. A., Aebersold, P. M., Cornetta, K., Kasid, A., Morgan, R. A., Moen, R., Karson, E. M., Lotze, M. T., Yang, J. C., Topalian, S. L., Merino, M. J., Culver, K., Miller, A. D., Blaese, R. M., and Anderson, W. F., Gene transfer into humans: Immunotherapy of patients with advanced melanoma using tumor infiltrating lymphocytes modified by retroviral gene transduction, *N. Engl. J. Med.*, 323, 570, 1990.
92. Bunnell, B. A., Unpublished data, 1996.
93. Walker, R., Personal communication, 1996.
94. Blaese, R. M., Culver, K. W., Miller, A. D., Carter, C. S., Fleisher, T., Clerici, M., Shearer, G., Chang, L., Tolstoshev, P., Greenblatt, J. J., Rosenberg, S. A., Klein, H., Berger, M., Mullen, C. A., Ramsey, W. J., Muul, L., Morgan, R. A., and Anderson, W.F., T lymphocyte-directed gene therapy for ADA$^-$SCID: Initial trial results after four years, *Science*, 270, 475, 1995.
95. Vaishnav, Y. N. and Wong-Staal, F., The biochemistry of AIDS, *Annu. Rev. Biochem.*, 60, 577, 1991.
96. Frankel, A. D., Activation of HIV transcription by Tat, *Curr. Opin. Genet. Dev.*, 2, 293, 1992.
97. Berkhout, B., Silverman, R. H., and Jeang, K. T., Tat trans-activates the human immunodeficiency virus through a nascent RNA target, *Cell*, 59, 273, 1989.
98. Cullen, B. R., Does HIV-1 Tat induce a change in viral initiation rights?, *Cell*, 73, 417, 1992.
99. Laspia, M. F., Rice, A. P., and Mathews, M. B., HIV-1 tat protein increases transcriptional initiation and stabilizes elongation, *Cell*, 59, 283, 1989.
100. Walker, R., A study of the safety and survival of the adoptive transfer of genetically marked syngeneic lymphocytes in HIV-infected identical twins, *Hum. Gene Ther.*, 4, 659, 1993.
101. VandenDriessche, T., Chuah, M. K. L., and Morgan, R. A., Gene therapy for acquired immune deficiency syndrome, *AIDS Updates*, DeVita, V. T., Hellman, S., and Rosenberg, S. A., Eds., J. B. Lippincott, Philadelphia, PA, 1994, 7 (4):1-14.

Chapter 11

Use of Antisense RNA Expression Vectors In Neurobiology

Genoveva Davidkova, Sui-Po Zhang, Long-Wu Zhou, Robert A. Nichols, and Benjamin Weiss

CONTENTS

0-8493-8552-0/97/$0.00+$.50

I. INTRODUCTION

A variety of tools have been employed to investigate neurobiological processes. These include behavioral manipulations, surgical interventions, neurotoxins, naturally occurring neurotransmitters and neuromodulators, and a variety of synthetic pharmacological agents. In all these studies, one is confronted with the fundamental problem of selectivity, and in the case of pharmacological tools, the additional problem of the design and synthesis of these agents. An understanding of the genetic basis that governs neurobiological events has ushered in a new era in experimental biology and offers the opportunity to make giant strides in controlling hitherto uncontrollable events.

The enormous progress in the cloning and sequencing of genes involved in neurobiological events and the elucidation of the identity, sites, and mechanisms of action of transcription modulators, such as activators, enhancers, and repressors has allowed the development of new and important strategies to study and alter biological events. These strategies have opened an opportunity for using a far more rational and selective approach to neuropharmacology. This new approach targets one of the several sites between gene transcription and protein synthesis.

One potential site for targeting involves those sites on the DNA with which transcription modulators interact. Nucleotides having the same sequence as these sites ("sense sequences") can now be designed. Use of these synthetic sequences in this competitive "sense" strategy would result in an alteration of the interaction of transcription modulators with their target DNA on a specific gene. Using an "antisense" strategy, nucleotides can also be designed either to interact with specific sequences on the gene forming a triple helix (triplex) or, through complementary Watson-Crick base pairing, to target the specific RNA encoding a particular protein under study.

Two general means of delivering antisense compounds have been developed. First is the use of antisense oligodeoxynucleotides, which, by forming DNA:RNA hybrids with target mRNA, may inhibit the translation of proteins. These agents can be directly administered *in vitro* or into living organisms. The other involves the use of vectors carrying DNA sequences encoding RNA that is antisense to the targeted mRNAs. These latter agents, when expressed in cells, inhibit translation by forming RNA:RNA hybrids.

This review will consider the advantages and disadvantages of the different antisense approaches to inhibit gene expression and will provide examples of the application of these novel tools in studying certain neurobiological processes, concentrating our attention largely on the use of antisense RNA-generating plasmid vectors. In particular, it will include examples from our laboratory on the use of antisense RNA expression plasmid vectors, one *in vitro* in tissue culture to study cellular growth and differentiation by altering the function of calmodulin, and the other, *in vivo* in mouse brain to study the actions and potential therapeutic applications of these agents in reversing behaviors associated with excessive dopaminergic activity.

Following delivery into cells, the antisense RNA can be continuously expressed by viral-based or nonviral plasmid-based vectors. The main merit in using antisense RNA expression vectors is the possibility of achieving persistent inhibition of gene expression after a single application of these agents. While there are abundant reports on the use of antisense oligodeoxynucleotides in neurobiology, there are relatively few studies on the use of antisense RNA expressed from plasmid vectors in neuronal cells. This might be due to the slow or nondividing nature of primary nerve cells, which has created technical difficulties in the culturing, transfection, and selection of stably transfected cells.

II. COMPARISON BETWEEN THE USE OF CONVENTIONAL PHARMACOTHERAPIES AND ANTISENSE STRATEGY

Intracellularly generated antisense RNA and antisense oligodeoxynucleotides hybridize to the complementary endogenous mRNA and act by one of several possible mechanisms to prevent the synthesis of the protein product.[1-4] Both the expression of antisense RNA by means of nonviral plasmid vectors and the use of antisense oligodeoxynucleotides share several advantages over traditional pharmacological antagonists (Table 1). In particular, antisense approaches have the potential for high specificity, being able to discriminate minute differences in mRNA structure. In addition, these agents can be readily targeted to the mRNAs for cell-surface receptors as well as specific intracellular proteins. In contrast, conventional pharmacotherapeutic drugs are often limited in their ability to act on intracellular sites, many of these compounds being hydrophilic, and those that penetrate cells often lack specificity for particular intracellular proteins. Moreover, inhibiting the synthesis of neuroreceptors using antisense oligomers would not be expected to cause receptor upregulation, a major complication arising from the use of traditional pharmacological antagonists.[5-8] Another advantage of the antisense compounds (oligodeoxynucleotides and antisense RNA) is the relative ease with which they can be designed and synthesized on the basis of limited knowledge of a portion of the gene sequence.

It is important to note that not all antisense oligodeoxynucleotides are specific and that some, particularly those that have been chemically modified to form phosphorothioates in order to increase their nuclease resistance, have been shown to have nonspecific, sequence-independent effects or non-antisense, sequence-specific effects (see Chapter 4). Therefore, as in all studies, strict controls should be performed to determine not only their specificity of action but also their mechanism of action.[9]

TABLE 1

Comparison Between Antisense Strategies and Conventional Pharmacological Treatment

Advantages of an Antisense Strategy
A. Rational and relative ease of designing antisense agents
B. Relative ease of synthesizing antisense agents
C. Capable of highly specific targeting of both cell surface receptors and intracellular proteins
D. Easier to develop proper controls
E. No upregulation of inhibited receptors
Advantages of Conventional Pharmacotherapy
A. More readily penetrate tissues, especially blood-brain barrier
B. May have a more rapid onset, especially if target protein has a long half-life
C. More shallow dose-response curve, which may provide a greater therapeutic index
D. Better acceptance among clinicians

III. COMPARISON BETWEEN THE PROPERTIES OF ANTISENSE RNA EXPRESSION VECTORS AND ANTISENSE OLIGODEOXYNUCLEOTIDES

In some instances the use of vector-expressed antisense RNA may have important advantages over the use of antisense oligodeoxynucleotides (Table 2). The duration of action of antisense RNA generated continuously inside the cell may be far longer than that of antisense oligodeoxynucleotides.[9] This might be of special importance, for example, if the antisense RNA has to be administered intracerebrally for therapeutic purposes. The longer duration of action might be beneficial in studies of processes that take place over a long period of time, such as neurite outgrowth and cell differentiation.[10,11] The antisense RNA produced by a plasmid vector might be less toxic than oligodeoxynucleotides, especially the phosphorothioate derivatives, which have the propensity to bind nonspecifically to proteins and have been shown to have toxic effects after repeated administration at high doses.[12-14] The antisense expression vector's RNA may be delivered into the nervous system with a greater efficiency than antisense oligodeoxynucleotides, as certain viral vectors, particularly herpesvirus, exhibit neurotropism. Finally, the antisense RNA can be selectively targeted to[15-17] and expressed[18-21] only in certain cell types.

TABLE 2

Advantages of Antisense RNA Expression Vectors Over Antisense Oligodeoxynucleotides

Antisense RNA Expression Vectors
A. Are longer lasting
B. May be less toxic (especially nonviral vectors)
C. May be able to penetrate tissues better (especially viral vectors)
D. Are able to express the antisense RNA in specific cell types through the use of tissue-specific transcription factors
E. Are able to express the antisense RNA at specific times through the use of inducible promoters

IV. VECTOR SYSTEMS FOR THE TRANSFECTION OF NERVE CELLS, CHARACTERISTICS OF NONVIRAL PLASMID VECTORS AND ADVANTAGES OVER VIRAL VECTORS AS VEHICLES FOR DELIVERY AND EXPRESSION OF ANTISENSE RNA

In discussing the vector systems suitable to deliver antisense RNA to cells of the nervous system, a distinction has to be made between the transfection of established neuronal cell lines, which are relatively homogeneous populations of dividing cells, and primary neuronal cultures or nerve tissue *in vivo*, which are, under most circumstances, a nonhomogeneous population of nondividing and dividing cells. While many eukaryotic expression vectors and transfection methods have been developed for established cell lines originating from cells of the nervous system,[22-25] primary neurons in culture and nerve tissue *in vivo* have been relatively difficult to transfect. In addition, unique vector requirements exist for the *in vivo* transfection of tumors of the nervous system, which are comprised of rapidly dividing cells.

Several viral and nonviral vector systems have been employed for the delivery of recombinant DNA to primary cultures of nerve cells or established neural cell lines *in vitro* and to primary nerve tissue *in vivo*. The characteristics and the relative merits of these nonviral and viral vectors are summarized in Table 3. Specific examples of the use of some of these vectors are discussed below.

TABLE 3

Relative Merits of Viral and Nonviral Plasmid Vectors in Gene Therapy

	Nonviral Vectors		Viral Vectors
A.	Little or no immunogenic properties	A.	Adenoviral vectors are immunogenic
B.	Do not produce potentially toxic viral proteins	B.	Viral vectors may produce toxic viral proteins
C.	Do not integrate into genomic DNA • No genomic alterations • Not permanent	C.	Adeno-associated viral and retroviral vectors integrate into genomic DNA • Possibility that integration produces gene inactivation or neoplasms
D.	Variable degree of penetration into different cell types	D.	Likely to penetrate cells easily • Herpes virus exhibits neurotropism
E.	Effective in cells with different potential for division	E.	Certain viral vectors are effective only in dividing cells
		F.	Difficulty in producing high titers

A. Viral Vectors

Among the viral vectors, the use of herpes simplex virus-based (HSV-1) vectors has been most extensively explored for their ability to deliver recombinant DNA to the nervous system. Their main advantage is the neurotropism of HSV-1, as HSV-1-based vectors infect neurons with very high efficiency.[26-29] The usefulness of these vectors, however, has been often limited by the neurotoxicity of HSV-1.[30,31] Retroviral,[32-34] adenoviral,[35-37] and adeno-associated vectors[38] have also been used as vehicles to deliver foreign genes into the nervous system, but with certain limitations. The majority of the retroviral vectors are effective only in dividing cells.[34] Adenoviral vectors are often immunogenic which limits their repeated administration.[39] Adeno-associated viral vectors set constraints on the size of the cloned genetic material.[40] Additional safety concerns arise from the inherent pathogenicity of viruses,[34,40] in spite of the use of nonreplicative viruses, and from the possibilities for insertional inactivation of genes or neoplastic transformation due to vector integration into the genome.[41-43] Other disadvantages of the viral-based vectors are the technical difficulties that exist in the production of high-titer viral vectors for *in vivo* use (Table 3).

That the nonviral plasmid vectors remain episomal *in vivo* may, in some cases, be viewed as a disadvantage since this would result in a relatively transient expression. However, unlike most cells, mature brain cells show little or no proliferative activity, and therefore the plasmid vectors, although not being incorporated into the genome of nerve cells, would be expected to have a relatively long duration of action.

B. Nonviral Vectors

The use of nonviral plasmid vectors obviates most of the aforementioned disadvantages and *in vivo* safety concerns of viral-based vectors (see Table 3). Direct injection into the central nervous system (CNS) of nonviral plasmid vectors harboring genes has been reported in several studies.[44-48] These studies have, however, explored the possibility of expressing foreign "sense" genes in brain; there are few if any reports on the *in vivo* use of nonviral plasmid vectors generating antisense RNA.

The plasmids used to express foreign genes have either been directly injected into the brain[44-47] or brain tumors,[48] or have been administered intracerebroventricularly.[49] The expression of these transfected genes has lasted from several days[44,47] up to several weeks.[45,46,49] Nonviral plasmid vectors, however, have not been widely used *in vivo* due to the relative difficulty with which they penetrate into cells. Some transfection procedures which are effective for cells in culture, such as transfection with calcium phosphate/DNA precipitates[22,50,51] and electroporation,[23,52,53] and particle-mediated gene transfer into neuronal slices,[54] are not applicable *in vivo*, because of the potential cytotoxicity of these methods and the limited tissue accessibility. To overcome these problems, methods have been devised for the more efficient introduction of nonviral plasmid vector DNA into cells *in vivo*: direct injection of naked plasmid DNA into tissues,[55-57] cationic lipid-mediated transfection,[25,48,58-63] and complexing of the plasmid DNA with ligands which bind to cell surface receptors.[15,16,48,64] We will discuss in greater detail the cationic lipid-mediated approach, since it has been found to be a very effective and relatively nontoxic means for introducing nonviral plasmid vector DNA into a variety of cell types, both *in vitro* and *in vivo*, and has been the most widely used approach to introduce nonviral plasmid vectors into the central nervous system.

C. Cationic Lipid-Mediated Delivery of Plasmid DNA

A number of different cationic lipid formulations have been used to transfect nonviral plasmid DNA *in vivo*, each varying in their cytotoxicity and transfection-enhancing ability.[44,47-49,65,66] In addition, for each individual cell type, the optimal type of lipid and ratio of lipid-to-plasmid DNA needs to be determined.[47,67] For example, in studies using a D_2 antisense vector we have found that a greater degree of inhibition of D_2 dopamine-mediated function (determined in behavioral studies) is achieved using the cationic lipid DOTAP as compared to lipofectin.[68,69]

A schematic representation of the postulated mechanism of delivery of plasmid vectors expressing antisense RNA into cells by means of cationic lipids and the possible mechanisms by which the antisense RNA produced by the vector inhibits the synthesis of specific proteins is shown in Figure 1. It has been proposed that a

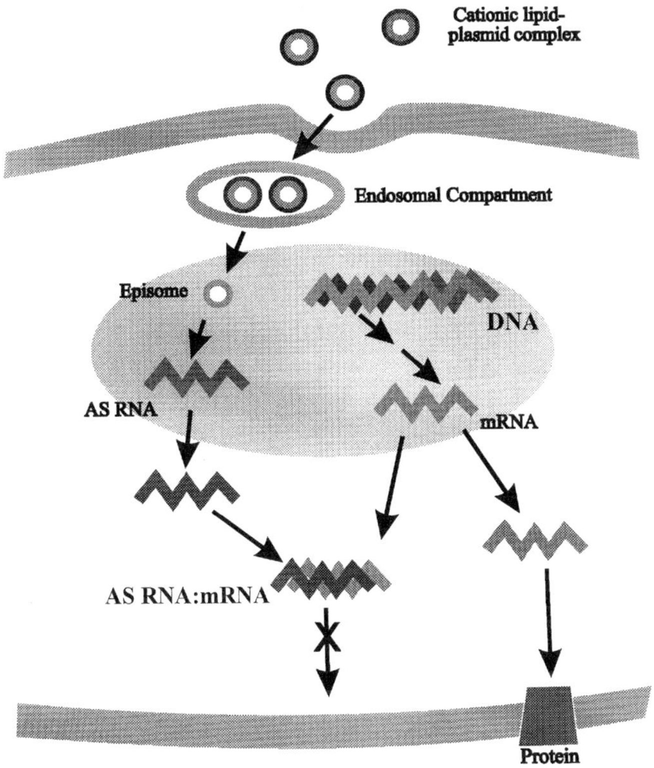

FIGURE 1
Schematic representation of the inhibition of specific proteins by means of antisense RNA delivered by a nonviral plasmid DNA-cationic liposome vector. A stable lipid-plasmid DNA complex can be formed *in vitro* when positively charged cationic lipids interact spontaneously with negatively charged DNA molecules. These complexes are then endocytosed and enter the cell. Once in the cytosol, the cationic lipid-complexed DNA can either escape lysosomal degradation, and the DNA can enter the cell nucleus and be expressed (episome), or the complexes can be delivered into the lysosome where the DNA may be degraded (not shown). The antisense RNA produced from the vector can hybridize to the targeted RNA either in the nucleus or in the cytoplasm and can act by one of several different possible mechanisms to inhibit the expression of the specific protein.

stable lipid-plasmid DNA complex can be formed spontaneously *in vitro* by the interaction between cationic lipids and the negatively charged DNA molecules. When administered, these complexes enter the cell, probably by a pinocytotic mechanism, forming an endosomal compartment. The mechanism by which the plasmid DNA reaches the nucleus is not well understood, but it has been suggested that the cationic lipids could act by preventing the delivery of DNA to the lysosomes. This would allow the DNA molecules to remain intact for a relatively long period of time and, therefore, be available for transfer from the endosomes to the cytosol and, perhaps, from the cytosol to the nucleus.[60,63] This concept is supported by studies involving microinjection of plasmid DNA or plasmid DNA expression vectors into primary rat myotubes in culture. They indicated that, although the plasmid DNA, even when uncomplexed with lipids, enters postmitotic nuclei and is expressed, the majority of the uncomplexed plasmid DNA is sequestered by cytoplasmic elements such as lysosomes.[56]

Unlike the DNA in viral vectors, most of the nonviral plasmid DNA found in the nucleus apparently is not integrated into the DNA but rather is expressed episomally.[70,71] The expressed antisense RNA then can interact with complementary sites on the target mRNA, either in the nucleus or in the cytoplasm, thereby inhibiting the processing of the mRNA and reducing the synthesis of the target protein.

V. OVERVIEW OF THE EXPRESSION OF NONVIRAL PLASMID VECTORS IN NEUROBIOLOGY

Nonviral plasmid vectors producing antisense RNA have been employed to study a wide variety of both nonmalignant and malignant processes that take place in the nervous system. A summary of these studies is presented in Table 4. In these studies antisense RNA was used to inhibit the function of receptors for neurotransmitters and neuropeptides (e.g., the receptors for D_2 dopamine, δ opioids, vasoactive intestinal peptide), neuronal and glial structural proteins (e.g., tau, glial fibrillary acidic protein, β-amyloid precursor protein), hormones, enzymes, and proteins involved in signal transduction processes in the nervous system (e.g., growth hormone, transglutaminase, multifunctional DNA repair enzyme, Gsα, protein kinase Cα, proenkephalin, calmodulin), oncogenes, and tumor suppressor genes (*n-myc, c-fos, bcl-2, DCC*) and growth factors (insulin-like growth factor I, (IGF-I); vascular endothelial growth factor, VEGF). The purposes of these studies have been to elucidate basic questions in neurobiology and to develop approaches for treating neuropsychiatric and oncologic conditions. The majority of these studies have been performed *in vitro* using established continuous cell lines or primary cultures of neuronal or glial cells. In some, an indirect *in vivo* approach has been used, whereby established cell lines have been initially transfected *in vitro* with antisense RNA expressing plasmid vectors, followed by transplantation of the antisense transfectants into animals.[61,62,72] This has been performed to determine whether inhibiting the expression of certain growth factors (IGF-I, VEGF) by means of antisense RNA inhibits the *in vivo* tumorigenicity of the antisense-transfected cells.[61,72] Studies from our laboratory using a direct *in vivo* antisense RNA approach to inhibit the expression of D_2 dopamine receptors in mouse brain are discussed below (see Section V.1A.2).

In the aforementioned studies, nonviral plasmid vectors with either constitutive (cytomegalovirus; CMV, SV40)[22,23,68,69] or inducible (MMTV, metallothionein)[24,61,62] promoters have been employed. A potential improvement of the nonviral plasmid vectors, which would be especially beneficial for the purposes of therapy using antisense RNA, would be to include cell-specific promoters in the vectors in order to selectively express the antisense RNA in restricted cell types. Examples of suitable tissue-specific promoters that have been used to selectively express genes in the nervous system include the promoters for preproenkephalin,[18] glial fibrillary acidic protein,[73,74] myelin basic protein,[73,75,76] and neuron-specific enolase.[77]

Similar to the studies using antisense oligodeoxynucleotides, the experiments using plasmid vectors to produce antisense RNA require appropriate controls. This is especially necessary because the specific mechanisms of action of antisense RNA have not yet been completely elucidated. Although several possible mechanisms have been shown to exist (e.g., interference with RNA splicing, inhibition of RNA export from the nucleus, blocking of translation, RNA-RNA duplexes), it is difficult to determine exactly which mechanism(s) operate in each specific case. The most commonly used control for nonspecific effects in *in vitro* studies has been an "empty" plasmid vector without an insert.[68,69,78] Transfection with a plasmid vector containing the recombinant sequence in the sense orientation has also been used,[11,79] as well as monitoring for nonspecific changes in the RNA levels of a "housekeeping" gene.[80] The *in vivo* experiments require additional controls to demonstrate the specificity of

TABLE 4

Effects of Antisense RNA Expression Vectors on the Levels and Function of Proteins in Neuronal Cells

Gene products	Cell type	Vector type	Stable or transient	Method of transfection	Function	Target protein	Target mRNA	Ref.
Neuroreceptors:								
Dopamine D_2 receptors	Human embryonic kidney cells (HEK293)	pCEP4	Stable	Lipofectin		Decrease	Decrease	69
Dopamine D_2 receptor	striatum	pCR3	Stable	DOTAP	Inhibits D_2 dopamine behavior	Decrease		68, 69
Opioid receptors:								
δ	Neuro-blastoma NG108-15 cells	pSVL	Stable	Calcium phosphate	Reduces [^{3}H] dipren-orphine binding	Decrease		22
Neuronal and glial structural proteins:								
tau	Pheo-chromo-cytoma PC 12 cells	pHβ Apr	Stable	Lipofectin	Slows neurite out-growth	Decrease		78
GFAP	Astro-cytoma, U251 MG, and U343 MG-A	pSV2 neo	Stable	Electro-poration	Increases cell growth	Decrease		23
β-APP	Pheo-chromo-cytoma PC12 cells	pJ7Ω	Stable		Inhibits neurite out-growth	Decrease		112
Hormones, enzymes, and proteins:								
Growth hormone	Pituitary tumor cells, GH_12C_1 and GH_3	pBSV neo	Transient	Electro-poration	Inhibits growth hormone produc-tion, Increases prolactin mRNA	Decrease	Decrease	80
Transglu-taminase	Neuro-blastoma SK-N-BE(2) cells	pSG5	Stable	Calcium phosphate	Decreases apoptosis			50
APEX nuclease	Glioma cells, C6 and KMG4	pA BWN	Stable	Calcium phosphate	Increases sensitivity to DNA damaging agents	Decrease		134
PKCα	Glio-blastoma U-87 cells	pRSV	Stable	Lipofectin	Inhibits cell growth	Decrease		25

TABLE 4 (CONTINUED)

Effects of Antisense RNA Expression Vectors on the Levels and Function of Proteins in Neuronal Cells

Gene products	Cell type	Vector type	Stable or transient	Method of transfection	Function	Target protein	Target mRNA	Ref.
Gsα	Pituitary tumor GH3 cells	pMThG H-111	Transient	Electro-poration	Decreases cAMP	Decrease	Decrease	52
Proenke-phalin	Neuro-blastoma NG 108-15 cells	pSVLSV 40	Stable	Calcium phosphate	Decreases opioid receptors	Decrease	Increase	135
Calmodulin	Pheo-chromo-cytoma PC12 cells	pMT-CB6+	Stable	Lipofectin	Induces neurite out-growth	Decrease	No change	11
GAP-43	Pheo-chromo-cytoma PC12 cells	pMA (–) Mneo	Stable	Electro-poration	Inhibits evoked dopamine and VIP release	Decrease		24
Oncogenes and tumor suppressor genes:								
n-myc	Neuro-blastoma IMR-32 cells	pREP3	Stable	Electro-poration	Inhibits neurite out-growth	Decrease		136
c-fos	Primary cultured bovine chromaffin cells	pSVsof	Transient	DOGS	No effect on neurite growth	Decrease		10
bcl-2	Embryonic chicken neurons	pM5G	Transient	Micro-injection	Kills BDNF-depend-ent neurons			117
DCC	Pheo-chromo-cytoma PC12 cells	pMA (–) Mneo	Stable	Electro-poration	Inhibits neurite out-growth	No change		79
Growth factors and growth-factor receptors:								
IGF-I	Neuro-blastoma C6/B104 cells	Episo-mal vector pAntiI GF-I	Stable	Lipofectin	Inhibits cell growth	Decrease	Decrease	62
IGF-I Receptor	Glio-blastoma C6 cells	Vector with HSP 70 pro-moter	Stable	Calcium phosphate	Inhibits cell growth	Decrease		115
IGF-I	Glio-blastoma C6 cells	Episo-mal vector pAntiI GF-I	Stable	Lipofectin	Inhibits cell growth	Decrease		61

TABLE 4 (CONTINUED)

Effects of Antisense RNA Expression Vectors on the Levels and Function of Proteins in Neuronal Cells

Gene products	Cell type	Vector type	Stable or transient	Method of transfection	Function	Target protein	Target mRNA	Ref.
VEGF	Glio-blastoma C6 cells	pEF-BOS	Stable	Calcium phosphate	Inhibits cell growth	Decrease	Decrease	72

Note: GAP, growth-associated protein; CaM, calmodulin; cAMP, adenosine 3′:5′-cyclic monophosphate; DOTAP, 1,2-dioleoyl-3-trimethylammonium propane; NE, norepinephrine; IGF-1, insulin-like growth factor-I; VIP, vasoactive intestinal peptide; *DCC*, deleted in colorectal cancer (tumor suppressor gene); DOGS, dioctadecylamidoglycylspermine; VEGF, vascular endothelial growth factor; PK-Cα, protein kinase Cα; β-APP receptor, β-amyloid precursor protein.

the functional changes produced by administering antisense RNA-producing plasmid vectors to animals. This issue will be discussed in detail later.

The following sections are not intended to completely review all the neurobiological studies performed thus far with antisense RNA produced by nonviral plasmid vectors (most of these studies are summarized in Table 4). Instead, we will describe only a few examples of the application of nonviral plasmid vectors producing antisense RNA *in vitro* and *in vivo* to demonstrate the diversity of neurobiological problems being addressed using this antisense RNA methodology and the different strategies which have been employed to deliver and express antisense RNA in cells originating from the nervous system. (See also Chapters 9 and 10.)

A. Antisense RNA To Neuroreceptors

1. In Vitro *Studies: VIP Receptors; Opioid Receptor-Associated Protein*

Cellular transfection with the mammalian expression vector pRc/CMV, producing antisense RNA to a newly cloned human receptor for the neuroendocrine mediator, vasoactive intestinal peptide (VIP), has been employed to characterize the binding and signal transduction events associated with the action of VIP.[81] VIP receptors are found in the CNS and peripheral nervous system, and in this study the colon carcinoma cell line HT-29, which bears VIP receptors, was used as a model. When the antisense orientation of the newly cloned VIP receptor clone was introduced into HT-29 cells, there was a 50% suppression of the specific binding of ^{125}I-VIP and of VIP-induced increases in the levels of cyclic AMP, relative to untransfected cells, thus confirming the identity of the receptor.

In another study, a plasmid vector producing antisense RNA was used to investigate the functional role of the opioid-binding cell adhesion molecule (OBCAM).[22] The NG108-15 neuroblastoma X glioma cells, which express a homogenous population of δ opioid receptors, were used as a model system. NG108-15 cells were stably transfected with plasmid pSVL containing either antisense or sense sequences derived from a portion of the rat cDNA for OBCAM. [^{3}H] Diprenorphine binding was greatly reduced in the antisense-transfected cells relative to the nontransfected cells, supporting the notion that OBCAM is part (or a subunit) of an opioid receptor.

As just described, continuous cell lines have provided valuable information about the function of neuroreceptors. Whenever possible, however, validation of the results obtained *in vitro* on cultured cells should be performed *in vivo*. As an example of the *in vivo* use of a nonviral plasmid vector producing antisense RNA, the results of targeting an individual subtype of the dopamine receptor will be described. This approach is compared to our experience with the *in vivo* use of antisense oligodeoxynucleotides to the individual subtypes of the dopamine receptor.

2. *In Vivo Study: Antisense RNA to the D_2 Dopamine Receptor*

Dopamine mediates a number of biological actions in the CNS, and several brain disorders are thought to be due to an alteration in the function of one of the several subtypes of dopamine receptors.[82,83] These disorders have been treated with a variety of pharmacological agents that block the actions of dopamine by preventing the interaction of dopamine with the receptor proteins. However, these drugs are relatively nonselective in that they interact not only with more than one of the five currently described isoforms of the dopamine receptor,[84-86] but also with receptors for several other neurotransmitters.[87] An alternative strategy to interfere with the actions of individual subtypes of the dopamine receptors is to inhibit the synthesis of receptor proteins through the use of antisense nucleic acids targeted to the transcripts encoding the different receptor subtypes.

Earlier studies showed that oligonucleotides antisense to the D_1 or D_2 dopamine receptor mRNAs, when injected into the cerebral ventricles of mice or rats, rapidly penetrated into brain cells[88] and specifically inhibited the biological actions mediated by these individual isoforms of the dopamine receptor[89-93] by inhibiting their synthesis.[2,88,94] However, although these actions were selective, they were also relatively short-lasting; responses returned to normal within a few days after cessation of treating the animals with the antisense oligonucleotides.[91,92] Moreover, in order to demonstrate an antisense effect, the oligonucleotides had to be administered either repeatedly[91,92] or continuously.[95] This regimen of repeated administration of oligonucleotides into brain, combined with their short duration of action, would likely render this strategy less attractive as a therapeutic regimen.

To obviate these problems and to produce a long-lasting blockade of functions mediated by the D_2 dopamine receptor, an expression vector housing a DNA sequence that generates antisense RNA targeted to the transcript encoding the D_2 dopamine receptor was injected into the corpus striatum of mice. The D_2 antisense sequence was chosen to encompass a region within the third cytoplasmic loop which has the least sequence homology to the remaining dopamine receptor subtypes. The uptake of plasmid DNA into cells was facilitated by complexing the plasmid to the cationic lipid DOTAP. Several assays were performed to establish that this is a suitable system to deliver and express a foreign DNA sequence in mouse brain. The expression of the plasmid *in vivo* was initially verified using the reporter plasmid CMV-β-gal in which the *Escherichia coli* β-galactosidase gene is driven by a CMV immediate-early promoter.[96] This plasmid, complexed with DOTAP, was injected into the corpus striatum of mice, and six days later the activity of β-galactosidase in the injected brains was determined by an *in situ* histochemical assay with the substrate 5-bromo-4-chloro-3-indolyl β-D galactoside.[69] The results showed positively stained cells in the corpus striatum, demonstrating that the procedure for administering the vector allows expression of a gene under the control of the CMV promoter (Figure 2). Next, the uptake of the D_2 antisense plasmid in brain was confirmed by PCR amplification of DNA isolated from the injected striata and identifying a band which corresponds to the cloned D_2 antisense insert in the polylinker of the vector.[69]

Thereafter, we determined the biological consequences and the duration of action of this D_2 antisense vector in mice, using *in vivo* model systems of altered or normal dopaminergic neurotransmission. One of the model systems employs mice with unilateral lesions of the corpus striatum induced by injecting the neurotoxin

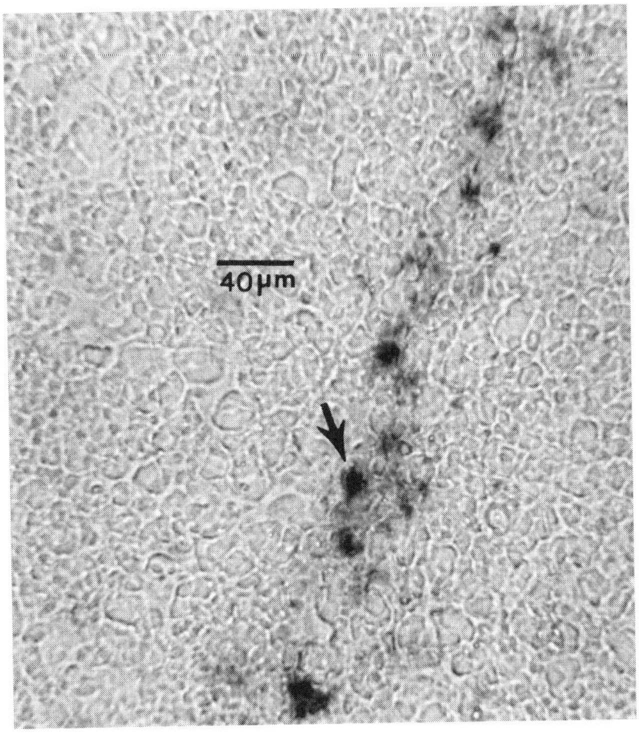

FIGURE 2
Expression of β-galactosidase vector injected with DOTAP in mouse brain. Mice were administered a single injection (5 µl) of pCMV β-galactosidase reporter vector[96] complexed with DOTAP (25 µg DNA/10 µg DOTAP) into the corpus striatum. Control mice received DOTAP alone. Six days later 30-µm cryostat sections of the brains were examined for β-galactosidase expression using a histochemical β-galactosidase assay. Positively stained cells (arrow) were seen on the injected side along the course of the injection track and in the striatal cells. No such staining was seen in mice receiving DOTAP alone. The results demonstrated that the procedure for administering the vector allows expression of a gene which was inserted downstream of the plasmid's CMV promoter. Scale bar, 40 µm.

6-hydroxydopamine.[97,98] This treatment renders the mice dopaminergically supersensitive, due to increased levels of dopamine receptors in the lesioned striatum.[5,99] As a result, the animals rotate in a direction contralateral to the lesioned side when challenged with parenteral injections of either D_1 or D_2 dopamine receptor agonists.[100-102] This model has proven useful for studying the behavioral effects of antisense oligonucleotides directed to the D_1 and D_2 receptor subtypes.[90-92]

6-Hydroxydopamine lesioned mice were administered a single intrastriatal injection of the D_2 antisense vector.[69] Periodically thereafter, the mice were given parenteral injections of the D_2 dopamine receptor agonist quinpirole, which produces a contralateral rotational behavior in this system.[103] The results showed that quinpirole produced a marked contralateral rotational behavior in animals injected with the empty, control vector (vector without an insert). However, rotations induced by quinpirole were significantly (p <0.01) inhibited after a single intrastriatal injection of the D_2 antisense vector pCR3-D_2AS (D_2AS vector). This inhibitory effect was still apparent 27 days after the injection (Figure 3).

To determine the specificity of the D_2 antisense effect, the mice were challenged with the D_1 dopamine agonist SKF 38393, which also produces contralateral rotational activity in this system.[103] The results showed that mice treated with the D_2 antisense expression vector had a reduced response to the D_2 dopamine receptor agonist quinpirole, but evidenced no significant change in their response to the D_1

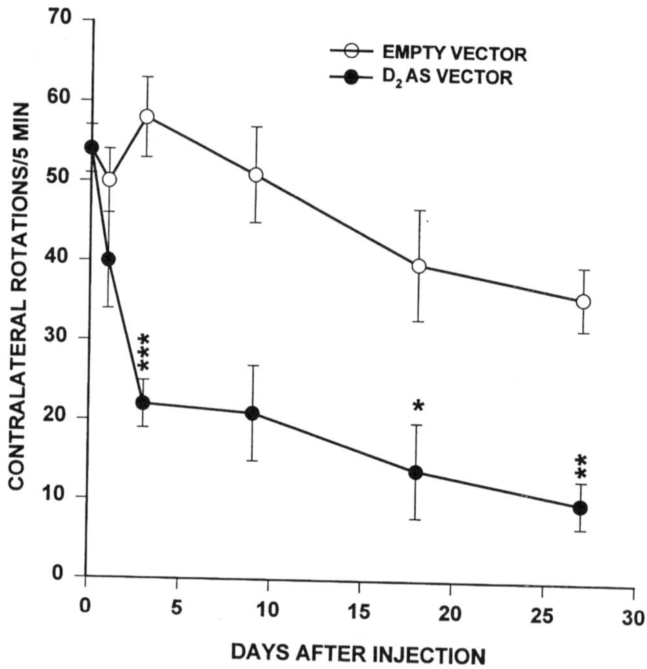

FIGURE 3
Intrastriatal injection of a D_2 antisense plasmid vector inhibits quinpirole-induced rotations in 6-hydroxydopamine lesioned mice. A D_2 antisense RNA plasmid expression vector (pCR3-D_2AS) was designed as follows. Starting with total mouse RNA and D_2 receptor sequence-specific primers, a 322-bp sequence of the mouse D_2 receptor cDNA was inserted by PCR cloning in the antisense orientation relative to the CVM promoter of vector pCR3 (Invitrogen). Mice with unilateral intrastriatal lesions induced by 6-hydroxydopamine (6-OHDA) were given a single intrastriatal injection of the D_2 antisense vector (pCR3-D_2AS) or an empty vector (pCR3) at day zero. The injections of 6-OHDA and D_2 antisense vector were made in the same striatum. Contralateral rotational behavior induced by the D_2/D_3 dopamine receptor agonist quinpirole (5 μmol/kg, subcutaneously) was measured at various times after the injection of the D_2 antisense or empty vector. Each point represents the mean value from 8 to 16 mice. Statistical analyses were performed by a two-way analysis of variance (ANOVA), followed by multiple comparisons using the Neuman-Keuls test. The results showed that rotational behavior induced by quinpirole was significantly inhibited after a single intrastriatal injection of the D_2 antisense plasmid vector, and that this inhibitory effect lasted for about one month. * = $p < 0.05$; ** = $p < 0.01$; and *** = $p < 0.001$ compared with values from mice treated with the empty vector.

dopamine agonist SKF 38393,[69] indicating that the antisense effect was specific for the D_2 subtype of dopamine receptors.

Use of another *in vivo* model confirmed the initial findings that a single intrastriatal injection of a D_2 antisense plasmid vector produces long-lasting changes in D_2 dopamine receptor-mediated behaviors. The rationale for using this model was that inhibition of D_2 dopamine receptors in mouse striatum produces a cataleptic behavioral effect.[88] If the D_2 antisense vector inhibited D_2 receptors, then the administration of this vector into the corpora striata of mice should induce catalepsy. Thus, mice were administered single bilateral intrastriatal injections of the D_2 antisense plasmid vector or the empty vector in DOTAP. Within one week after the injections, cataleptic behavior appeared in the D_2 antisense vector-treated, and not in the empty vector-treated mice, an effect that remained statistically significant for at least four weeks (Figure 4).

The studies using the two different *in vivo* models indicate that a nonviral plasmid vector, expressing antisense RNA to the D_2 dopamine receptor, reduces the levels of D_2, but not D_1, dopamine receptors and produces long-term, specific

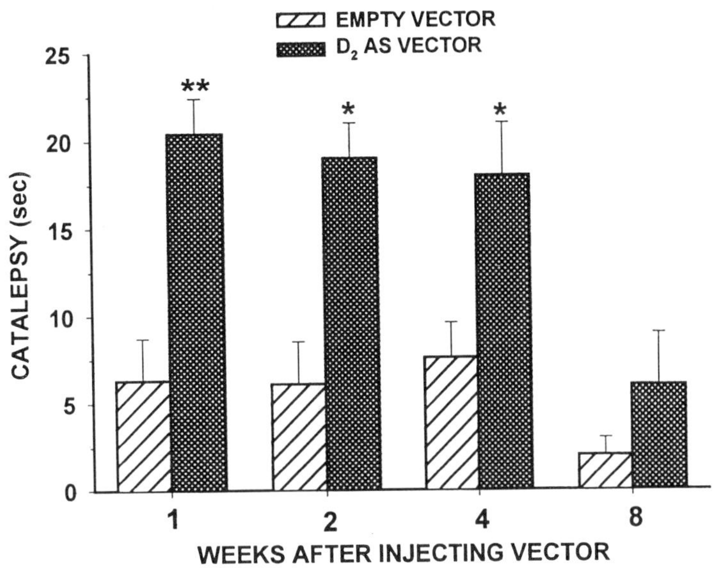

FIGURE 4
A single bilateral intrastriatal injection of a D_2 antisense plasmid vector induces persistent catalepsy in normal mice. Mice were injected bilaterally into the corpus striatum with the D_2 antisense vector (pCR3-D_2AS) or empty vector (pCR3) complexed with DOTAP (25 µg DNA/10 µg DOTAP). Catalepsy was determined at various times thereafter. Statistical analyses among the different animal groups were performed using a two-way analysis of variance (ANOVA) followed by multiple comparisons using the Neuman-Keuls test. * = p <0.05; and ** = p <0.01 compared with the corresponding values for empty vector-treated mice. The results showed that treatment of normal mice with the D_2 antisense vector induced catalepsy which lasted for at least 4 weeks.

inhibition of the behavioral responses mediated by the D_2 dopamine receptor subtype. This suggests that this agent may provide a novel pharmacological tool to study and, perhaps, treat disorders associated with hyperactivity in the D_2 dopaminergic system.

For example, long-term treatment with antipsychotic drugs often results in serious and debilitating motor disturbances, termed tardive dyskinesia.[8,104] These side effects appear to be due to an upregulation of D_2 dopamine receptors in the nigrostriatal system induced by long-term inhibition of these receptors by neuroleptic agents.[5-7] Using plasmid vectors producing D_2 dopamine receptor antisense RNA in the corpus striatum, it might be possible to reduce the levels of these D_2 dopamine receptors in this region of the brain and, thereby, reverse the symptoms of tardive dyskinesia. In addition, D_2 and D_3 dopaminergic hyperactivity in the mesolimbic areas of the brain is thought to be responsible for some of the symptoms associated with schizophrenia,[105,106] and blockade of these receptors is believed to be responsible for the antipsychotic effects of the classical neuroleptic agents.[107] Inhibition of the synthesis of D_2 or D_3 dopamine receptors in the limbic regions of the brain may, therefore, reverse some of the symptoms of schizophrenia. In order to avoid the motor disturbances associated with dopaminergic blockade, however, it would be important to inhibit these dopamine receptors in the limbic, but not in the nigrostriatal, system. Selective targeting of dopaminergic neurons in the limbic regions might possibly be achieved by coating the dopamine receptor antisense vector-lipid complex with ligands that selectively target cell-surface proteins which are highly expressed in limbic regions, and selective expression of the antisense RNA might be achieved by incorporating promoters into the vector that are preferentially activated in cells of the limbic system.[108-110]

B. Antisense RNA to Structural Proteins: GAP-43, tau, LBP110, and GFAP

The PC12 pheochromocytoma cells have been frequently used as an *in vitro* model to study the functions of neuronal structural proteins. They are suitable for this purpose because PC12 cells share many of the properties of neuronal cells and differentiate in response to nerve growth factor (NGF). Unlike primary cultured neurons, however, PC12 cells are relatively easy to transfect using methods such as lipofection[111] or electroporation.[24,79] The PC12 cell line has also been used as a model of neuronal cells in studies from our laboratory aimed at investigating the role of calmodulin in neuronal development (described later).

An antisense strategy has been employed to investigate the role of the neuronal growth-associated protein (GAP-43), a neuron-specific protein found at particularly high levels in axonal growth cones and in regions of the brain displaying pronounced synaptic plasticity.[24] Transfection with a pMAMneo expression plasmid, containing the entire coding region of the human GAP-43 cDNA in the antisense orientation, caused changes in the K^+-evoked and A23187 calcium ionophore-evoked dopamine release from PC12 cells. These changes were correlated with a reduction in the levels of GAP-43 in the antisense transfectants, and they were not observed in the control cells transfected with an empty vector or in untransfected PC12 cells. These results implicate GAP-43 in calcium-dependent release of neurotransmitters.

Antisense transfection analysis has been used to investigate the role of the microtubule-associated protein tau in several aspects of neuronal behavior: microtubule assembly, neurite outgrowth, and neuritic stability.[78] PC12 cells have been stably transfected with plasmid vectors containing tau cDNA in the antisense or sense orientation, or, as a control, with the empty vector. Immunoblotting showed that all of the control (empty vector) transfectants expressed tau at levels comparable to non-NGF-treated wild-type PC12 cells, whereas the antisense- and sense-expressing transfectants had reduced and increased levels of tau, respectively. Transfectants underexpressing tau exhibited reduced numbers of microtubules and slower neurite outgrowth, whereas stable transfectants overexpressing tau accumulated more microtubule mass and extended neurites more rapidly than the control cells. Furthermore, tau overexpressing cells were markedly more resistant to neuritic degeneration induced by the microtubule depolymerizing agent nocodazole when compared to tau underexpressing or to parental PC12 cells. These observations suggested that tau plays a crucial role in the development and maintenance of neuronal cells.

In another study, the identity and function of a 110-kDA membrane-associated laminin-binding protein (LBP110) from brain was characterized using transfection of PC12 cells with antisense β-amyloid precursor protein (APP) RNA.[112] APP and LBP110 have been reported to have similar distributions, particularly after injury to the brain. PC12 cells transfected with antisense APP RNA produced less APP and LBP110, as determined by Western blot analyses, and formed fewer processes when cultured on either laminin or the laminin A chain site (IKVAV peptide) when compared to controls. Thus, it was concluded that LBP110 is a member of the APP family and that APP plays a role in neurite outgrowth.

The role of the astrocyte-specific cytoskeletal protein, glial-fibrillary acidic protein (GFAP), in cell growth has been studied using an antisense RNA strategy. Antisense RNA vector transfection was chosen over the use of oligodeoxynucleotides in order to study the effects of continuous and long-term suppression of the synthesis of GFAP on the formation of filaments in human astrocytoma cells. Human astrocytoma U 251 MG cells were transfected by electroporation with a mammalian expression plasmid pSV2neo containing a fragment of the GFAP cDNA in the antisense orientation.[23] GFAP-negative stably transfected cells were identified by indirect immunofluorescent analysis. The cells transfected with an empty vector as control retained an astrocytic phenotype. In contrast, the antisense-transfected cells exhibited marked morphological differences from the astrocytic phenotype, the cells being epithelioid-like and devoid of long processes. In addition to changes in the morphology, the antisense transfectants had an enhanced growth and invasive potential over the controls, suggesting that GFAP may play a role in the regulation of certain aspects of tumor growth.

C. Antisense RNA to Growth Factors and Growth Factor Receptors: IGF-I, IGF-I Receptor, and VEGF

IGF-I and the IGF-I receptor have been extensively studied using an antisense RNA strategy. This is due to the important role IGF-I plays in cellular maturation in the CNS and the association of certain CNS tumors and congenital malformations with high levels of IGF-I.[113] The studies described below have both theoretical and practical implications for the gene therapy of gliomas. In one series of studies, cultured C6 glioma cells were stably transfected with an extrachromosomally replicating vector bearing an inducible metallothionein promoter and an antisense sequence to IGF-I. This vector was chosen to bypass the limitations of integrating vectors and to produce sufficient quantities of antisense RNA.[62] After induction of the promoter with $ZnSO_4$, the stable C6 glioma transfectants accumulated high levels of IGF-I antisense transcript, which dramatically decreased the levels of IGF-I mRNA and protein and, consequently, the tumorigenicity of the cells. As a control, B-104 neuroblastoma cells, derived originally from the same tumor but not expressing IGF-I, were also transfected. When injected subcutaneously or intracerebrally, the control (untransfected) C6 cells formed tumors.[62] Subcutaneous injection of rats with the antisense-transfected C6 cells prevented the formation of both subcutaneous tumors and brain tumors induced by nontransfected C6 cells.[62] In contrast, the transfection of IGF-I antisense RNA in B-104 cells did not result in the suppression of the tumorigenicity of B-104 cells. The antisense-transfected cells also caused regression of established brain glioblastomas when injected at a point distal to the tumor, an effect which resulted from a glioma-specific immune response involving $CD8^+$ lymphocytes.[61] These studies demonstrated a role of IGF-I in the tumorigenicity of gliomas and suggested a novel antisense approach to the treatment of these tumors.

The role of the IGF-I receptor in the tumorigenicity of glioma cells was also demonstrated in other studies using antisense RNA transfection analysis. Sell et al.[114] showed that human T98G cells transfected with a mammalian expression vector producing antisense RNA to the IGF-I receptor were characterized by a reduced ability to form colonies in soft agar with colony formation in agar being an indication of tumorigenicity. The study of Resnicoff et al.[115] demonstrated that the IGF-I receptor plays a critical role in the growth, clonogenicity, and tumorigenicity of glioblastoma cells, using rat C6 glioblastoma cells stably transfected with an expression plasmid that has a fragment of the IGF-R I cDNA in the antisense orientation driven by an inducible *Drosophila* heat shock promoter HSP70.

Another growth factor expressed in gliomas is vascular endothelial growth factor (VEGF), an endothelial cell-specific mitogen that promotes angiogenesis in solid tumors, including brain tumors.[116] After transfection of rat C6 glioma cells with a eukaryotic expression vector bearing an antisense VEGF cDNA, a reduction in the levels of VEGF in culture under hypoxic conditions was observed.[72] When implanted subcutaneously into nude mice, the growth of the antisense-VEGF transfectants was inhibited when compared to the control cells, thus providing support for the potential role of VEGF antiangiogenic gene therapy.

This latter study, in which an inducible promoter was used to express VEGF antisense RNA, as well as other studies using inducible promoters, illustrates that the ability to generate antisense RNA and to observe an antisense effect only under certain conditions can add an additional level of specificity to the antisense effect.

D. Antisense RNA to Oncogenes and Tumor Suppressor Genes: *c-fos, bcl-2, and DCC*

The intracellular signals underlying the differentiation of adult bovine chromaffin cells in response to histamine were investigated using antisense RNA to *c-fos*.[10] This study was undertaken because *c-fos* has been implicated in the differentiation of PC12 cells and because treatment of bovine chromaffin cells with histamine has been shown to rapidly induce cell flattening, attachment, and neurite outgrowth, as well as to produce time-dependent increases in *c-fos* mRNA.[10] Primary cultures of adult bovine chromaffin cells were transfected with an expression vector directing the synthesis of *c-fos* mRNA under the control of an SV40 promoter, using a polycationic lipid dioctadecylamidoglycylspermine (DOGS) as a DNA carrier. The efficiency of the *c-fos* antisense RNA to prevent the expression of the endogenous *c-fos* mRNA was determined by monitoring *c-fos* immunoreactivity. Administration of histamine to cells in which maximum decreases in *c-fos* immunoreactivity were achieved by transfection with the vector directing the synthesis of *c-fos* mRNA did not alter the neurite outgrowth response of these cells. These results suggested that the histamine-induced differentiation in bovine chromaffin cells is independent of increased levels of *c-fos*.

Antisense RNA to the proto-oncogene product *bcl-2* has been used to study the intracellular mechanisms governing cell survival and cell death and to determine whether Bcl-2 participates in the neurotrophin survival response.[117] In this study, two kinds of embryonic chicken neurons, the neurons of the terminal mesencephalic nucleus (TMN) and the ciliary ganglion neurons, which respond to different trophic factors, were used to explore the Bcl-2-sensitive and -insensitive cell death pathways. Both types of neurons die after being deprived of certain trophic factors. TMN neurons can be supported by brain-derived neurotrophic factor (BDNF) or ciliary neurotrophic factor (CTNF) and are rescued by Bcl-2 overexpression following BDNF, but not by CTNF deprivation.[118] Ciliary neurons are supported by CTNF, growth promoting activity (GPA), or basic fibroblast growth factor (bFGF), but they are not rescued by Bcl-2 overexpression after trophic factor deprivation.[118] Microinjection of TMN neurons with plasmid constructs that express RNA antisense to different regions of the chicken *bcl-2* mRNA resulted in an inhibition of the survival response of these neurons to BDNF.[117] Thus, the antisense constructs caused an abrupt decrease in the number of neurons growing in the presence of BDNF, cell death being manifested by chromatin condensation and nuclear fragmentation. Such changes were not observed in the cultures that were microinjected with the vector control. In contrast, *bcl-2* antisense RNA did not inhibit the survival response of TMN neurons to CNTF, nor did it alter the survival response of ciliary neurons to CNTF, GPA, or bFGF. These findings suggested that Bcl-2 participates in the neurotrophin survival response and demonstrate the existence of alternative Bcl-2-independent survival mechanisms in neurons.

The relationship between tumor suppressor genes and neuronal differentiation was addressed using antisense RNA to the tumor suppressor gene "deleted in colon cancer" (*DCC*) and the PC12 cell line as a model.[79] *DCC* expression has been detected in many normal tissues, including brain and colonic mucosa, but its expression is absent or greatly reduced in most colonic carcinomas.[119] When exposed to NGF for several days, PC12 cells exhibit morphological changes, such as the extension of long neurites, and biochemical changes, such as a transient expression of immediate-early genes as well as *DCC*. PC12 cells were stably transfected with a dexamethasone-inducible vector that produces antisense RNA to *DCC*. Both the *DCC* antisense RNA expression vector and the control vector (containing the *DCC* sequence in the sense orientation) transfectants exhibited typical morphological differentiation after 7 days of treatment with NGF. Addition of dexamethasone to the control cultures did not interfere with the action of NGF. The *DCC* antisense RNA expression vector transfectants, on the other hand, showed a pronounced inhibition of NGF-induced differentiation when treated with dexamethasone. The NGF-induced activation of the immediate-early genes *c-fos* and *egr-1* was not affected in the *DCC* antisense RNA transfectants treated with dexamethasone. These results suggested that persistent *DCC* expression is necessary to maintain the normal differentiation response of neuronal cells by a mechanism which does not involve the immediate-early genes *c-fos* and *egr-1*.

E. Antisense RNA to Hormones and Enzymes: Growth Hormone, Transglutaminase

In order to study the regulation of hormone synthesis in differentiated rat pituitary tumor cells, an approach employing the expression of antisense RNA to inhibit the production of rat growth hormone (GH) was utilized.[80] An expression vector that carried an inverted insert of the rat growth hormone (rGH) cDNA downstream of the SV40 promotor was used to transfect two different GH-producing rat pituitary cell lines, $GH_1 2C_1$ and GH_3. This resulted in a specific inhibition of the production of growth hormone which was parallelled by a decrease in the levels of GH mRNA and an increase in the levels of prolactin mRNA. In contrast, the levels of β-actin mRNA and Gsα mRNA were unaltered. The changes in the levels of GH and GH mRNA and prolactin mRNA were not induced in the cells transfected with a control, empty vector.

The role of tissue transglutaminase (tTG) in apoptosis was studied using the neural crest-derived neuroblastoma cell line SK-N-BE and overexpression of tTG or expression of an antisense RNA to tTG.[50] Cells transfected with a full-length tTG cDNA under the control of a constitutive promoter showed a drastic reduction in proliferative capacity, parallelled by a large increase in the death rate of the cells. The dying tTG-transfected cells exhibited both cytoplasmic and nuclear changes characteristic of cells undergoing apoptosis. In agreement with these findings, transfection of these neuroblastoma cells with the same expression vector which contained segments of the human tTG cDNA in the antisense orientation resulted in a pronounced decrease in both the spontaneous and retinoic acid-induced apoptosis. These results indicated that the tTG participates in events that take place during apoptotic cell death.

F. Antisense RNA to Calmodulin

An antisense strategy using transfection with a eukaryotic expression plasmid has been employed in order to inhibit the functions of calmodulin, a ubiquitous Ca^{2+}-binding protein, which participates in many intracellular processes, including Ca^{2+}-

dependent regulation of cyclic nucleotide metabolism, Ca^{2+} transport, protein phosphorylation-dephosphorylation cascades, ion transport, cytoskeletal function, and cell proliferation.[120,121] Because the levels of calmodulin[122] and calmodulin mRNA[123,124] are found in high concentrations in the CNS, modulation of its levels presents a difficult challenge, especially to the use of antisense oligodeoxynucleotides. Moreover, in addition to participating in normal processes in the nervous system, higher than normal levels of calmodulin are found in several tumors, including gliomas.[125] Thus, high-level expression of antisense RNA using plasmid vectors offered the best opportunity to substantially alter the levels of calmodulin in order to investigate the role of calmodulin in the proliferation and differentiation of nerve cells.

PC12 cells were again employed as an *in vitro* model of neuronal cells.[11] In this study PC12 cells were stably transfected using lipofectin with an eukaryotic expression vector containing the cDNA for calmodulin gene I in the sense or antisense orientation relative to the metallothionein promoter (Figure 5). The empty vector was used as a control. An inducible promoter was chosen because calmodulin has been shown to be essential for cell viability,[126,127] and PC12 cells stably transfected with the calmodulin antisense construct with a constitutively active promoter might not survive.

Stable colonies from the cells transfected with control vector or with calmodulin sense vector appeared approximately 12 to 14 days after the beginning of selection with the antibiotic geneticin, whereas calmodulin antisense colonies did not appear until after 27 to 30 days. The antisense-transfected colonies were smaller in size and significantly fewer in number than the colonies from cells transfected with control vector or with the calmodulin sense construct. The results are consistent with a previously established role for calmodulin in cellular proliferation,[128,129] extended here to include nerve cell proliferation.[11] The PC12 cells stably transfected with the calmodulin sense gene evidenced increased levels of calmodulin and calmodulin mRNA, whereas the PC12 cells stably transfected with the calmodulin antisense construct showed reduced levels of calmodulin. This suggests that the calmodulin antisense RNA might be acting by preventing the translation of the targeted protein. Reducing the levels of calmodulin by expression of antisense calmodulin mRNA resulted in a marked inhibition of cell proliferation, whereas increasing the levels of calmodulin by overexpressing calmodulin mRNA resulted in an acceleration of cell proliferation (Figures 6 and 7). The antisense-transfected PC12 cells having reduced levels of calmodulin evidenced spontaneous outgrowth of long, stable, and highly branched neuritic processes. In contrast, PC12 cells in which calmodulin was overexpressed evidenced no apparent changes in cell morphology (Figures 6 and 7).

These results indicated that, by reducing the levels of calmodulin in PC12 cells, it is possible to inhibit cell proliferation and to induce terminal differentiation. Accordingly, they suggested that the use of a calmodulin antisense RNA produced by an expression vector may provide a possible approach to limit the growth and induce differentiation of tumors of the nervous system. Indeed, drugs with anti-calmodulin activity have been effective at inhibiting the growth and inducing differentiation of glioma cells.[130,131] However, these drugs are relatively nonspecific in their action because they interact with other intracellular targets such as protein kinase C.[132] The use of calmodulin antisense RNA produced by a plasmid expression vector would provide a more selective approach to inhibit calmodulin in gliomas. The selectivity of this approach could be further enhanced by delivering the plasmid with cationic lipids which are coated with an antibody that will bind to antigens expressed specifically on glioma cells. Selectivity could be increased even further by engineering the plasmid vector to contain a tissue-specific promoter such as the glial fibrillary acidic promoter which would be active only in glial-derived cells. In addition, an extrachromosomally

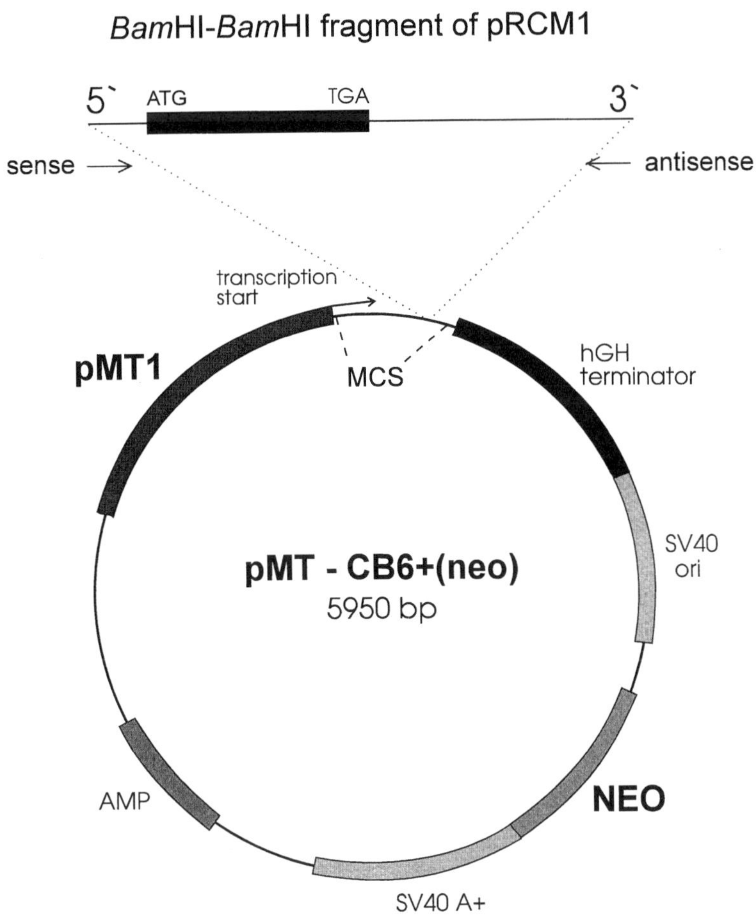

FIGURE 5
Schematic representation of the vectors expressing calmodulin sense or antisense RNA. Vectors generating rat calmodulin sense or antisense RNA were constructed using standard molecular cloning methodology.[133] A 1.4-kb *Bam*H1-*Bam*H1 restriction fragment from pRCM1 (expression plasmid containing the 1.4 kb full-length calmodulin gene I cDNA; donated by Dr. Hiroshi Nojima, Osaka University, Osaka, Japan) was subcloned in the sense or antisense orientation in the expression plasmid pMT-CB6+(neo) (generously supplied by Dr. Frank Rauscher III, The Wistar Institute, Philadelphia, PA). The orientation of the calmodulin inserts was ascertained by restriction enzyme analysis and nucleic acid sequencing. Shown are the elements of the resultant calmodulin sense and antisense vectors: 0.48 kb calmodulin coding region (black rectangle), initiation codon (ATG), termination codon (TGA), sheep metallothionein promoter (pMT1), neomycin/geneticin resistance gene (NEO), ampicillin resistance gene (AMP), multiple cloning site (MCS), human growth hormone transcription termination signal (hGH), SV40 replication origin (SV40 ori), and SV40 polyadenylation signal (SV40 A+). The depicted calmodulin sense or antisense vectors were used to increase and decrease the expression of calmodulin, respectively. The empty cloning vector was used as a control. (Reprinted from Davidkova, G. et al., *Neuroscience*, 75, 1003, 1996, with kind permission from Elsevier Science Ltd, The Boulevard, Langford Lane, Kidlington OX5 16B, UK.)

replicating nonviral plasmid (for example, the commercially available plasmid pCEP4, containing an EBV origin of replication) could be used in order to produce sufficient amounts of calmodulin antisense RNA in rapidly dividing tumor cells.

VI. CONCLUSIONS

Antisense RNA produced continuously inside the cell by means of both viral and nonviral plasmid expression vectors has been shown to inhibit the synthesis of

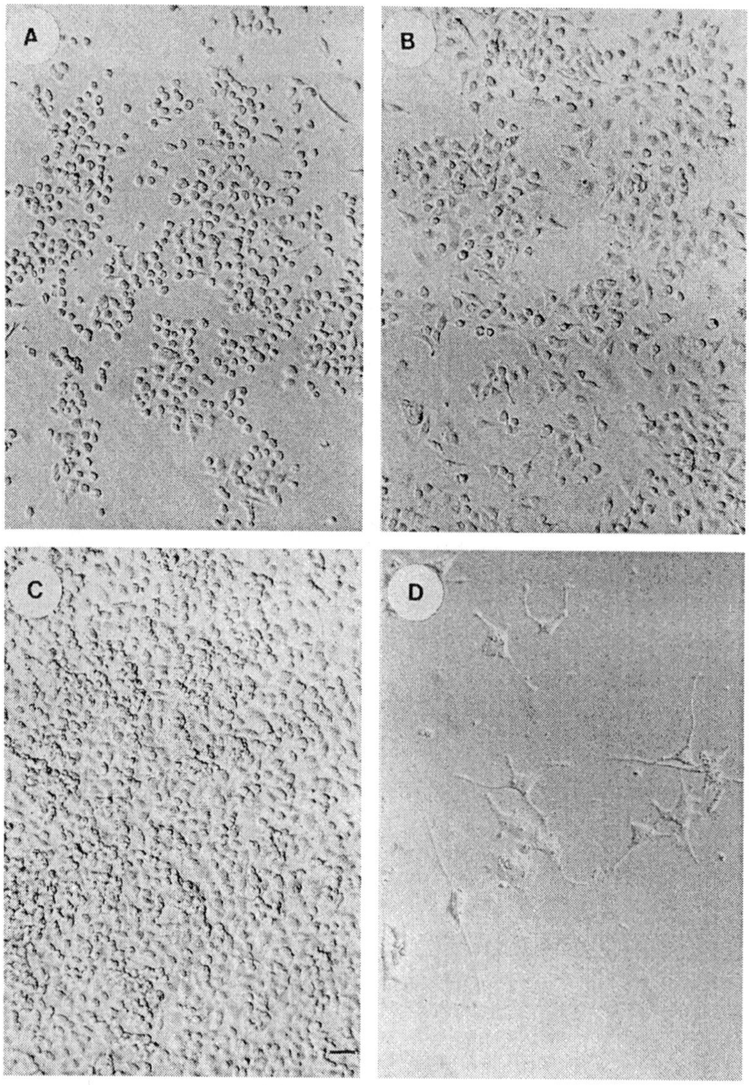

FIGURE 6
Effect of altering the levels of calmodulin using vectors expressing calmodulin sense or antisense RNA on the proliferation and differentiation of PC12 cells. PC12 cells were stably transfected with vectors expressing calmodulin sense or antisense RNA (the structure of the vectors is depicted in Figure 5). Untransfected PC12 cells and PC12 cells stably transfected with the empty, calmodulin sense or calmodulin antisense vectors were subcultured onto collagen-coated 24-well tissue culture dishes at a density of 2×10^4 cells/cm^2 and were grown for 8 days. (A) Untransfected parental PC12 cells; (B) cells transfected with the empty, control vector; (C) cells transfected with the calmodulin sense vector; and (D) cells transfected with the calmodulin antisense vector. The figure shows that, when compared with the parental cells (A) or with the empty vector transfected cells (B), cells transfected with the calmodulin sense vector (C) exhibited an increased rate of cellular proliferation, whereas cells transfected with the calmodulin antisense vector (D) exhibited a reduced rate of proliferation and an increase in differentiation, as evidenced by an increase in neurite outgrowth. Scale bar = 100 μm. (Reprinted from Davidkova, G. et al., *Neuroscience*, 75, 1003, 1996, with kind permission from Elsevier Science Ltd, The Boulevard, Langford Lane, Kidlington OX5 16B, UK.)

a variety of neuronal proteins, including receptors for neurotransmitters, neuronal and glial structural proteins, growth factors and their receptors, oncogenes, and tumor suppressor genes. The use of antisense RNA expression vectors has not only

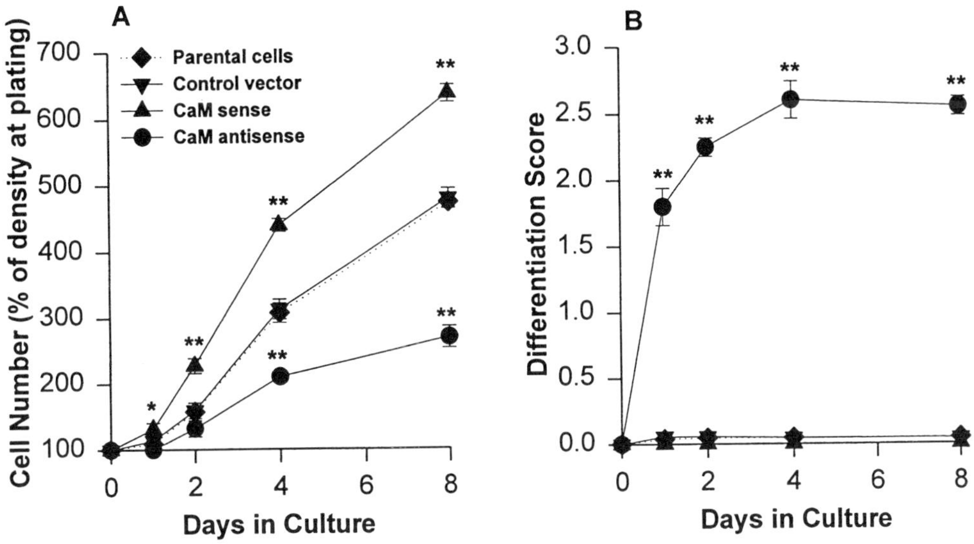

FIGURE 7
Quantitative analysis of the effects of overexpressing or underexpressing calmodulin on the proliferation and differentiation of PC12 cells. Untransfected parental PC12 cells and cells transfected with control vector, or the calmodulin gene I sense or antisense constructs were plated (5×10^4 cells/cm^2) onto collagen-coated 24-well plates at day 0. The cell numbers (A) as determined by direct counting, and the differentiation score (B), as determined by the degree of neurite outgrowth, were measured at days 1, 2, 4, and 8. These data show significant increases in cell growth in calmodulin sense transfectants and significant decreases in cell growth in calmodulin antisense transfectants. They also show that calmodulin antisense transfectants exhibited a statistically significant increase in cellular differentiation when compared with that seen in parental cells, or in cells transfected with the control (empty) vector or calmodulin sense vector. *p <0.05 and **p <0.01 compared with the values obtained from parental cells or cells tranfected with control vector at the corresponding time-points. (Reprinted from Davidkova, G. et al., *Neuroscience*, 75, 1003, 1996, with kind permission from Elsevier Science Ltd, The Boulevard, Langford Lane, Kidlington OX5 16B, UK.)

aided in elucidating the function of these proteins, but also has suggested their potential for treating a variety of diseases of the nervous system. We have summarized some of these studies and have provided examples from our laboratory showing that the *in vivo* administration of a nonviral antisense RNA expression vector directed to the D_2 subtype of the dopamine receptor can produce long-term and specific inhibition of D_2 dopamine receptor-mediated behaviors, suggesting the possibility of using this approach to study and treat disorders associated with dopaminergic hyperactivity. We have also shown that the application of an antisense RNA expression vector directed to the calmodulin transcripts in the PC12 pheochromocytoma cell line can inhibit their proliferation, suggesting the potential for using this approach to treat certain malignancies.

The use of vectors generating antisense RNA has several advantages over conventional pharmacotherapy and over the use of antisense oligodeoxynucleotides. In particular, antisense RNA-generating vectors can be engineered not only to be selectively targeted to a specific mRNA in cells, but also to be targeted to specific cell types. In addition, they can be designed to be expressed in only certain cell types through the use of inducible cell-specific promoters. If all these goals can be achieved, the use of antisense RNA expression vectors may hold the promise for developing a novel, highly selective, and effective pharmacotherapeutic regimen.

ACKNOWLEDGMENTS

This work was supported by grants MH42148 and NS30724 awarded by the National Institutes of Health and funds by START Technologies.

REFERENCES

1. Zon, G., Brief overview of control of genetic expression by antisense oligonucleotides and in vivo applications, *Mol. Neurobiol.*, 10, 219, 1995.
2. Weiss, B., Zhang, S.-P., and Zhou, L.-W., Antisense strategies in dopamine receptor pharmacology, *Life Sci.*, 10, 433, 1996.
3. Munroe, S. H., Antisense RNA inhibits splicing of pre-mRNA *in vitro*, *EMBO J.*, 7, 2523, 1988.
4. Hildebrandt, M. and Nellen, W., Differential antisense transcription from the *Dictyostelium* EB4 gene locus: Implications on antisense-mediated regulation of mRNA stability, *Cell*, 69, 197, 1992.
5. Burt, D. R., Creese, I., and Snyder, S. S., Antischizophrenic drugs: chronic treatment elevates dopamine receptors binding in brain, *Science*, 196, 326, 1977.
6. Owen, F., Cross, A. J., Waddington, J. L., Poulter, M., Gamble, S. J., and Crow, T. J., Dopamine-mediated behavior and 3H-spiperone binding to striatal membranes in rats after nine months haloperidol administration, *Life Sci.*, 26, 55, 1980.
7. Creese, I. and Snyder, S. H., Receptor adaptations to centrally acting drugs, *Annu. Rev. Pharmacol.*, 21, 357, 1981.
8. Ebadi, M. and Hama, Y., Dopamine, GABA, cholecystokinin and opioids in neuroleptic-induced tardive dyskinesia, *Neurosci. Biobehav. Rev.*, 12, 179, 1988.
9. Weiss, B., Davidkova, G., and Zhang, S.-P., Antisense strategies in neurobiology, *Neurochem. Int.*, in press, 1997.
10. Demeneix, B. A., Kley, N., and Loeffler, J. P., Differentiation to a neuronal phenotype in bovine chromaffin cells is repressed by protein kinase C and is not dependent on c-fos oncoproteins, *DNA Cell Biol.*, 9, 335, 1990.
11. Davidkova, G., Zhang, S.-P., Nichols, R. A., and Weiss, B., Reduced level of calmodulin in PC12 cells induced by stable expression of calmodulin antisense RNA inhibits cell growth and induces neurite outgrowth, *Neuroscience*, 75, 1003, 1996.
12. Gura, T., Antisense has growing pains, *Science*, 270, 575, 1995.
13. Srivasta, G. S., Batt, M., Schuette, J., Carlson, R., Fitchett, J., Lee, C., and Cole, D. L., Quantitative capillary gel electrophoresis (QCGE) assay of phosphorothioate oligonucleotide in pharmaceutical formulations, *J. Chromatogr.*, 680, 469, 1994.
14. Nielsen, P. E., Egholm, M., and Buchard, O., Sequence-specific transcription arrest by peptide nucleic acid bound to the DNA template strand, *Gene*, 149, 139, 1994.
15. Wang, C. Y. and Huang, L., pH-sensitive immunoliposomes mediate target-cell-specific delivery and controlled expression of a foreign gene in mouse, *Proc. Natl. Acad. Sci. U.S.A.*, 84, 7851, 1987.
16. Wang, C. Y. and Huang, L., Highly efficient DNA delivery mediated by pH-sensitive immunoliposomes, *Biochemistry*, 28, 9508, 1989.
17. Yoshida, J. and Mizuno, M., Simple preparation and characterization of cationic liposomes associated with a monoclonal antibody against glioma-associated antigen (immunoliposomes), *J. Lipos. Res.*, 5, 981, 1995.
18. Kaplitt, M. G., Kwong, A. D., Kleopoulos, S. P., Mobbs, C. V., Rabkin, S. D., and Pfaff, D. W., Preproenkephalin promoter yields region-specific and long-term expression in adult brain after direct *in vivo* gene transfer via a defective herpes simplex viral vector, *Proc. Natl. Acad. Sci. U.S.A.*, 91, 8979, 1994.
19. Vile, R. G. and Hart, I. R., *In vitro* and *in vivo* targeting of gene expression to melanoma cells, *Cancer Res.*, 53, 962, 1993.
20. Schinke, M., Bohm, M., Bricca, G., Ganten, D., and Bader, M., Permanent inhibition of angiotensinogen synthesis by antisense RNA expression, *Hypertension*, 27, 508, 1996.
21. Hart, I., Tissue specific promoters in targeting systemically delivered gene therapy, *Semin. Oncol.*, 23, 154, 1996.
22. Ann, D., Hasegawa, J., Ko, J.-L., Chen, S.-T., Lee, N., and Loh, H., Specific reduction of δ-opioid receptor binding in transfected NG108-15 cells, *J. Biol. Chem.*, 267, 7921, 1992.

23. Rutka, J. T., Hubbard, S. L., Fukuyama, K., Matsuzawa, K., Dirks, P., and Becker, L., Effects of antisense glial fibrillary acidic protein complementary DNA on the growth, invasion and adhesion of human astrocytoma cells, *Cancer Res.*, 54, 3267, 1994.
24. Ivins, K., Neve, K., Feller, D., Fidel, S., and Neve, R., Antisense GAP-43 inhibits the evoked release of dopamine from PC12 cells, *J. Neurochem.*, 60, 626, 1993.
25. Ahmad, S., Toshihiro, M., Martuza, R., and Glazr, R., Antisense expression of protein kinase C α inhibits the growth and tumorigenicity of human glioblastoma cells, *Neurosurgery*, 35, 904, 1994.
26. Federoff, H., Geschwind, M., Geller, A., and Kessler, J. A., Expression of nerve growth factor in vivo from a defective herpes simplex virus 1 vector prevents effects of axotomy on sympathetic ganglia, *Proc. Natl. Acad. Sci. U.S.A.*, 89, 1636, 1992.
27. Geller, A., A system, using neural cell lines, to characterize HSV-1 vectors containing genes which affect neuronal physiology or neuronal promoters, *J. Neurosci. Methods*, 36, 91, 1991.
28. Fink, D. J., DeLuca, N. A., Goins, W. F., and Glorioso, J. C., Gene transfer to neurons using herpes simplex virus-based vectors, *Annu. Rev. Neurosci.*, 19, 265, 1996.
29. During, M., Naegele, J., O'Malley, K., and Geller, A. I., Long-term behavioral recovery in Parkinsonian rats by an HSV vector expressing tyrosine hydroxylase, *Science*, 266, 1399, 1994.
30. Pakzaban, P., Geller, A. I., and Isacson, O., Effect of exogenous nerve growth factor on neurotoxicity of and neuronal gene delivery by a herpes simplex amplicon vector in the rat brain, *Hum. Gene Ther.*, 5, 987, 1994.
31. Sabel, B. A., Vick, A., and Hoellt, V., Neurotoxic reactions of CNS following gene transfer with defective herpes simplex virus (HSV-1) vector, *Neuroreport*, 6, 2447, 1995.
32. Naldini, L., Blomer, U., Gallay, P., Ory, D., Mulligan, R., Gage, F., Verma, I., and Trono, D., *In vivo* gene delivery and stable transduction of nondividing cells by a lentiviral vector, *Science*, 272, 263, 1996.
33. Boviatsis, E. J., Chase, M., Wei, M., Tamiya, T., Hurford, R. K., Jr., Kowall, N. W., Tepper, R. I., Breakfield, X. O., and Chiocca, E. A., Gene transfer into experimental brain tumors mediated by adenovirus, herpes-simplex-virus (HSV) and retrovirus vectors, *Hum. Gene Ther.*, 5, 183, 1994.
34. Kramm, C., Sena-Esteves, M., Barnett, F., Rainov, N., Schuback, D., Yu, J., Pechan, P., Paulus, W., Antonio Chiocca, E., and Breakfield, X. O., Gene therapy for brain tumors, *Brain Pathol.*, 5, 345, 1995.
35. Davidson, B., Allen, E., Kozarsky, K., Wilson, J. M., and Roessler, B., A model system for *in vivo* gene transfer into the central nervous system using an adenoviral vector, *Nature Genet.*, 3, 219, 1993.
36. Ikari, H., Zhang, L., Chernak, J. M., Mastrangeli, A., Kato, S., Kuo, H., Crystal, R. G., Ingram, D. K., and Roth, G. S., Adenovirus-mediated gene transfer of dopamine D_2 receptor cDNA into rat striatum, *Mol. Brain Res.*, 34, 315, 1995.
37. Perez-Cruet, M. J., Trask, T. W., Chen, S.-H., Goodman, J. C., Woo, S. L. C., Grossman, R. G., and Shine, H. D., Adenovirus-mediated gene therapy of experimental gliomas, *J. Neurosci. Res.*, 39, 506, 1994.
38. Kaplitt, M., Leone, P., Samulski, R., Xiao, X., Pfaff, D., O'Malley, K., and During, M. J., Long-term gene expression and phenotypic correction using adeno-associated virus vectors in the mammalian brain, *Nature Genet.*, 8, 148, 1994.
39. Byrnes, A., MacLaren, R. E., and Charlton, H. M., Immunological instability of persistent adenovirus vectors in the brain: peripheral exposure to vector leads to renewed inflammation, reduced gene expression, and demyelination, *J. Neurosci.*, 16, 3045, 1996.
40. Smith, A. E., Viral vectors in gene therapy, *Annu. Rev. Microbiol.*, 49, 807, 1995.
41. Hilleman, M., DNA vectors. Precedents and safety, *Ann. NY Acad. Sci.*, 772, 1, 1995.
42. Kurth, R., Risk potential of the chromosomal insertion of foreign DNA, *Ann. NY Acad. Sci.*, 772, 140, 1995.
43. FDA, Addendum to the Points to Consider in Human Somatic Cell and Gene Therapy (1991), *Hum. Gene Ther.*, 7, 1181, 1996.
44. Ono, T., Fujino, Y., Tsuchiya, T., and Tsuda, M., Plasmid DNAs directly injected into mouse brain with lipofectin can be incorporated and expressed by brain cells, *Neurosci. Lett.*, 117, 259, 1990.
45. Roessler, B. J. and Davidson, B., Direct plasmid mediated transfection of adult murine brain cells *in vivo* using cationic liposomes, *Neurosci. Lett.*, 167, 5, 1994.
46. Cao, L., Zheng, Z.-C., Zhao, Y.-C., Jiang, Z.-H., Liu, Z.-G., Chen, S.-D., Zhou, C.-F., and Liu, X.-Y., Gene therapy of Parkinson disease model rat by direct injection of plasmid DNA-lipofectin complex, *Hum. Gene Ther.*, 6, 1497, 1995.
47. Schwartz, B., Benoist, C., Abdallah, B., Scherman, D., Behr, J.-P., and Demeneix, B. , Lipospermine-based gene transfer into the newborn mouse brain is optimized by a low lipospermine/DNA charge ratio, *Hum. Gene Ther.*, 6, 1515, 1995.

48. Yagi, K., Hayashi, Y., Ishida, N., Ohbayashi, M., Ohishi, N., Mizuno, M., and Yoshida, J., Interferon-beta endogenously produced by intratumoral injection of cationic liposome-encapsulated gene: cytocidal effect on glioma transplanted into nude mouse brain, *Biochem. Mol. Biol. Int.*, 32, 167, 1994.
49. Li-Xin, Z., Min, W., and Ji-Sheng, H., Suppression of audiogenic epileptic seizures by intracerebral injection of a CCK gene vector, *Neuroreport*, 3, 700, 1992.
50. Melino, G., Annicchiarico-Petruzzelli, M., Piredda, L., Candi, E., Gentile, V., Davies, P. J., and Piacentini, M., Tissue transglutaminase and apoptosis: sense and antisense transfection studies with human neuroblastoma cells, *Mol. Cell. Biol.*, 14, 6584, 1994.
51. Loyter, A., Scangos, G., Juricek, D., Keene, D., and Ruddle, F. H., Mechanisms of DNA entry into mammalian cells. II. Phagocytosis of calcium phosphate DNA co-precipitate visualized by electron microscopy, *Exp. Cell Res.*, 139, 223, 1982.
52. Paulssen, R. H., Paulssen, E., Gautvik, K., and Gordeladze, J., The thyroliberin receptor interacts directly with a stimulatory guanine-nucleotide-binding protein in the activation of adenyl cyclase in GH3 rat pituitary tumor cells, *Eur. J. Biochem.*, 204, 413, 1992.
53. Neumann, E., Schaefer-Ridder, M., Wang, Y., and Hofschneider, P. H., Gene transfer into mouse lyoma cells by electroporation in high electric fields, *EMBO J.*, 1, 841, 1982.
54. Lo, D., McAllister, K., and Katz, L., Neuronal transfection in brain slices using particle-mediated gene transfer, *Neuron*, 13, 1263, 1994.
55. Ledley, F., Nonviral gene therapy: the promise of genes as pharmaceutical products, *Hum. Gene Ther.*, 6, 1129, 1995.
56. Dowty, M. E., Williams, P., Zhang, G., Hagstrom, J. E., and Wolff, J. A., Plasmid DNA entry into postmitotic nuclei of primary rat myotubes, *Proc. Natl. Acad. Sci. U.S.A.*, 92, 4572, 1995.
57. Cooper, M. J., Noninfectious gene transfer and expression systems for cancer gene therapy, *Semin. Oncol.*, 23, 172, 1996.
58. Goyal, L. and Huang, L., Gene therapy using DC-Chol liposomes, *J. Lipos. Res.*, 5, 49, 1995.
59. Trivedi, R. and Dickson, G., Liposome-mediated gene transfer into normal and dystrophin-deficient mouse myoblasts, *J. Neurochem.*, 64, 2230, 1995.
60. Felgner, P., Tsai, Y., Sukhu, L., Wheeler, C., Manthorpe, M., Marshall, J., and Cheng, S., Improved cationic lipid formulations for *in vivo* gene therapy, *Ann. NY Acad. Sci.*, 772, 126, 1995.
61. Trojan, J., Johnson, T. R., Rudin, S. D., Ilan, J. U., Tykocinski, M., and Ilan, J., Treatment and prevention of rat glioblastoma directed by immunogenic antisense IGF-1 tumor transfectants, *Science*, 259, 94, 1993.
62. Trojan, J., Blossey, B. K., Johnson, T. R., Rudin, S. D., Tykocinski, M., Ilan, J. U., and Ilan, J., Loss of tumorigenicity of rat glioblastoma directed by episome-based antisense cDNA transcription of insulin-like growth factor I, *Proc. Natl. Acad. Sci. U.S.A.*, 89, 4874, 1992.
63. Felgner, P. L., Gadek, T. R., Holm, M., Roman, R., Chan, H. W., Wenz, M., Northrop, J. P., Ringold, G. M., and Danielson, M., Lipofection: A novel highly efficient lipid mediated DNA transfection procedure, *Proc. Natl. Acad. Sci. U.S.A.*, 84, 7413, 1987.
64. Trubetskoy, V. S., Torchilin, V. P., Kennel, S., and Huang, L., Cationic liposomes enhance targeted delivery and expression of exogenous DNA mediated by N-terminal modified poly(L-lysine)-antibody conjugate in mouse lung endothelial cells, *Biochim. Biophys. Acta*, 1131, 311, 1992.
65. Lappalainen, K., Jaaskelainen, I., Syrjanen, K., Urtti, A., and Syrjanen, S., Comparison of cell proliferation and toxicity assays using two cationic liposomes, *Pharm. Res.*, 11, 1127, 1994.
66. Jiao, S., Ascadi, G., Jani, A., Felgner, P. L., and Wolff, J. A., Persistence of plasmid DNA expression in rat brain cells *in vivo*, *Exp. Neurol.*, 115, 400, 1992.
67. Harrison, G. S., Wang, Y., Tomczak, J., Hogan, C., Shpall, E. J., Curiel, T. J., and Felgner, P. L., Optimization of gene transfer using cationic lipids in cell lines and primary CD4+ and CD34+ hematopoietic cells, *BioTechniques*, 19, 816, 1995.
68. Zhou, L.-W., Davidkova, G., Zhang, S.-P., and Morabito, M., Biochemical and behavioral effects of a D_2 dopamine receptor antisense RNA vector transfected in mouse brain, *Soc. Neurosci.*, 22, 1318, 1996.
69. Davidkova, G., Zhou, L.-W., Zhang, S.-P., Morabito, M., and Weiss, B., Transfection of D_2 dopamine receptor antisense RNA plasmid vector *in vitro* and *in vivo*, *Soc. Neurosci.*, 22, 1319, 1996.
70. Zhu, N., Liggitt, D., Liu, Y., and Debs, R., Systemic gene expression after intravenous DNA delivery into adult mice, *Science*, 261, 209, 1993.
71. Wolff, J. A., Malone, R. W., Williams, P., Chong, W., Ascadi, G., Jani, A., and Felgner, P. L., Direct gene transfer into mouse muscle *in vivo*, *Science*, 247, 1465, 1990.
72. Saleh, M., Stacker, S. A., and Wilks, A. F., Inhibition of growth of C6 glioma cells *in vivo* by expression of antisense vascular endothelial growth factor sequence, *Cancer Res.*, 56, 393, 1996.

73. Miyao, Y., Shimizu, K., Moriuchi, S., Yamada, M., Nakahira, K., Nakajima, K., Nakao, J., Kuriyama, S., Tsujii, T., and Mikoshiba, K., Selective expression of foreign genes in glioma cells: use of the mouse myelin basic gene promoter to direct toxic gene expression, *J. Neurosci. Res.*, 36, 472, 1993.
74. Masood, K., Besnard, F., Su, Y., and Brenner, M., Analysis of a segment of the human glial fibrillary acidic protein gene that directs astrocyte-specific transcription, *J. Neurochem.*, 61, 160, 1993.
75. Miskimins, R., Knapp, L., Dewey, M. J., and Zhang, X., Cell and tissue-specific expression of a heterologous gene under control of the myelin basic protein gene promoter in transgenic mice, *Dev. Brain Res.*, 65, 217, 1992.
76. Wrabetz, L., Shumas, S., Grinspan, J., Feltri, M. L., Bozyczko, D., McMorris, F. A., Pleasure, D., and Kamholz, J., Analysis of the human MBP promoter in primary cultures of oligodendrocytes: positive and negative cis-acting elements in the proximal MBP promoter mediate oligodendrocyte-specific expression of MBP, *J. Neurosci. Res.*, 36, 455, 1993.
77. Ridet, J.-L. and Privat, A. , Gene therapy in the central nervous system: Direct versus indirect gene delivery, *J. Neurosci. Res.*, 42, 287, 1995.
78. Esmaeli-Azad, B., McCarty, J. H., and Feinstein, S., Sense and antisense transfection analysis of tau function: Tau influences net microtubule assembly, neurite outgrowth and neuritic stability, *J. Cell Sci.*, 107, 869, 1994.
79. Lawlor, K. and Narayanan, R., Persistent expression of the tumor suppressor gene DCC is essential for neuronal differentiation, *Cell Growth Differ.*, 3, 609, 1992.
80. Paulssen, R., Paulssen, E., Alestrom, P., Gordeladze, J., and Gautvik, K. M., Specific antisense RNA inhibition of growth hormone production in differentiated rat pituitary tumor cells, *Biochem. Biophys. Res. Commun.*, 171, 293, 1990.
81. Sreedharan, S., Robichon, A., Peterson, K., and Goetzl, E., Cloning and expression of the human vasoactive intestinal peptide receptor, *Proc. Natl. Acad. Sci. U.S.A.*, 88, 4986, 1991.
82. Smith, M., Wolf, A. D., Brodie, J., Arnett, C. D., Barouche, F., Shine, C.-Y., Fowler, J. S., Russel, J. A., MacGregor, R. R.,Wolkin, A., Angrist, A., Rotrosen, J., and Peselow, E., Serial [18F] *N*-methylspiroperidol PET studies to measure changes in antipsychotic drug D_2 receptor occupancy in schizophrenic patients, *Biol. Psychiatr.*, 23, 653, 1988.
83. Lublin, H., Gerlach, J., and Peacock, L., Effect of D_1 and D_2 agonists in primates withdrawn from long-term treatment with haloperidol: The potential role of dopamine D_1 receptors in dyskinesia, *Clin. Neuropharmacol.*, 15, 448, 1992.
84. Malmberg, A., Jackson, D. M., Eriksson, A., and Mohell, N., Unique binding characteristics of antipsychotic agents interacting with human dopamine D_{2A}, D_{2B}, and D_3 receptors, *Mol. Pharmacol.*, 43, 749, 1993.
85. Sokoloff, P. and Schwartz, J.-C., Novel dopamine receptors half a decade later, *Trends Pharmacol. Sci.*, 16, 270, 1995.
86. Tang, L., Todd, R. D., Heller, A., and O'Malley, K. L., Pharmacological and functional characterization of D_2, D_3 and D_4 dopamine receptors in fibroblast and dopaminergic cell lines, *J. Pharmacol. Exp. Ther.*, 268, 495, 1994.
87. Peroutka, S. J. and Snyder, S., Relationship of neuroleptic drug effects at brain dopamine, serotonin, alpha-adrenergic, and histamine receptors to clinical potency, *Am. J. Psychiatr.*, 137, 1518, 1980.
88. Qin, Z.-H., Zhou, L.-W., Zhang, S.-P., Wang, Y., and Weiss, B., D_2 dopamine receptor antisense oligodeoxynucleotide inhibits the synthesis of a functional pool of D_2 dopamine receptors, *Mol. Pharmacol.*, 48, 730, 1995.
89. Zhang, S.-P., Zhou, L.-W., Morabito, M., Lin, R. C. S., and Weiss, B., Uptake and distribution of fluorescein-labeled D_2 dopamine receptor antisense oligodeoxynucleotide in mouse brain, *J. Mol. Neurosci.*, 7, 13, 1996.
90. Weiss, B., Zhou, L.-W., Zhang, S.-P., and Qin, Z.-H., Antisense oligodeoxynucleotide inhibits D_2 dopamine receptor-mediated behavior and D_2 messenger RNA, *Neuroscience*, 55, 607, 1993.
91. Zhou, L.-W., Zhang, S.-P., Qin, Z.-H., and Weiss, B., *In vivo* administration of an oligodeoxynucleotide antisense to the D_2 dopamine receptor mRNA inhibits D_2 dopamine receptor-mediated behavior and the expression of D_2 dopamine receptors in mouse striatum, *J. Pharmacol. Exp. Ther.*, 1994.
92. Zhang, S.-P., Zhou, L.-W., and Weiss, B., Oligodeoxynucleotide antisense to the D_1 dopamine receptor mRNA inhibits D_1 dopamine receptor-mediated behaviors in normal mice and in mice lesioned with 6-hydroxydopamine, *J. Pharmacol. Exp. Ther.*, 271, 1462, 1994.
93. Zhou, L.-W., Zhang, S.-P., and Weiss, B., Intrastriatal administration of an oligodeoxynucleotide antisense to the D_2 dopamine receptor mRNA inhibits D_2 dopamine receptor-mediated behavior and D_2 dopamine receptors in normal mice and in mice lesioned with 6-hydroxydopamine, *Neurochem. Int.*, 29, 583, 1996.

94. Weiss, B., Zhou, L.-W., and Zhang, S.-P., Dopamine antisense oligodeoxynucleotides as potential novel tools for studying drug abuse, *Antisense Strategies for the Study of Receptor Mechanisms*, Raffa, R.B. and Porreca, F., Eds., R.G. Landes Publishing, Georgetown, TX, 1996, 71.
95. Zhang, M. and Creese, I., Antisense oligodeoxynucleotide reduces brain dopamine D_2 receptors: Behavioral correlates, *Neurosci. Lett.*, 161, 223, 1993.
96. Spaete, R. and Mocarski, E., Regulation of cytomegalovirus gene expression: α and β promoters are trans activated by viral functions in permissive human fibroblasts, *J. Virol.*, 56, 135, 1985.
97. Ungerstedt, U., Postsynaptic supersensitivity after 6-hydroxydopamine induced degeneration of the nigrostriatal dopamine system, *Acta Psychiatr. Scand. Suppl.*, 367, 69, 1971.
98. Von Voigtlander, P. F. and Moore, K. E., Turning behavior of mice with unilateral 6-hydroxydopamine lesions in the striatum: effects of apomorphine, l-dopa, amantadine, amphetamine and other psychomotor stimulants, *Neuropharmacology*, 12, 451, 1973.
99. Savasta, M., Dubois, A., Feuerstein, C., Manier, M. and Scatton, B., Denervation supersensitivity of striatal D_2 dopamine receptors is restricted to the ventro- and dorsolateral regions of the striatum, *Neurosci. Lett.*, 74, 180, 1987.
100. Thornburg, J. E. and Moore, K. E., Supersensitivity to dopamine agonists following unilateral 6-hydroxydopamine-induced striatal lesions in mice, *J. Pharmacol. Exp. Ther.*, 192, 42, 1975.
101. Arnt, J., Hyperactivity induced by stimulation of separate dopamine D_1 and D_2 receptors in rats with bilateral 6-OHDA lesions, *Life Sci.*, 37, 717, 1985.
102. Weiss, B., Zhou, L.-W., Chen, J. F., Szele, F., and Bai, G., Distribution and modulation of the D_2 dopamine receptor mRNA in mouse brain: Molecular and behavioral correlates, *Adv. Biosci.*, 77, 9, 1990.
103. Qin, Z.-H., Chen, J. F., and Weiss, B., Lesions of mouse striatum induced by 6-hydroxydopamine differentially alter the density, rate of synthesis, and level of gene expression of D_1 and D_2 dopamine receptors, *J. Neurochem.*, 62, 411, 1994.
104. Casey, D. E., Neuroleptic drug-induced extrapyramidal syndromes and tardive dyskinesia, *Schizophr. Res.*, 4, 109, 1991.
105. Carlsson, A. and Piercey, M., *Dopamine Receptor Subtypes in Neurological and Psychiatric Diseases, Clinical Neuropharmacology, Vol. 18, Suppl. 1*, Raven Press, New York, 1995, S215.
106. Seeman, P., Dopamine receptors and the dopamine hypothesis of schizophrenia, *Synapse*, 1, 133, 1987.
107. Creese, I., Burt, D. R., and Snyder, S. H., Dopamine receptor binding predicts clinical and pharmacological potencies of antischizophrenic drugs, *Science*, 192, 481, 1976.
108. Zacco, A., Cooper, V., Chantler, P. D., Fisher-Hyland, S., Horton, H.-L., and Levitt, P., Isolation, biochemical characterization and ultrastructural analysis of the limbic system-associated membrane protein (LAMP), a protein expressed by neurons comprising functional neural circuits, *J. Neurosci.*, 10, 73, 1990.
109. Levitt, P., A monoclonal antibody to limbic system neurons, *Science*, 223, 229, 1984.
110. Pimenta, A., Zhukareva, V., Barbe, M. F., Reinoso, B., Grimley, C., Henzel, W., Fisher, I., and Levitt, P., The limbic system-associated membrane protein is an Ig superfamily member that mediates selective neuronal growth and axon targeting, *Neuron*, 15, 287, 1995.
111. Muller, S., Sullivan, P., Clegg, D., and Feinstein, S., Efficient transfection and expression of heterologous genes in PC12 cells, *DNA Cell Biol.*, 9, 221, 1990.
112. Kibbey, M., Jucker, M., Weeks, B., Neve, R., Van Nostrand, W., and Kleinman, H., β-Amyloid precursor protein binds to the neurite-promoting IKVAV site of laminin, *Proc. Natl. Acad. Sci. U.S.A.*, 90, 10150, 1993.
113. Sturm, M. A., Conover, C. A., Pham, H., and Rosenfeld, R. G., Insulin-like growth factor receptors and binding protein in rat neuroblastoma cells, *Endocrinology*, 124, 388, 1989.
114. Sell, C., Rubini, M., Rubin, R., Liu, J.-P., Efstratiadis, A., and Baserga, R., Simian virus 40 large tumor antigen is unable to transform mouse embryonic fibroblasts lacking type 1 insulin-like growth factor receptor, *Proc. Natl. Acad. Sci. U.S.A.*, 90, 11217, 1993.
115. Resnicoff, M., Sell, C., Rubini, M., Coppola, D., Ambrose, D., Baserga, R., and Rubin, R., Rat glioblastoma cells expressing an antisense RNA to the insulin-like growth factor-1 (IGF-1) receptor are nontumorigenic and induce regression of wild-type tumors, *Cancer Res.*, 54, 2218, 1994.
116. Plate, K. H. and Risau, W., Angiogenesis in malignant gliomas, *Glia*, 15, 339, 1995.
117. Allsopp, T., Kiselev, S., Wyatt, S., and Davies, A. M., Role of bcl-2 in the brain-derived neurotrophic factor survival response, *Eur. J. Neurosci.*, 7, 1266, 1995.
118. Allsopp, T. E., Wyatt, S., Paterson, H. F., and Davies, A. M., The proto-oncogene bcl-2 can selectively rescue neurotrophic factor-dependent neurons from apoptosis, *Cell*, 73, 295, 1993.
119. Fearon, E. R., Cho, K. R., Nigro, J. M., Kern, S. E., Simons, J. W., Ruppert, J. M., Hamilton, S. R., Preisinger, A. C., Thomas, G., Kinzler, K., and Vogelstein, B., Identification of a chromosome 18q gene that is altered in colorectal cancers, *Science*, 247, 49, 1988.

120. Thermos, K. and Weiss, B., Calmodulin: function and pharmacological regulation, *Spasmophilia: Calcium Metabolism and Cell Physiology*, Agnoli, A., Canonico, P., Milhaud, G., and Scapagini, U., Eds., Libby, London, 1985, 26.
121. Means, A. R., Calcium, calmodulin and cell cycle regulation, *FEBS Lett*, 347, 1, 1994.
122. Zhou, L.-W., Moyer, J. A., Muth, E. A., Clark, B., Palkovits, M., and Weiss, B., Regional distribution of calmodulin activity in rat brain, *J. Neurochem.*, 44, 1657, 1985.
123. Roberts-Lewis, J., Cimino, M., Krause, II, R. G., Tyrell, Jr., D. F., Davis, L. G., Weiss, B., and Lewis, M., Anatomical localization of calmodulin mRNA in the rat brain with cloned cDNA and synthetic oligonucleotide probes, *Synapse*, 5, 247, 1990.
124. Cimino, M., Chen, J., and Weiss, B., Ontogenetic development of calmodulin mRNA in rat brain using *in situ* hybridization histochemistry, *Dev. Brain Res.*, 54, 43, 1990.
125. Kitajima, S., Sano, M., Kato, K., Seto-Oshima, A., and Mizutani, A., Changes in calmodulin and S-100 protein in C6 glioma cells as a result of cellular differentiation induced by forskolin, *Acta Histochem.*, 19, 365, 1986.
126. Weiss, B., Prozialeck, W. C., Cimino, M., Barnette, M. S., and Wallace, T. C., Calmodulin and cell functions, *Ann. NY Acad. Sci.*, 356, 319, 1980.
127. Means, A. R., Van Berkum, M. F. A., Bagchi, I., Lu, K. B., and Rasmussen, C. D., Regulatory functions of calmodulin, *Pharmacol. Ther.*, 50, 255, 1991.
128. Chafouleas, J., Bolton, W. E., Hidaka, H., Boyd, A. E., and Means, A. R., Calmodulin and the cell cycle: Involvement in regulation of cell cycle progression, *Cell*, 28, 41, 1982.
129. Sasaki, Y. and Hidaka, H., Calmodulin and cell proliferation, *Biochem. Biophys. Res. Commun.*, 104, 451, 1982.
130. Hait, W. N., Gesmonde, J., and Lazo, J., Effect of anti-calmodulin drugs on the growth and sensitivity of C6 rat glioma cells to bleomycin, *Anticancer Res.*, 14, 1711, 1994.
131. Marushige, Y., Marushige, K., and Koestner, A., Chemical control of growth and morphological characteristics of anaplastic glioma cells, *Anticancer Res.*, 9, 1729, 1989.
132. Schatzman, R. C., Raynor, R., and Kuo, J. F., *N*-(6-Aminohexyl)-5-chloro-1-naphthalenesulfonamide (W-7), a calmodulin antagonist, also inhibits phospholipidsensitive calcium-dependent protein kinase, *Biochim. Biophys. Acta*, 755, 144, 1983.
133. Sambrook, J., Fritsch, E. F., and Maniatis, T., *Molecular Cloning: A Laboratory Manual*, 2nd ed., Cold Spring Harbor Press, Cold Spring Harbor, New York,1989,
134. Ono, Y., Furuta, T., Ohmoto, T., Akiyama, K., and Seki, S., Stable expression in rat glioma cells of sense and antisense nucleic acids to a human multifunctional DNA repair enzyme, APEX nuclease, *Mutat. Res. DNA Repair*, 315, 55, 1994.
135. Arany, I., Zhang, X., Loh, H., and Lee, N., Antisense proenkephalin cDNA transfection decreases opioid binding in NG 108-15 cells, *Mol. Brain Res.*, 16, 295, 1992.
136. Whitesell, L., Rosolen, A., and Neckers, L. M., Episome-generated N-myc antisense RNA restricts the differentiation potential of primitive neuroectodermal cell lines, *Mol. Cell. Biol.*, 11, 1360, 1991.

INDEX

B

C

N

O

P

W

X

Y